P9-DMZ-857

POCKET GUIDE

to

Nutritional Assessment
and Care

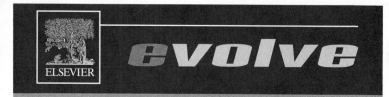

ELSEVIER

evolve

•• To access your Student Resources, visit:
http://evolve.elsevier.com/Moore/nutritional/

Evolve® Student Resources for Moore: *Pocket Guide for Nutritional Assessment and Care,* Sixth edition, offer the following features:

NOTE: Instructors also have access to student material.

- **Appendix A: Dietary Reference Intakes**
  Nutrition recommendations from the National Academy of Sciences for different life-stages.

- **Appendix B: Functions and Dietary Sources of Some Important Nutrients**
  Learn the signs and symptoms of nutritional deficiencies and their dietary sources for prevention and correction.

- **Appendix C: Dietary Fiber in Common Foods**
  Discover the amount of fiber in selected food sources you see every day.

- **Appendix D: Growth Charts (United States)**
  The most recent growth charts from the Centers for Disease Control and Prevention.

- **Appendix E: Triceps Skinfold (TSF) Measurements for Caucasians and African Americans in Millimeters**
  A resource that helps you estimate body fat percentage.

- **Appendix F: Laboratory Reference Values**
  Conveniently verify reference ranges for some of the most commonly ordered laboratory tests.

- **Appendix G: Drug-Nutrient Interactions**
  Find out more about the adverse effects of medications on nutritional status.

- **Appendix H: Selected Nutrition Resources**
  Practical links to nutrition information, resources, and tools for patient education and further study.

- **Appendix I: Modified Diets**
  Special diets recommended to improve the wellness of patients with health concerns.

- **Appendix J: Food Safety Guidelines**
  Reduce the risk of food-borne illnesses with these guidelines.

POCKET GUIDE

to

Nutritional Assessment and Care

Mary Courtney Moore, RN, RD, PhD
Research Associate Professor
Department of Molecular Physiology and Biophysics
Vanderbilt University
School of Medicine
Nashville, Tennessee

Sixth Edition

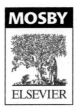

MOSBY

ELSEVIER

MOSBY
ELSEVIER

11830 Westline Industrial Drive
St. Louis, Missouri 63146

POCKET GUIDE TO NUTRITIONAL
ASSESSMENT AND CARE

ISBN: 978-0-323-05265-8

Notice

Knowledge and best practice in this field are constantly changing. As new research and experience broaden our knowledge, changes in practice, treatment and drug therapy may become necessary or appropriate. Readers are advised to check the most current information provided (i) on procedures featured or (ii) by the manufacturer of each product to be administered, to verify the recommended dose or formula, the method and duration of administration, and contraindications. It is the responsibility of the practitioner, relying on their own experience and knowledge of the patient, to make diagnoses, to determine dosages and the best treatment for each individual patient, and to take all appropriate safety precautions. To the fullest extent of the law, neither the Publisher nor the Editors/Authors assume any liability for any injury and/or damage to persons or property arising out of or related to any use of the material contained in this book.

The Publisher

Library of Congress Cataloging-in Publication Data
Moore, Mary Courtney.
Pocket guide to nutritional assessment and care / Mary Courtney Moore. —6th ed.
  p. ; cm.
Rev. ed. of: Pocket guide to nutritional care / Mary Courtney Moore. 4th ed. c2001.
Includes bibliographical references and index.
ISBN 978-0-323-05265-8 (pbk. : alk. paper)
1. Diet therapy—Handbooks, manuals, etc. 2. Nutrition—Handbooks, manuals, etc. 3. Nursing—Handbooks, manuals, etc. I. Moore, Mary Courtney. Pocket guide to nutritional care. II. Title. III. Title: Nutritional assessment and care.
[DNLM: 1. Diet Therapy—Handbooks. 2. Nutrition Assessment—Handbooks. 3. Nutrition Physiology—Handbooks. WB 39 M823p 2009]
RM219.M585 2009
615.8'54—dc22

2008008744

Acquisitions Editor: Yvonne Alexopoulos
Developmental Editor: Heather Bays
Publishing Services Manager: Jeff Patterson
Senior Project Manager: Anne Konopka
Book Designer: Kimberly Denando

Working together to grow
libraries in developing countries
www.elsevier.com | www.bookaid.org | www.sabre.org
ELSEVIER   BOOK AID International   Sabre Foundation

Printed in Canada.
Last digit is the print number: 9 8 7 6 5 4 3 2 1

REVIEWERS

Jessie Pavlinac, MS, RD, CSR, LD
Clinical Nutrition Manager
Food & Nutrition Services
Oregon Health & Science University
Portland, Oregon

J. Scott Peterson, MSN, BSN
Instructor of On-line Nutrition
Hill College
Hillsboro, Texas

Tracy Stopler, MS, RD
President
Nutrition E.T.C., Inc.
Plainview, New York;
Adjunct Professor
Nutrition and Human Performance
Adelphi University
Garden City, New York

Alyce Thomas, RD
Perinatal Nutrition Consultant
St. Joseph's Regional Medical Center
Paterson, New Jersey

Ruth Leyse-Wallace, PhD, RD
Author
Alpine, California;
Relief Clinical Dietitian
Sharp Mesa Hospital
San Diego, California

Janet E. Willis, BSN, MSN, RN
Senior Professor
Harrisburg Area Community College
Harrisburg, Pennsylvania

Beth Wolfgram, MS, RD, CD, CSCS
Nutrition Consultant and Personal Fitness Trainer
Salt Lake City, Utah;
Professor
University of Utah
Salt Lake City, Utah

Pocket Guide to Nutritional Assessment and Care is designed to be a brief yet comprehensive resource for clinical practitioners. Many of the features of previous editions have been retained:

- Emphasis on performing a thorough nutrition assessment as a basis for planning nutrition interventions and teaching
- Overview of cultural and ethnic impacts on nutrition
- Focus on overweight and obesity and their contribution to diabetes, prediabetes, and other health problems
- Application of enteral and parenteral nutrition support wherever appropriate
- Drug-nutrient interactions information included in relevant chapters, as well as being detailed in Appendix G on Evolve
- Reliance on evidence-based practice

This edition of the book has been revised to highlight key changes in nutrition and make it an integral key to practice. **The following are new to this edition:**

- Key recommendations from the *Dietary Guidelines for Americans 2005*
- Expanded coverage of the metabolic syndrome and of physical fitness in adults and children
- Utilization and description of the MyPyramid plan in diet and lifestyle planning
- Integration of the Nutrition Care Process developed by the American Dietetic Association into every chapter to help identify and address nutritional concerns
- Separate listing of medications that can impair control of glucose and lipid levels
- Increased emphasis on limiting sodium intake to help control hypertension and prevent or treat ischemic heart disease

My hope is that this sixth edition of *Pocket Guide to Nutritional Assessment and Care* will be a timely and useful reference for health professionals and that it will serve to improve the care of their patients.

Mary Courtney Moore

CONTENTS

APPENDIXES (on Evolve available at http://evolve.elsevier. com/Moore/nutritional)

NUTRITION FOR HEALTH PROMOTION

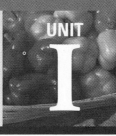

The following chapters introduce normal nutrition. Included in the discussion are a summary of the required nutrients, an explanation of nutrition guidelines, an overview of digestion and absorption, a description of the process of nutrition assessment, and a discussion of nutrition needs and concerns throughout the life cycle. These chapters provide a basis for understanding the role of nutrition in health promotion and prevention of disease.

NUTRITION AND HEALTH: OVERVIEW

Good nutrition and physical fitness are key elements of a healthy lifestyle. More than 40 nutrients are known to be essential for human health. All these nutrients are found in foods and beverages, but some skill and planning may be required to choose a diet adequate in all nutrients. Appendix B on Evolve summarizes the roles, major food sources, and symptoms of deficiency of nutrients known to be essential.

Healthy People Initiative

Healthy People is an ongoing project aimed at increasing the years of healthy life and decreasing disparities in health care among Americans. The initiative identifies the most significant and controllable health issues for Americans and focuses on public and private sector attempts to address them. The current summary (*Healthy People 2010;* available at http://www.health.gov/healthypeople/) emphasizes the importance of nutrition-related measures—increasing physical activity and prevention of overweight/obesity—in reducing the prevalence of chronic disease. Thus the need for education about nutrition and a healthy lifestyle is a high priority among Americans.

The *Steps to a Healthier US Cooperative Agreement Program* (Steps Program), one component of *Healthy People*, is a national program coordinated by the U.S. Department of Health and Human Services and the Centers for Disease Control and Prevention (CDC). The *Steps Program* funds communities to implement chronic disease prevention and health promotion programs that target three major chronic diseases—diabetes, obesity, and asthma and their underlying risk factors of physical inactivity, poor nutrition, and tobacco use. The U.S. government provides a number of resources for laypeople and professionals designed to encourage healthy behaviors (available at www.healthfinder.gov).

Dietary Reference Intakes

A careful estimate of the nutrient needs of the population provides a basis for setting nutrition policy, monitoring the adequacy of the food supply, and educating the public about proper diet. Prompted by the growing recognition of the role of nutrition in health promotion and prevention of chronic diseases, over the last decade U.S. and Canadian nutritionists have developed guidelines called the **Dietary Reference Intakes (DRIs)**. The DRIs are used in regulating the fortification of foods (addition of nutrients, as in vitamin D fortification of milk) and the composition of diet supplements; setting goals and budgets for food assistance programs for low-income families, schools, and the elderly; planning menus for individuals in the military and in many institutions; determining what nutrition information should be supplied on food labels; and similar purposes.

Various types of guidelines have been set, depending on the nutrient. Either a **Recommended Dietary Allowance (RDA)** or an **Adequate Intake (AI)** is specified for each nutrient. An RDA (see Appendix A on Evolve), which is estimated to meet the needs of almost all (97% to 98%) of the healthy population, is assigned when nutrient needs are well established. An AI is assigned when nutrient needs cannot be quantified as precisely, but the recommendation is believed to cover the needs of the population. The RDA or AI for a nutrient provides a goal that the individual should strive to achieve. The **Estimated Average Requirement (EAR)** is the average daily nutrient intake that is believed to meet the requirements of one half the healthy individuals in a life stage or gender group. The EAR is used for setting the RDA and also for evaluating the adequacy of food intake of groups. Finally, the **Tolerable Upper Intake Level (UL)** is given for most nutrients and is defined as the upper limit of intake associated with a low risk of adverse effects in almost all members of a population. The DRIs are updated regularly. The most current information can be found in the Food and Nutrition section at http://www.iom.edu.

Guides for Wise Food Choices

The DRIs are useful for health care professionals, the food industry, and government agencies involved in food and health policy, but most individuals would find them hard to translate into appropriate food choices. The *Dietary Guidelines for Americans* and **MyPyramid** have been developed to help the public choose foods wisely. Nutritional labeling of foods is designed to make it easier to know what nutrients are in foods.

Dietary Guidelines for Americans

The *Dietary Guidelines for Americans 2005* are intended to help Americans over the age of 2 years improve their health and reduce the risks of chronic disease. The guidelines, intended primarily for use by policymakers, health care providers, nutritionists, and nutrition educators, provide a basis for planning nutrition policy and education. The guidelines are summarized in Box 1-1.

Text continued on p. 11.

Box 1-1   Dietary Guidelines for Americans

Adequate Nutrients Within Calorie Needs

Key Recommendations

- Consume a variety of nutrient-dense foods and beverages within and among the basic food groups while choosing foods that limit the intake of saturated and *trans* fats, cholesterol, added sugars, salt, and alcohol.
- Meet recommended intakes within energy needs by adopting a balanced eating pattern, such as the USDA Food Guide or the DASH Eating Plan.

Key Recommendations for Specific Population Groups

- *People over age 50 years.* Consume vitamin B_{12} in its crystalline form (i.e., fortified foods or supplements). See Chapter 5.
- *Women of childbearing age who may become pregnant.* Eat foods high in heme-iron and/or consume iron-rich plant foods or iron-fortified foods with an enhancer of iron absorption, such as vitamin C–rich foods.
- *Women of childbearing age who may become pregnant and those in the first trimester of pregnancy.* Consume adequate synthetic folic acid daily (from fortified foods or supplements) in addition to food forms of folate from a varied diet.
- *Older adults, people with dark skin, and people exposed to insufficient ultraviolet band radiation (i.e., sunlight).* Consume extra vitamin D from vitamin D–fortified foods and/or supplements.

Continued

Box 1-1   Dietary Guidelines for Americans—cont'd

Weight Management

Key Recommendations

- To maintain body weight in a healthy range, balance calories from foods and beverages with calories expended.
- To prevent gradual weight gain over time, make small decreases in food and beverage calories and increase physical activity.

Key Recommendations for Specific Population Groups

- *Those who need to lose weight.* Aim for a slow, steady weight loss by decreasing calorie intake while maintaining an adequate nutrient intake and increasing physical activity. The BMI chart inside the back cover provides a guide to estimate healthy weights for adults.
- *Overweight children.* Reduce the rate of body weight gain while allowing growth and development. Consult a health care provider before placing a child on a weight-reduction diet. General guidelines to healthy weights for children can be found at Appendix D on Evolve.
- *Pregnant women.* Ensure appropriate weight gain as specified by a health care provider.
- *Breastfeeding women.* Moderate weight reduction is safe and does not compromise weight gain of the nursing infant.
- *Overweight adults and overweight children with chronic diseases and/or on medication.* Consult a health care provider about weight loss strategies before starting a weight-reduction program to ensure appropriate management of other health conditions.

Physical Activity

Key Recommendations

- Engage in regular physical activity and reduce sedentary activities to promote health, psychologic well-being, and a healthy body weight.
  - To reduce the risk of chronic disease in adulthood: Engage in at least 30 minutes of moderate-intensity physical activity, above usual activity, at work or home on most days of the week.

Box 1-1   Dietary Guidelines for Americans—cont'd

- For most people, greater health benefits can be obtained by engaging in physical activity of more vigorous intensity or longer duration.
- To help manage body weight and prevent gradual, unhealthy body weight gain in adulthood: Engage in approximately 60 minutes of moderate- to vigorous-intensity activity on most days of the week while not exceeding caloric intake requirements.
- To sustain weight loss in adulthood: Participate in at least 60 to 90 minutes of daily moderate-intensity physical activity while not exceeding caloric intake requirements. Some people may need to consult with a health care provider before participating in this level of activity.
- Achieve physical fitness by including cardiovascular conditioning, stretching exercises for flexibility, and resistance exercises or calisthenics for muscle strength and endurance.

Key Recommendations for Specific Population Groups

- *Children and adolescents.* Engage in at least 60 minutes of physical activity on most, preferably all, days of the week.
- *Pregnant women.* In the absence of medical or obstetric complications, incorporate 30 minutes or more of moderate-intensity physical activity on most, if not all, days of the week. Avoid activities with a high risk of falling or abdominal trauma.
- *Breastfeeding women.* Be aware that neither acute nor regular exercise adversely affects the mother's ability to successfully breastfeed.
- *Older adults.* Participate in regular physical activity to reduce functional declines associated with aging and to achieve the other benefits of physical activity identified for all adults.

Food Groups to Encourage

Key Recommendations

- Consume a sufficient amount of fruits and vegetables while staying within energy needs. Two cups of fruit and 2½ cups of vegetables per day are recommended for a reference 2000-calorie intake, with higher or lower amounts depending on the calorie level.

Continued

Box 1-1   Dietary Guidelines for Americans—cont'd

Food Groups to Encourage

Key Recommendations

- Choose a variety of fruits and vegetables each day. In particular, select from all five vegetable subgroups (dark green, orange, legumes, starchy vegetables, and other vegetables) several times per week.
- Consume 3 or more ounce equivalents of whole-grain products per day, with the rest of the recommended grains coming from enriched or whole-grain products. In general, at least half the grains should come from whole grains.
- Consume 3 cups per day of fat-free or low-fat milk or equivalent milk products.

Key Recommendations for Specific Population Groups

- *Children and adolescents.* Consume whole-grain products often; at least half the grains should be whole grains. Children 2 to 8 years should consume 2 cups per day of fat-free or low-fat milk or equivalent milk products. Children 9 years of age and older should consume 3 cups per day of fat-free or low-fat milk or equivalent milk products.

Fats

Key Recommendations

- Consume less than 10% of calories from saturated fatty acids and less than 300 mg/day of cholesterol, and keep *trans* **fatty acid** consumption as low as possible.
- Keep total fat intake between 20% to 35% of calories, with most fats coming from sources of polyunsaturated and mono-unsaturated fatty acids, such as fish, nuts, and vegetable oils.
- When selecting and preparing meat, poultry, dry beans, and milk or milk products, make choices that are lean, low fat, or fat free.
- Limit intake of fats and oils high in saturated and/or *trans* fatty acids, and choose products low in such fats and oils.

Key Recommendations for Specific Population Groups

- *Children and adolescents.* Keep total fat intake between 30% to 35% of calories for children 2 to 3 years of age and between 25% to 35% of calories for children and adolescents 4 to 18 years of age, with most fats coming from sources of

Box 1-1   Dietary Guidelines for Americans—cont'd

polyunsaturated and monounsaturated fatty acids, such as fish, nuts, and vegetable oils.

Carbohydrates

Key Recommendations

- Choose fiber-rich fruits, vegetables, and whole grains often.
- Choose and prepare foods and beverages with little added sugars or caloric sweeteners, such as amounts suggested by the USDA Food Guide and the DASH Eating Plan.
- Reduce the incidence of dental caries by practicing good oral hygiene and consuming sugar- and starch-containing foods and beverages less frequently.

Sodium and Potassium

Key Recommendations

- Consume less than 2300 mg (approximately 1 tsp of salt) of sodium per day.
- Choose and prepare foods with little salt. At the same time, consume potassium-rich foods, such as fruits and vegetables.

Key Recommendations for Specific Population Groups

- *Individuals with hypertension, blacks, and middle-aged and older adults.* Aim to consume no more than 1500 mg of sodium per day, and meet the potassium recommendation of 4700 mg/day with food (approximately 8 to 10 servings of fruits, vegetables, low-fat dairy products, and meats).

Alcoholic Beverages

Key Recommendations

- Those who choose to drink alcoholic beverages should do so sensibly and in moderation—defined as the consumption of up to one drink per day for women and up to two drinks per day for men.
- Alcoholic beverages should not be consumed by some individuals, including those who cannot restrict their alcohol intake, women of childbearing age who may become pregnant, pregnant and lactating women, children and adolescents, individuals taking medications that can interact with alcohol, and those with specific medical conditions.

Continued

Box 1-1   Dietary Guidelines for Americans—cont'd

Alcoholic Beverages

Key Recommendations

■ Alcoholic beverages should be avoided by individuals engaging in activities that require attention, skill, or coordination, such as driving or operating machinery.

Food Safety

Key Recommendations

■ To avoid microbial food-borne illness:
  ■ Clean hands, food contact surfaces, and fruits and vegetables. Meat and poultry should not be washed or rinsed.
  ■ Separate raw, cooked, and ready-to-eat foods while shopping, preparing, or storing foods.
  ■ Cook foods to a safe temperature to kill microorganisms.
  ■ Chill (refrigerate) perishable food promptly, and defrost foods properly.
  ■ Avoid raw (unpasteurized) milk or any products made from unpasteurized milk, raw or partially cooked eggs or foods containing raw eggs, raw or undercooked meat and poultry, unpasteurized juices, and raw sprouts.

Key Recommendations for Specific Population Groups

■ *Infants and young children, pregnant women, older adults, and those who are immunocompromised.* Do not eat or drink raw (unpasteurized) milk or any products made from unpasteurized milk, raw or partially cooked eggs or foods containing raw eggs, raw or undercooked meat and poultry, raw or undercooked fish or shellfish, unpasteurized juices, and raw sprouts.

■ *Pregnant women, older adults, and those who are immunocompromised*: Only eat luncheon meats and frankfurters that have been reheated to steaming hot.

For more information on food safety, see Appendix J on Evolve and www.fightbac.org.

From U.S. Department of Health and Human Services (USDHHS) and U.S. Department of Agriculture (USDA): *Dietary guidelines for Americans, 2005*, ed 6, Washington, DC, 2005, U.S. Government Printing Office.
BMI, Body mass index; *DASH*, Dietary Approaches to Stop Hypertension; *USDA*, United States Department of Agriculture.

MyPyramid

MyPyramid (Figure 1-1) is a simple tool for helping individuals to ensure a varied diet. A personalized version, based on an individual's age, height, weight, and activity level, is available on-line at www.mypyramid.gov. The website also includes a "tracker" program in which the individual can record and store daily dietary intake and physical activity for a personalized evaluation. According to the U.S. Department of Agriculture (USDA), the emphasis in teaching individuals to use the MyPyramid plan should be on

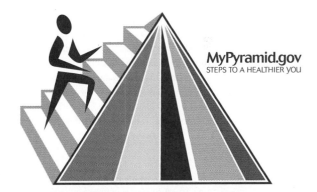

GRAINS Make half your grains whole	VEGETABLES Vary your veggies	FRUITS Focus on fruits	MILK Get your calcium-rich foods	MEAT & BEANS Go lean with protein
Eat at least 3 oz. of whole-grain cereals, breads, crackers, rice, or pasta every day	Eat more dark-green veggies like broccoli, spinach, and other dark leafy greens	Eat a variety of fruit	Go low-fat or fat-free when you choose milk, yogurt, and other milk products	Choose low-fat or lean meats and poultry
1 oz. is about 1 slice of bread, about 1 cup of breakfast cereal, or 1/2 cup of cooked rice, cereal, or pasta	Eat more orange vegetables like carrots and sweet potatoes	Choose fresh, frozen, canned, or dried fruit	If you don't or can't consume milk, choose lactose-free products or other calcium sources such as fortified foods and beverages	Bake it, broil it, or grill it
	Eat more dry beans and peas like pinto beans, kidney beans, and lentils	Go easy on fruit juices		Vary your protein routine – choose more fish, beans, peas, nuts, and seeds
For a 2,000-calorie diet, you need the amounts below from each food group. To find the amounts that are right for you, go to MyPyramid.gov.				
Eat 6 oz. every day	Eat 2 1/2 cups every day	Eat 2 cups every day	Get 3 cups every day; for kids aged 2 to 8, it's 2	Eat 5 1/2 oz. every day

Figure 1-1

MyPyramid. A guide to daily food intake and physical activity.
(From U.S. Department of Agriculture and U.S. Department of Health and Human Services: *My Pyramid.* Available at http://www.mypyramid.gov. Accessed July 25, 2007.)

(1) variety—consume foods from all the food groups and sub-groups (e.g., dark green vegetables, orange vegetables, and legumes); (2) proportionality—eat more of certain food groups (vegetables, fruits, whole grains, and fat-free or low-fat milk products) and less of others (foods high in saturated or *trans* fats, added sugars, cholesterol, salt, and alcohol); (3) moderation—particularly in energy intake; and (4) activity—be physically active every day. Table 1-1 provides recommended amounts of food from each group for 12 different energy levels. Table 1-2 lists suggested energy intakes based on age and activity level.

Dietary Approaches to Stop Hypertension (DASH)

A diet plan that was originally designed to be part of the therapy for hypertension has proven to be a healthful and practical plan for the general population. The DASH plan is consistent with MyPyramid, but it provides more emphasis on the importance of fruits and vegetables; beneficial fats and oils; and nuts, seeds, and legumes in the diet and more guidance in limiting intake of saturated fat, cholesterol, salt, and sweets. The DASH plan for different calories levels is summarized briefly in Table 1-3 and described in more detail in Chapter 14 (see Table 14-1).

Nutrition Labeling

Nutrition labeling is required on almost all processed foods, meat, and poultry (Figure 1-2). Similar information also appears near fresh produce and fish in many markets. This labeling is a valuable source of information for the consumer who is trying to choose a healthful diet or modify his or her diet (e.g., reduce fat or sodium intake) and is a useful tool for health care professionals engaged in educating their patients about nutrition. The total energy (kilocalorie, or kcal) content and kilocalories from fat must appear on the label to help consumers meet the dietary guidelines recommending no more than 30% of kilocalories from fat. Also included on the label are the amounts of total fat, saturated fat, *trans* fat, cholesterol, sodium, total carbohydrate, fiber, sugars, and protein. Information about most macronutrients is expressed in both units of weight (g or mg) and % **Daily Value (DV).** Labels must express DV in relation to a 2000-kcal diet, a caloric level that meets the energy needs of many adults. For example, fat should provide no more than 30% of the total kilocalorie intake (approximately 600 kcal, or 65 g/day for the person consuming 2000 kcal). A food that provides 12 g of fat in one serving provides nearly 20% of the fat included in a 2000-kcal diet. Food labels may contain information about DVs for other caloric intakes, if there is room. Polyunsaturated and monounsaturated fat and potassium content of foods is optional. Various vitamins and minerals appear on the label, depending on the food's nutritional composition. *Trans* fat content is included to guide consumers in keeping their intake of *trans* fats as low as possible. A shortened form of the food label may be used on small food packages. Major types of allergens found in the product must also be listed under or next to the ingredient list. These include milk, eggs, fish (e.g., bass, flounder, cod), crustacean shellfish (e.g., crab, lobster, shrimp), tree nuts (e.g., almonds, walnuts, pecans), peanuts, wheat, and soybeans.

New standards for labeling products "gluten free" will make it easier for individuals with celiac disease, or gluten-sensitive enteropathy, to avoid gluten-containing foods. Some examples of foods that would not be able to use the term *gluten free* on labeling include wheat, rye, barley, spelt, kamut, triticale, farina, vital gluten, semolina, and malt vinegar.

The U.S. Food and Drug Administration (FDA) has created guidelines to make food labels more informative for consumers who want to choose a healthful diet. These guidelines include definitions for the use of specific terms, such as *low fat* and *light,* in food labeling (Box 1-2), as well as a description of 14 types of health claims (relationships between diet and specific diseases) that can be included on food labels (Box 1-3).

Cultural Influences on Nutrition

Not all food choices are made because of nutritional considerations, of course. Economic constraints, peer pressure, persuasive advertising, and convenience are just a few of the factors influencing food choices. Cultural practices, including those shaped by national, ethnic, or religious background, can exert strong influences on eating patterns.

Immigrants and their families gradually adopt the typical American diet, especially as new generations are born in North America. This transition occurs both because it may be difficult or expensive to obtain particular foods and because of a desire to fit in with the dominant culture. Cultural, ethnic, and personal views about health and wellness and the role of diet also influence food patterns. Nevertheless, it is helpful to be aware of some characteristic cultural food practices. Appreciation of distinct cultural food habits helps the health

Table 1-1   MyPyramid Food Intake Patterns

Calorie Level[*]	Daily Amount of Food from Each Group											
	1000	1200	1400	1600	1800	2000	2200	2400	2600	2800	3000	3200
Fruits[†] (cups)	1	1	1.5	1.5	1.5	2	2	2	2	2.5	2.5	2.5
Vegetables[‡] (cups)	1	1.5	1.5	2	2.5	2.5	3	3	3.5	3.5	4	4
Grains[§] (oz eq)	3	4	5	5	6	6	7	8	9	10	10	10
Meat and beans[∥] (oz eq)	2	3	4	5	5	5.5	6	6.5	6.5	7	7	7
Milk[¶] (cups)	2	2	2	3	3	3	3	3	3	3	3	3
Oils[#] (tsp)	3	4	4	5	5	6	6	7	8	8	10	11
Discretionary calorie allowance[**]	165	171	171	132	195	267	290	362	410	426	512	648

From the U.S. Department of Agriculture, Center for Nutrition Policy and Promotion: *MyPyramid food intake patterns.* Available at http://www.mypyramid.
gov/downloads/MyPyramid_Food_Intake_Patterns.pdf. Accessed March 2, 2007.

[*]Calorie levels are set across a wide range to accommodate the needs of different individuals. Table 1-2 can be used to help assign individuals to the food intake pattern at a particular calorie level.

[†]Fruit group includes all fresh, frozen, canned, and dried fruits and fruit juices. In general, 1 cup (240 ml) of fruit or 100% fruit juice or ½ cup of dried fruit
can be considered as 1 cup from the fruit group.

†Vegetable group includes all fresh, frozen, canned, and dried vegetables and vegetable juices. In general, 1 cup of raw or cooked vegetables or vegetable juice or 2 cups of raw leafy greens can be considered as 1 cup from the vegetable group.

§Grains group includes all foods made from wheat, rice, oats, cornmeal, and barley, such as bread, pasta, oatmeal, breakfast cereals, tortillas, and grits. In general, 1 slice of bread, 1 cup of ready-to-eat cereal, or ½ cup of cooked rice, pasta, or cooked cereal can be considered as 1 ounce equivalent from the grain group. At least one half of all grains consumed should be whole grains.

‖Meat and beans group: In general, 1 oz (30 g) of lean meat, poultry, or fish, 1 egg, 1 tablespoon (15 ml) peanut butter, ¼ cup cooked dry beans, or ½ oz of nuts or seeds can be considered as 1 ounce equivalent from the meat and beans group.

¶Milk group includes all fluid milk products and foods made from milk that retain their calcium content, such as yogurt and cheese. Foods made from milk that have little or no calcium, such as cream cheese, cream, and butter, are not part of the group. Most milk group choices for adults and children over age 2 years should be fat free or low fat. In general, 1 cup of milk or yogurt, 1½ oz of natural cheese, or 2 oz of processed cheese can be considered as 1 cup from the milk group.

#Oils are fats that are liquid at room temperature and may come from plant sources, such as canola, corn, olive, soybean, and sunflower oil, or from some fatty fish. Some foods are naturally high in oils, such as nuts, olives, some fish (e.g., sardines, herring, salmon, mackerel), and avocados. Foods that are mainly oil include mayonnaise, certain salad dressings, and soft margarine.

**Discretionary calorie allowance is the remaining amount of calories in a food intake pattern after accounting for the calories needed for all food groups—using forms of foods that are fat free or low fat and with no added sugars (i.e., if whole milk is consumed, rather than fat free, this will use a portion of the discretionary allowance).

Table 1-2   Estimated Daily Calorie Needs

	Calorie Range		
	Sedentary*	→	Active
Children 2-3 yr	1000	→	1400
Females (yr)			
4-8	1200	→	1800
9-13	1600	→	2200
14-18	1800	→	2400
19-30	2000	→	2400
31-50	1800	→	2200
51+	1600	→	2200
Males (yr)			
4-8	1400	→	2000
9-13	1800	→	2600
14-18	2200	→	3200
19-30	2400	→	3000
31-50	2200	→	3000
51+	2000	→	2800

From U.S. Department of Agriculture, Center for Nutrition Policy and Promotion: *MyPyramid food intake patterns.* Available at http://www.mypyramid.gov/downloads/ *MyPyramid_Food_Intake_Patterns*.pdf. Accessed March 2, 2007.
*Sedentary means a lifestyle that includes only the light physical activity associated with typical day-to-day life. Active means a lifestyle that includes physical activity equivalent to walking more than 3 mi/day at 3 to 4 mi/hr, in addition to the light physical activity associated with typical day-to-day life.

care professional to demonstrate respect for both the individual and the culture and to be aware of food habits that may need modification. It may be possible to use cultural pride to reinforce or promote healthier eating habits. It is important to remember that not all members of a particular cultural or ethnic group follow the same food practices. For dietary practices associated with religious affiliation, the likelihood of following specific dietary rules is greatest among people with the strongest religious beliefs.

Some cultural, religious, or ethnic food practices that are prevalent in the United States are summarized in Table 1-4. Native Americans are not included in the table because the eating patterns of such a diverse group are not easily categorized. Alcoholism is a serious problem among most Native American groups, however,

Table 1-3 The DASH Eating Plan Daily Servings for 1600-, 2000-, 2600-, and 3100-Calorie Levels*

Food Group	Caloric Intake			
	1600	2000	2600	3100
Grains†	6	6-8	10-11	12-13
Vegetables	3-4	4-5	5-6	6
Fruits	4	4-5	5-6	6
Fat-free or low-fat milk and milk products	2-3	2-3	3	3-4
Lean meats, poultry, and fish	3-6	6 or fewer	6	6-9
Nuts, seeds, and legumes	3/wk	4-5/wk	1	1
Fats and oils	2	2-3	3	4
Sweets and added sugars	0	≤5/wk	≤2	≤2

From U.S. Department of Health and Human Services: *Your guide to lowering your blood pressure with DASH: the DASH eating plan*, Washington, DC, 2006 (revised), National Institute of Health (NIH), National Heart, Lung, and Blood Institute (NHLBI). *DASH*, Dietary Approaches to Stop Hypertension.
*See Table 14-1 for more information on the DASH eating plan.
†Whole grains are recommended for most grain servings as a good source of fiber and nutrients.
The number of daily servings can be modified to suit individuals with different energy needs.

and diabetes is increasingly common among many tribal groups, particularly those in the Southwest.

Two types of vegetarian diets are described in the table, but many others exist, including pescovegetarians, who avoid animal products except fish, and individuals who avoid red meats but eat all other animal products. Thus the term *vegetarian* tells little about food intake, and the health care provider will need to get more information in order to assess the diet and determine whether intervention and education are needed. A vegetarian food guide pyramid has been developed to aid in diet planning (Messina et al., 2003). The pyramid is similar to the MyPyramid plan described previously, but it suggests five servings of legumes, nuts, or other protein sources and eight servings of calcium-rich foods daily. One-half cup

Text continued on p. 22.

Macaroni & Cheese

Nutrition Facts

Serving Size 1 cup (228g)
Servings Per Container 2

1. Start Here ➡

2.

Amount Per Serving

Calories 250   Calories from fat 110

	% Daily Value*
Total Fat 12g	18%
Saturated Fat 3g	15%
Trans Fat 3g	
Cholesterol 30mg	10%
Sodium 470mg	20%
Total Carbohydrate 31g	10%
Dietary Fiber 0g	0%
Sugars 5g	
Protein 5g	
Vitamin A	4%
Vitamin C	2%
Calcium	20%
Iron	4%

3. Limit These Nutrients

4. Get Enough of These Nutrients

5. Quick Guide to % DV:

5% or Less Is Low

20% or More Is High

* Percent Daily Values are based on a 2,000 calorie diet. Your Daily Values may be higher or lower depending on your calorie needs:

	Calories:	2,000	2,500
Total Fat	Less than	65g	80g
Sat Fat	Less than	20g	25g
Cholesterol	Less than	300mg	300mg
Sodium	Less than	2,400mg	2,400mg
Total Carbohydrate		300g	375g
Dietary Fiber		25g	30g

6. Footnote

Figure 1-2

Sample nutrition label. To read the label, note the following: (1) the serving size and number of servings in the package, and how the serving size compares with the amount you usually eat or plan to eat; all nutrition information on the label is based on the stated serving size; (2) the total calories (kcal) and fat kcal per serving; (3) the food components that should be limited in the diet: total fat, saturated fat, *trans* fat, cholesterol, and sodium; (4) nutrients that should be encouraged in the diet; (5) the % DV provided by this serving size; and (6) the footnote showing that the % Daily Values (DVs) are based on a 2000-kcal diet. Some food components, such as *trans* fats, do not have a DV; *trans* fats contribute to elevation of low-density lipoprotein (LDL or "bad") cholesterol. A DV for protein is needed only if some claim such as "high protein" is made for the product. In the Nutrition Facts label shown, certain sections are colored to help focus on those areas that are explained in detail. These colors do not appear on actual food labels.

(From U.S. Food and Drug Administration: *How to understand and use the Nutrition Facts label*. Available at www.cfsan.fda.gov/~dms/foodlab.html. Accessed July 25, 2007.)

Some Terms Used on Food Labels and Their Definitions

Free: Contains none, or an insignificant amount, of a particular component (fat, saturated fat, cholesterol, sodium, sugars, or calories).

Good Source or High: Good source: contains 10% to 19% of the Daily Value for a particular nutrient. High (or "rich in" or "excellent source of"): contains 20% or more of the Daily Value for a particular nutrient.

Lean or Extra Lean: Lean: contains <10 g fat, <4 g saturated fat, and <95 mg cholesterol per serving and per 100 g. Extra lean: contains <5 g fat, <2 g saturated fat, and <95 mg cholesterol per serving and 100 g. Used in describing the fat content of meat, poultry, seafood, and game.

Light or Lite: Contains one-third fewer calories or one half the fat of the reference food.* A low-calorie, low-fat food can also be referred to as "light in sodium" if it contains 50% or less sodium than that reference food.

Reduced or Less: Contains at least 25% fewer calories or less of a particular nutrient (sugar, fat, cholesterol, saturated fat, or sodium) per serving than the reference food.

Low: Contains only a small amount of a particular food component, e.g., per serving (or per 50 g, if the normal serving size is 30 g or 2 tablespoons or less); low calorie means 40 calories or less, low fat means 3 g fat or less, low saturated fat means 1 g or less, low cholesterol means 20 mg or less, and low sodium means 140 mg or less. "Very low," applies only to sodium, means 35 mg or less per serving.

More: Contains at least 10% more of a nutrient per serving than the reference food.

Healthy: Low in fat and saturated fat and contains limited amounts of cholesterol and sodium. In addition, if it is a single-item food, it must provide at least 10% of one or more of vitamins A or C, iron, calcium, protein, or fiber (unless it is a raw, frozen, or canned fruit or vegetable or certain cereal grains that do not naturally provide at least 10% of one of the nutrients).

Adapted from U.S. FDA CFSAN: *A food labeling guide,* 1994, rev. 1999 and 2004. Available at www.cfsan.fda.gov/~dms/flg-6a.html. Accessed March 3, 2007.
*A reference food is a nonnutritionally altered version of the same food product (e.g., a regular chocolate cake mix would be the reference food for a chocolate cake mix labeled "low fat") or a dissimilar food that may generally be substituted for the labeled food (e.g., potato chips for pretzels).

Box 1-3   Health Claims Permitted on Food Labels*

Calcium and Reduction in the Risk of Osteoporosis

Foods or supplements must be "high" in calcium in a form readily absorbed and utilized in the body and must not contain more phosphorus than calcium. The claim must name the target group most in need of adequate calcium intakes (i.e., teens and young adult Caucasian and Asian women) and state the need for exercise and a healthy diet in addition to calcium.

Sodium and Reduction in the Risk of Hypertension (High Blood Pressure)

Foods must meet the criteria for "low sodium."

Dietary Fat and Reduction in Cancer Risk

Foods must meet the definition of "low fat," the claim must refer to total fat rather than any specific type of fat, and the claim must be limited to "some cancers" or "some types of cancers."

Dietary Saturated Fat and Cholesterol and Reduction in Risk of Coronary Heart Disease

Foods must meet the definition of "low saturated fat," "low cholesterol," and "low fat."

Fiber-Containing Grain Products, Fruits, and Vegetables and Reduction of Cancer Risk

Foods must meet the definition for "low fat" and, without fortification, be a "good source" of dietary fiber. The claim must not mention particular types of fiber.

Fruits, Vegetables, and Grain Products That Contain Fiber, Particularly Soluble Fiber, and Reduction in the Risk of Coronary Heart Disease

Food must meet the definition of "low saturated fat," "low cholesterol," and "low fat." It must contain, without fortification, at least 0.6 g soluble fiber per reference amount, and the soluble fiber amount must be listed.

Fruits and Vegetables and Reduction of Cancer Risk

Foods must meet the criteria for "low fat" and, without fortification, be a "good source" of fiber, vitamin A, or vitamin C.

Box 1-3   Health Claims Permitted on Food Labels*—cont'd

Folate and Reduction in the Risk of Neural Tube Defects

Foods must meet the criteria for "good source" of folate and must not provide more than 100% of the Daily Value for vitamins A and D because of their potential risk to fetuses.

Dietary Sugar Alcohol and Reduction in the Risk of Dental Caries

Foods or sugarless gums must meet the criteria for "sugar free"; must contain xylitol, sorbitol, mannitol, maltitol, isomalt, lactitol, hydrogenated starch hydrolysates, hydrogenated glucose syrups, erythritol, or a combination; must not lower plaque pH below 5.7 or promote tooth decay.

Dietary Soluble Fiber, Such as Found in Whole Oats and Psyllium Seed Husk, and Reduction in the Risk of Coronary Heart Disease

Foods must meet the definition of "low saturated fat," "low cholesterol," and "low fat." Foods that contain whole oats or psyllium must provide at least 0.75 or 1.7 g soluble fiber per serving, respectively, and soluble fiber content must appear on the label.

Soy Protein and Reduction of Risk of Coronary Heart Disease

Foods must contain at least 6.25 g soy protein per reference amount and meet the definition of "low saturated fat," "low cholesterol," and "low fat." The exception is that foods providing no added fat except that from soybeans are exempt from the "low fat" requirement.

Plant Sterols/Stanols and Reduction of Risk of Heart Disease

Foods must contain at least 0.65 g plant sterol esters or 1.7 g plant stanol esters per reference amount of spread, salad dressing, snack bars, or supplement; meet the definition of "low saturated fat" and "low cholesterol." Spreads and salad dressings that contain more than 13 g fat per 50 g of product must include on the label the statement "see nutrition information for fat content." The label must indicate that sterols or stanols should be consumed with at least two different meals daily.

Continued

Box 1-3   Health Claims Permitted on Food Labels*—cont'd

Whole Grain Foods and Reduction of Risk of Certain Cancers and Heart Disease

Foods must contain at least 50% whole grain by weight, and the dietary fiber content must be at least 3 g if the serving is 55 g, 2.8 g if the serving is 50 g, 2.5 g if the serving is 45 g, or 1.7 g if the serving is 35 g.

Potassium and Reduction in Risk of High Blood Pressure

The food must be a "good source" of potassium, "low sodium," "low saturated fat," and "low cholesterol."

Adapted from U.S. FDA CFSAN: *A food labeling guide—Appendix C, 1994, rev. 1999, 2000, 2001, 2002, and 2005.* Available at www.cfsan.fda.gov/~dms/flg-6c.html. Accessed February 14, 2007.
*The claims cannot state that a particular food or nutrient will prevent disease; "may" and "might" are the preferred terms. The claims must state that disease risk depends on many factors other than a particular food or nutrient. For example, regular exercise, in addition to calcium intake, reduces the risk of osteoporosis. To make a health claim on the label, the food must contain, without fortification, at least 10% of the Daily Value for one of six nutrients: vitamin C, vitamin A, iron, calcium, protein, or fiber. The claim cannot be made for individuals younger than 2 years of age, and it cannot quantify any degree of risk reduction.

(120 ml) of cow milk or 21 g (¾ oz) of cheese is one calcium-rich serving. Individuals who do not use dairy products can obtain one calcium serving by consuming alternatives such as 120 ml calcium-fortified juice; 28 g (1 oz) fortified breakfast cereal; 240 ml (1 cup) cooked greens, bok choy, okra, or broccoli (or 480 ml of the uncooked vegetables); or 60 ml (¼ cup) almonds.

Additional information is available online in the series *Cultural Diversity: Eating in America*, at http://ohioline.osu.edu/lines/food.html.

Physiologic Influences on Nutrition

During digestion, foods are broken down mechanically by chewing and by mixing motions in the stomach and small intestine. Most carbohydrates, proteins, and fats in the diet are too large to be absorbed even after this mechanical breakdown and must be further digested by enzymes in the lumen or brush border of the intestine (Figure 1-3).

Text continued on p. 32.

Table 1-4 Examples of Cultural, Religious, or Ethnic Food Practices

Characteristic Food Practices	Health Implications
African American*	
Cooking methods: Frying and barbecuing common; vegetables often boiled for prolonged periods and seasoned with fatback (salt pork); gravy often served.	*Positives:* Many different vegetables consumed.
	Concerns: Fat and sodium intake often high; many adults have little milk intake (lactose intolerance common); pica (eating nonfood items such as soil and clay) occurs especially among women and may inhibit iron absorption. Breastfeeding is less common than among Caucasians.
Foods enjoyed: Chicken, barbecue pork, ham, chitterlings (boiled or fried pig intestines), grits (coarsely ground corn that is boiled and usually served with cheese, butter, or margarine), greens, okra (boiled or fried), tomatoes, sweet and white potatoes, biscuits, cornbread, melons, peaches, pecans, and peanuts. Homemade pies and cakes are common.	*Prevalent nutrition-related problems:* Obesity, diabetes, hypertension, and heart disease; iron deficiency anemia among women.

*This diet is often referred to as African American "soul food," but many African Americans have Southern roots. These foods and cooking methods are also typical "home cooking" of Southern Caucasians.

Continued

Table 1-4   Examples of Cultural, Religious, or Ethnic Food Practices—cont'd

Characteristic Food Practices	Health Implications
Mexican American (also applies to some Central Americans)	
Cooking methods: Boiling, stewing; frying. *Foods enjoyed:* Dry beans (pinto, garbanzo, black beans; beans often mashed and cooked with lard), beef, pork, chicken, fish, goat, eggs, hot sausage, tripe (beef stomach), rice, corn or flour tortillas, posole (hominy), sweet pastries, cookies, candies (often candied fruits), chilies, pumpkin, chayote squash, corn, prickly pear cactus leaves (nopales), avocado, tomatoes, citrus, papaya, cilantro.	*Positives:* High in complex carbohydrates. *Concerns:* High fat intake; lard used in Mexico and by recent immigrants; margarine, oils, and mayonnaise widely used in the United States; little milk used by adults; sugar intake high. Nutrients most likely to be lacking in the diet include calcium, iron, vitamins A and C, folate. Breastfeeding is common in Mexico but not in U.S. immigrants. *Prevalent nutrition-related problems:* Diabetes, obesity, heart disease, and dental caries.
Puerto Rican	
Cooking methods: Frying, boiling, or simmering for prolonged periods with lard or salt pork for seasoning. *Foods enjoyed:* Cafe con leche (coffee with 2-5 oz milk), beans (especially red or white), rice, pork, chicken, eggs, viands (starchy vegetables: plantains, sweet potatoes, chayote squash), breadfruit, mango, avocado, corn,	*Positives:* Many fruits and vegetables used in Puerto Rico. High in complex carbohydrates. Breastfeeding is relatively common, and breast milk is perceived as nutritious for the infant. *Concerns:* High fat intake; adults consume milk mainly in coffee, and low-fat or skim milk is not

Continued

sofrito (relish of tomatoes, green peppers, chilies, onions, spices, and oil or lard).

Food beliefs: Diseases are categorized as hot or cold, and foods are divided into hot, cold, and cool; suitability of a food in sickness or postpartum depends on its category; malt beer believed to be nutritious, often given to children and lactating women.

commonly used; Sazon, a popular seasoning, is high in sodium.

Prevalent nutrition-related problems: Obesity, high blood pressure, diabetes, cardiovascular disease.

Southeast Asian (Vietnamese, Cambodian)

Cooking methods: Stir-frying, steaming.

Foods enjoyed: White rice, fish, duck, chicken, eggs, pork, tofu (soybean curd), chicken-rice noodle soup, green leafy vegetables, "cellophane" (bean starch) noodles, fruits, French bread and pastries, tea.

Positives: Low-fat cooking methods; limited intake of high-fat animal products; high complex carbohydrate and low sugar intakes. Breastfeeding is common among new immigrants

Concerns: Little milk product use among adults.

Prevalent nutrition-related problems: Osteoporosis among women, anemia, dental caries.

Table 1-4   Examples of Cultural, Religious, or Ethnic Food Practices—cont'd

Characteristic Food Practices	Health Implications
Japanese *Cooking methods:* Stir-frying, steaming, broiling, simmering. *Foods enjoyed:* Rice, noodles, many vegetables, fish, tofu and other soy products, pickles, green tea.	*Positives:* Traditional diet low in fat, high in complex carbohydrates, rich in vegetables. *Concerns:* Japanese diet ≈4 times as high in sodium as American; gastric cancer rate high in Japan, probably related to use of dried, smoked fish high in nitrates; little milk product intake among adults; raw fish (sashimi) consumed, potential for food poisoning and tapeworms.
Chinese *Cooking methods:* Broiling, steaming, frying, or simmering. *Foods enjoyed:* Rice, noodles, tofu and other soybean products, pork, chicken, many vegetables, tea.	*Positives:* Vegetables used often. *Concerns:* Sodium intake can be high; lactose intolerance common among adults.

Continued

Indian (Asian)

Cooking methods: Braising, pot roasting (dum), frying, tandoori (clay oven), curry (stew).

Foods enjoyed: Breads, rice, lamb or mutton, cauliflower, potatoes, cucumbers, peas, chickpeas, chicken and eggs, mango, melons, raisins, coconut, almonds, pistachios. Various spices are used in all types of cooking.

Positives: Most are vegetarians and eat a wide variety of vegetables and fruits.

Concerns: Vegetarians may have difficulty consuming enough vitamin B_{12}; yogurt and (in some areas of India) eggs are used and provide a reliable source of vitamin B_{12}; diets of children and pregnant and lactating women should be assessed for adequacy. Ghee (clarified butter) is used often and may result in a high intake of total and saturated fat.

Jewish

Cooking methods: Boiling, stewing, many meats salted; "kashruth," or Jewish food laws, are followed; milk products and meat are not combined in food preparation; utensils used to prepare or serve meat not used for milk products and vice versa; milk consumption must occur at least 3-6 hr after meat; "pareve" foods (e.g., fish, eggs, some margarines, breads) contain neither meat nor dairy products and may be used with either.

Positives: A wide variety of foods from all groups are included in the kashruth.

Concerns: Meats salted; fasting is practiced several times each year, but pregnant and nursing women and sick individuals are not required to fast.

Table 1-4   Examples of Cultural, Religious, or Ethnic Food Practices—cont'd

Characteristic Food Practices	Health Implications
Jewish	
Foods enjoyed: Milk, cheese, eggs, fish with scales and fins, wide variety of vegetables, fruits, and breads; beef, lamb, poultry must be slaughtered and prepared in kosher manner; packaged foods are marked with a K, circled U, or other symbol to indicate that they are kosher.	
Foods not used: Pork, horsemeat, or meat of any other four-footed animal that does not chew a cud and/or have split hooves; fish without fins and scales; shellfish; insects; reptiles; during Passover (8 days in spring), certain foods (e.g., bread products) must be "kosher for Passover" and no leavenings are used.	
Ovolactovegetarian (e.g., some Seventh-Day Adventists)	
Cooking methods: All.	*Positives:* Lower rates of certain cancers than general population; diet tends to be lower fat; provides all known nutrients.
Foods enjoyed: Milk and milk products, eggs, all fruits, vegetables, soy, and grain products; Seventh-Day Adventists use cereal-based beverages (Postum) and meat	*Concerns:* Iron and zinc intake must be assessed.

analogues made from soy or other vegetable proteins.

Foods not used: Meat, poultry, fish; Seventh-Day Adventists avoid caffeinated beverages.

Vegan (strict vegetarian)

Cooking methods: All, steaming and stir-frying popular.

Foods enjoyed: Grains (especially whole grains), fruits, vegetables, soy and fermented soy products, oils, nuts and seeds.

Foods not used: Any animal products (milk, eggs, cheese, yogurt, meat, fish, poultry); some avoid fortified and processed foods.

Positives: Tends to be low in fat and high in fiber, reducing risk of heart disease, obesity, and some cancers; combining grains, legumes, nuts, and seeds yields adequate protein.

Concerns: Vitamin B_{12} is found only in foods of animal origin, supplements, and fortified foods; fermented soy products (miso, tempeh) are not reliable sources of vitamin B_{12}; calcium intake often low; absorption of iron and zinc often poor; inadequate energy density for optimal growth in children.

Continued

Table 1-4   Examples of Cultural, Religious, or Ethnic Food Practices—cont'd

Characteristic Food Practices	Health Implications
Middle Eastern (Syria, Lebanon, Turkey, Jordan, Iraq, Iran, Greece, Israel, Egypt)	
Cooking methods: Meats cooked in a large amount of animal fat (butter or ghee, a clarified butter from sheep, goat, or camel milk) or oil (olive, sesame). *Foods enjoyed:* Breads, rice, pilaf, beans, lentils, yogurt, cheese, lamb, goat, olives, cucumbers, citrus, onions, tomatoes, eggplant, dates, figs, pomegranates, baklava (layered pastry with honey and nuts), seasonings of cinnamon, mint, and oregano. *Foods not used:* Muslims avoid alcohol and pork.	*Positives:* Fruit served for dessert except on special occasions; breads usually whole grain and rich in fiber; yogurt used in many foods; avoidance of alcohol-related health problems by Muslims. *Concerns:* High-fat cooking methods; females assigned lower status by some Middle Easterners, so quantity and variety of food may be less for females.

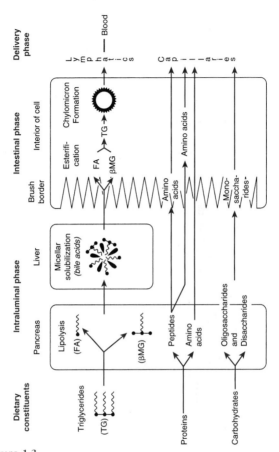

Figure 1-3
Digestion and absorption of triglycerides (fat), proteins, and carbohydrates. *FA*, Fatty acid; *MG*, monoglyceride; *TG*, triglyceride.
(From Silverman A, Roy CC: *Pediatric clinical gastroenterology*, ed 3, St Louis, 1983, Mosby.)

Digestion and Absorption
Energy-providing nutrients and the products of their digestion
Carbohydrates

Carbohydrates can be large, small, or intermediate in size. *Polysaccharides,* such as the starches, are the largest carbohydrates. They are found in grains, legumes, potatoes, and other vegetables. Polysaccharides are formed from many *monosaccharide* (glucose, fructose, mannose, or galactose) units, and they must be broken down into monosaccharides or small oligosaccharides so that they can be absorbed. *Dextrins* and *oligosaccharides* are compounds made up of chains of glucose molecules (usually 3 to 20 glucose units). They are formed during digestion of starch, and they are used commercially in the manufacturing of medical foods for enteral tube feedings and nutritional supplements. *Disaccharides* are sugars composed of two monosaccharides. Sucrose is a disaccharide composed of glucose and fructose. It is found in table sugar, brown sugar, maple syrup, and molasses. Lactose is a disaccharide found in milk and consisting of glucose and galactose. Maltose is a disaccharide consisting of two glucose molecules; maltose is not common in the diet, but it is produced during digestion of starch. In addition to being building blocks for larger carbohydrates, the monosaccharides glucose and fructose are found by themselves in foods such as honey and fruits. Monosaccharides and disaccharides are often called *simple sugars*.

Fiber consists of indigestible polysaccharides and lignins from plants. Although fiber is incompletely digested and absorbed, diets rich in fiber stimulate gastrointestinal transit, reduce the risk of coronary heart disease, and might decrease the likelihood of developing type 2 diabetes.

Proteins

Dietary *proteins* are compounds made up of hundreds of *amino acids*, or nitrogen-containing molecules. During the digestion of a protein, *polypeptides* (or compounds containing fewer than 100 amino acids) and *peptides* (shorter chains of amino acids) are formed from the protein. These intermediate products must be further digested into amino acids or dipeptides and tripeptides (compounds containing two or three amino acids) to be absorbed. After absorption the dipeptides and tripeptides are further digested to amino acids, which can be used for synthesis of body proteins.

Amino acids are either essential (required in the diet) or nonessential (formed in the body in sufficient amounts for the building of tissues). Proteins of high biologic value, such as those from meats and milk products, contain essential amino acids in amounts that are adequate for tissue repair and formation of new tissue. Proteins of lower biologic value, such as those from grains and nuts, tend to be limited in one or more essential amino acids; choosing a variety of different plant proteins improves the biologic value of the diet.

Lipids (fats) and fat-soluble vitamins

Most dietary fat, and most fat stored in the body, is in the form of *triglycerides* (Figure 1-4), consisting of a glycerol backbone esterified (bonded) to three fatty acids. Fatty acids can be saturated (with no carbon-carbon double bonds) or unsaturated (with one or more carbon-carbon double bonds). Triglycerides must be digested into smaller forms to be absorbed. A diglyceride is a molecule composed of glycerol bound to two fatty acids; it is produced during triglyceride digestion. A diglyceride is broken down further into a monoglyceride (a molecule composed of glycerol bound to one fatty acid), and these products can be absorbed. Fat-soluble vitamins are absorbed in a manner similar to other lipids.

Diets where the fat is primarily in the form of **monounsaturated** and **polyunsaturated fatty acids** are associated with the lowest risk of heart disease. The *Dietary Guidelines* recommend that less than 10% of energy intake should come from saturated fatty acids. **Omega-3 fatty acids** are **unsaturated fatty acids** obtained from fatty fish (e.g., salmon, herring, trout) and plant sources, such as canola oil, walnuts, and flaxseed; they tend to reduce inflammatory conditions associated with obesity, heart disease, and type 2 diabetes.

Process of digestion and absorption of macronutrients

Table 1-5 summarizes the major enzymes involved in digestion, the sites where they are released, and the products of their action. Most nutrients are absorbed in the duodenum, jejunum, and ileum (Figure 1-5); therefore, damage to or surgical removal of a

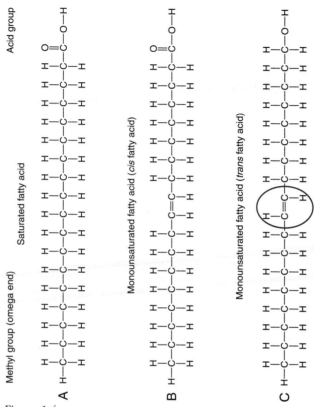

Figure 1-4
Structures of some common fatty acids and triglycerides.
Fatty acids containing only single bonds *(A)* are saturated.
Unsaturated fatty acids may be monounsaturated *(B)* or
polyunsaturated *(D and E).*

significant portion of the small intestine often leads to malabsorption of a nutrient or nutrients. Fat malabsorption is especially likely because fat and fat-soluble vitamin absorption is a
complicated process requiring adequate production of bile salts
and adequate bowel surface area for absorption (see Chapter 8).
Bile salts are reabsorbed in the ileum and reused, and therefore
an intact ileum is needed for normal fat absorption.

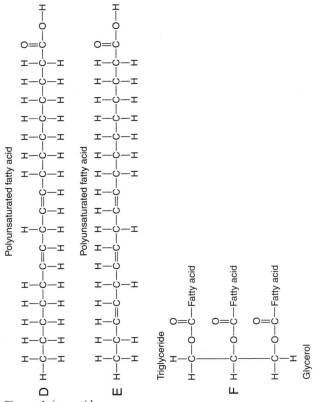

Figure 1-4, cont'd
Fatty acids are often described by the number of carbon atoms they contain and by the number and location of double bonds. One system is to count the carbon atoms starting at the methyl (or omega) end. Using this system, fatty acid D is an omega-6 fatty acid, and E is an omega-3 fatty acid. Most dietary fat is in the form of triglycerides *(F)*.

Vitamins and minerals

Most vitamins are absorbed by means of specific transporters in the small intestine, with most of the water-soluble vitamins (B complex and vitamin C) being absorbed in the jejunum and proximal ileum (see Figure 1-5). Vitamin B_{12} is an exception in that specific receptors are required for its absorption, and they are found only in the ileum.

Table 1-5   Summary of the Major Digestive Enzymes

Enzyme	Site of Production	Process of Digestion*
Carbohydrate Digestion		
Salivary amylase	Mouth	Starch → Oligosaccharides, dextrins, and maltose
Pancreatic amylase	Pancreas (released into intestine)	Starch → Oligosaccharides, dextrins, and maltose
"Brush border" enzymes	Small intestine	
Isomaltase, glucoamylase		Oligosaccharides and dextrins → Maltose and glucose
Lactase		Lactose → Glucose and galactose
Maltase		Oligosaccharides and maltose → Glucose
Sucrase		Sucrose → Glucose and fructose
Protein Digestion		
Pepsin	Stomach	Proteins → Peptides
Trypsin, chymotrypsin	Pancreas (released into small intestine)	Proteins, peptides → Smaller peptides

Carboxypeptidase	Pancreas (released into small intestine)	Peptides → Small peptides, amino acids
Aminopeptidase, dipeptidase	Intestine (brush border)	Peptides → Smaller peptides, amino acids
Various peptidases	Intestine (inside mucosal cell)	Tripeptides, dipeptides → Amino acids
Fat Digestion		
Milk lipase	Human milk	Triglycerides → Glycerol, fatty acids
Gastric lipase	Mouth; stomach	Triglycerides → Diglycerides, fatty acids
Pancreatic lipase	Pancreas (released into small intestine)	Fat → Diglycerides, monoglycerides, fatty acids

*Dextrins, short chains of glucose molecules; peptides, chains of linked amino acids; triglycerides, the form of most fat in the diet and consisting of a glycerol backbone with three fatty acids attached.

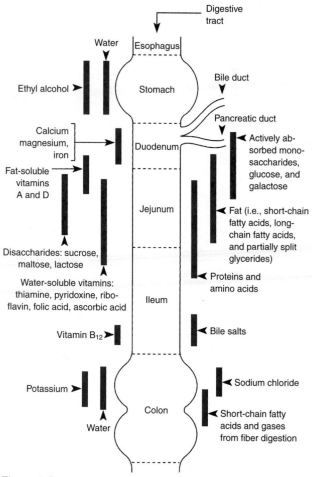

Figure 1-5
Sites of nutrient absorption.
(From Heimburger DC, Weinsier RL: *Handbook of clinical nutrition*, ed 3, St Louis, 1997, Mosby.)

Much of the calcium absorption occurs by means of a specific calcium-binding protein that requires vitamin D for its synthesis. Iron is absorbed best in an acid environment, and therefore iron absorption occurs primarily in the duodenum, before the chyme (partially digested food released from the stomach) has time to mix with alkaline secretions in the intestine. A transport protein, the divalent metal transporter, is responsible for iron absorption into the intestinal mucosa cells (enterocytes). The divalent metal transporter is not specific for iron and can also transport other minerals. Iron stores in the body are carefully regulated, since an excess can cause toxicity, particularly liver damage. If body iron stores are low, the absorbed iron is released from the enterocytes to be transported in the blood by ferritin, an iron-binding protein, to cells throughout the body. If iron stores are abundant, a large proportion of the absorbed iron remains in the enterocytes. Enterocytes have a short life span of approximately 3 to 5 days, after which they are sloughed off the intestinal mucosa. The iron contained in the enterocytes is shed from the body with other cell components. Very large doses of iron inhibit the absorption of zinc and copper.

Food Safety

Maintaining food safety and preventing food-borne illnesses is an important part of ensuring adequate nutritional intake. Guidelines for safe handling, storage, and preparation of foods are outlined in Appendix J on Evolve. In general, consumers should wash hands thoroughly before preparing foods; store foods properly; wash produce carefully; avoid cross-contamination of produce by raw meats, poultry, and fish; and cook meats to the recommended internal temperatures before serving. Additional information is available at www.foodsafety.gov.

Conclusion

Nutritional status has important effects on individual, national, and global health. Seven of ten Americans who die each year die of a chronic disease such as cancer, cardiovascular disease, or diabetes (CDC, 2007). Many of these deaths could have been prevented or delayed with optimal nutrition and lifestyle choices. Education of the public about wise nutrition and lifestyle choices, in a manner sensitive to ethnic, cultural, and physiologic considerations, and public policy decisions designed to encourage healthy choices are essential.

REFERENCES

Centers for Disease Control and Prevention (CDC): Chronic disease prevention. Available at http://www.cdc.gov/nccdphp/. Accessed November 21, 2007.

Messina V, Melina V, Mangels AR: A new food guide for North American vegetarians, *J Am Diet Assoc* 103:771, 2003.

SELECTED BIBLIOGRAPHY

Blitstein JL, Evans WD: Use of nutrition facts panels among adults who make household food purchasing decisions, *J Nutr Educ Behav* 38(6): 360, 2006.

Centers for Disease Control and Prevention: Prevalence of fruit and vegetable consumption and physical activity by race/ethnicity—United States, 2005, *MMWR Morb Mortal Wkly Rep* 56(13):301, 2007.

Drewnowski A: Concept of a nutritious food: toward a nutrient density score, *Am J Clin Nutr* 82(4):721, 2005.

Food and Nutrition Board, National Academy of Sciences, Institute of Medicine: *Dietary reference intakes for energy, carbohydrate, fiber, fat, fatty acids, cholesterol, protein, and amino acids (macronutrients)*, Washington, DC, 2002, National Academy Press.

Food and Nutrition Board, National Academy of Sciences, Institute of Medicine: *Dietary reference intakes: the essential guide to nutrient requirements*, Washington, DC, 2006, National Academy Press.

Murphy SP, Guenther PM, Kretsch MJ: Using the dietary reference intakes to assess intakes of groups: pitfalls to avoid, *J Am Diet Assoc* 106(10): 1550, 2006.

Schneeman BO: Gastrointestinal physiology and functions, *Br J Nutr* 88(suppl 2):159, 2002.

Russell RM: Setting dietary intake levels: problems and pitfalls, *Novartis Found Symp* 282:29, 2007.

U.S. Department of Health and Human Services (USDHHS) and U.S. Department of Agriculture (USDA): *Dietary guidelines for Americans, 2005*, ed 6, Washington, DC, 2005, U.S. Government Printing Office.

U.S. Department of Health and Human Services: *Healthy people 2010*, Washington, DC, 2000, U.S. Government Printing Office.

NUTRITION ASSESSMENT

An individual's nutritional status affects performance, well-being, growth and development, and resistance to illness. **Nutrition assessment** is the process used to evaluate nutritional status, identify disorders of nutrition, and determine which individuals need nutrition instruction and/or nutrition support.

Malnutrition

Malnutrition includes both undernutrition and overnutrition. It can result from inadequate intake; disorders of digestion, absorption, or assimilation; or excessive intake of nutrients.

Undernutrition

Protein-energy malnutrition

Protein-energy malnutrition (PEM) or **protein-calorie malnutrition (PCM)** is defined as undernutrition resulting from inadequate intake, digestion, or absorption of protein and/or energy (calories). Weight loss, fat loss, muscle wasting and weakness, impaired immune function, poor wound healing, and reduction of protein synthesis are characteristics of PEM. Two forms of PEM are termed *marasmus* and *kwashiorkor*. Marasmus describes a condition in which weight loss and wasting of muscle and fat are the predominant signs. It occurs when intake of energy nutrients is inadequate to meet the person's needs, such as under conditions of famine. Kwashiorkor, on the other hand, refers to a condition in which the most evident symptoms are related to impaired protein synthesis. Levels of serum proteins such as albumin, prealbumin or transthyretin (a protein participating in thyroxine transport), and retinol binding protein are reduced. These proteins are termed *visceral proteins* since they are produced by the liver. Serum oncotic pressure (a function of serum protein concentrations) falls in kwashiorkor, allowing edema and sometimes ascites to develop. In severe kwashiorkor, skin lesions, loss of hair pigmentation, and hepatomegaly (largely caused by fatty infiltration of the liver resulting from impaired ability to synthesize the lipoproteins that transport lipid from the liver to other tissues) are evident. Classically, kwashiorkor has been viewed as a disease occurring when energy intake is adequate or near adequate but protein intake is very low; it was first described in African infants weaned from human milk to a diet consisting almost entirely of cereal. It can occur in developed countries among children and adults with inadequate vegetarian or alternative diet patterns (Carvalho et al., 2001; Liu et al., 2001; Katz et al., 2005).

PEM occurs not only in developing countries but also among ill individuals in all nations when their intakes are inadequate to meet their needs for energy and tissue synthesis. It has been suggested that kwashiorkor among sick patients results at least partly from the presence of inflammation and/or inadequate antioxidant status and that the signs and symptoms of kwashiorkor are associated with elevated levels of the inflammatory **cytokines** (immunoregulatory proteins such as the interleukins, tumor necrosis factor, and interferon that are secreted by cells, especially those of the immune system) (Dülger et al., 2002; Fuhrman et al., 2004). In any case, inflammation and trauma can alter serum protein levels so that they are not reliable indicators of PEM (see the later section, "Biochemical or Laboratory Analyses").

Vitamin and mineral deficiencies

Vitamin and mineral deficiencies develop in a progressive manner, with depletion of tissue stores occurring first, followed by biochemical abnormalities (e.g., decrease in activity of enzymes requiring a particular vitamin or mineral), and finally the development of overt clinical signs and symptoms. The clinical signs and symptoms may be subtle and nonspecific (e.g., cracking skin may be a sign of deficiency of riboflavin or biotin or a sign of excess vitamin A intake). The most common nutritional disease in this category is iron deficiency anemia. Although individuals with severe iron deficiency may have pallor and spoon-shaped nails (Figure 2-1), there may be no overt signs. Suboptimal intakes of vitamins and minerals may result in adverse outcomes even if overt deficiency is not present. For example, inadequate folate intake among women in the childbearing years contributes to births of infants with neural tube defects, even though macrocytic anemia (which can be a nutritional deficiency disease resulting from folate deficiency) is not prevalent.

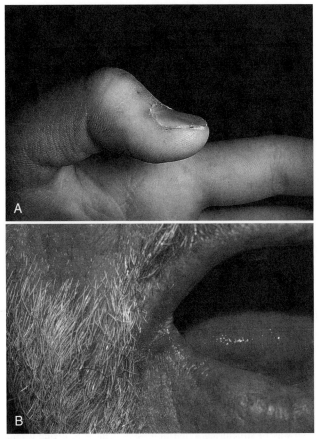

Figure 2-1
Examples of findings in malnourished states. **A**, Spoon-shaped
nails, or koilonychia. **B**, Cracking at the corners of the mouth,
or cheilosis ("cheilitis").
(**A** from Callen J et al: *Color atlas of dermatology*, ed 2, Philadelphia, 2000,
WB Saunders; **B** from Caucasian GM, Cox NH: *Diseases of the skin*, ed 2, London,
2006, Mosby.)

It is common for multiple vitamin and mineral deficits to be present or for these deficits to occur in conjunction with PEM. For example, the individual who consumes no animal products is at risk of deficiency of vitamin B_{12}, calcium, iron, and zinc; in addition, protein and energy intake may be suboptimal unless the diet is carefully planned.

Overnutrition

The most common forms of overnutrition, present in more than half of American adults, are overweight and obesity. Overweight and obesity refer to an excess of body fat, but for simplicity they are often defined as being 10% and 20%, respectively, greater than the ideal body weight. These conditions are associated with numerous health risks, including hypertension, heart disease, type 2 diabetes, stroke, gallbladder disease, osteoarthritis, sleep apnea and other respiratory disorders, and certain cancers.

Overnutrition can also occur with excessive intakes of fat-soluble vitamins and some minerals. For instance, excessive intake of vitamin A, especially an intake of 10 mg or more daily over a period of several months, can cause increased intracranial pressure, liver damage, bone and joint pain, and scaly skin. Water-soluble vitamins are usually excreted in the urine without ill effects, but very large amounts of these vitamins may also result in side effects. Megadoses of vitamin C (usually more than 1 g/day), for example, can cause diarrhea, false-negative results on tests for occult blood in the stool, and interference with anticoagulant therapy.

Assessment Procedures

One way of structuring a nutrition assessment is to divide it into four components:
A, anthropometric measurements
B, biochemical or laboratory analyses
C, clinical and physical assessment
D, diet or nutritional history

Anthropometric Measurements

Anthropometric measurements are measurements of the human body. Essential measurements include height (or length for children less than 2 to 3 years) and weight. Head circumference is included for children less than 2 years of age. A rough estimate of the ideal body weight (IBW) for adults may be obtained with these rules of thumb:

Women: IBW = 100 lb for the first 5 ft of height + 5 lb for every inch over 5 ft

Men: IBW = 106 lb for the first 5 ft of height + 6 lb for every inch over 5 ft

Using these equations, the desirable body weight is within 10% of the estimated IBW. These simple equations yield only rough estimates of IBW. Because of variations in body build and other factors, the values determined by these equations may not be very accurate for a particular individual.

The **body mass index (BMI)** is a simple tool for evaluating the appropriateness of weight for height (Box 2-1). It does not involve measurement of body composition, and thus it is not an accurate method for assessing the percentage of lean body mass or fat. However, the BMI correlates well with many measures of body fat content, as well as with risk of morbidity under a variety of conditions

---

Box 2-1   Body Mass Index (BMI)*

Calculating BMI

$$BMI = \frac{Weight\,(kg)}{Height^2\,(m)} \quad \text{or} \quad BMI = \frac{Weight\,(lb)}{Height^2\,(in)} \times 704.5$$

Example: An individual weighs 65 kg (143 lb) and is 1.7 m (5'7") tall. BMI = $65/(1.7)^2 = 22.5$ kg/m^2

Classification of BMI

Underweight: <18.5
Normal: 18.5-24.9
Overweight: 25.0-29.9
Obese: ≥30.0
Extreme obesity ≥40.0

Classification is from *Clinical guidelines on the identification, evaluation, and treatment of overweight and obesity in adults,* Washington, DC, 1998, National Heart, Lung, and Blood Institute (NHLBI) and National Institute of Diabetes and Digestive and Kidney Diseases (NIDDK).

*A nomogram for determining BMI without making any calculations can be found inside the back cover.

(Bogers et al., 2007; Campillo et al., 2004). In addition, it is quickly and easily performed in virtually any setting. A chart for determining BMI without making any calculations can be found inside the back cover of this book, and an automatic BMI calculator can be found at http://www.nhlbisupport.com/bmi/.

The Centers for Disease Control Website contains the standardized growth charts for children, showing percentile rankings of height and weight for age and weight for height, as well as BMI for age. In long-term undernutrition, children exhibit growth retardation, with height low in relation to expected height for age (length or height will be below the 5th percentile). Short stature is also found in endocrine and other disorders unrelated to nutrition in children. When short-term undernutrition has occurred, height may be normal for age but weight will be low for height. (Weight for height below the 5th percentile indicates undernutrition; see Appendix D on Evolve.) Overweight children have a weight for height or BMI that is above the 95th percentile. Those with a BMI between the 85th and 95th percentile are at risk for overweight.

Adjustments to ideal or desirable body weights

Certain physical body changes require adjustments to the ideal or desirable body weights. For amputees, reduce IBW by the following percentages, depending on the extremity lost: hand and forearm, 2.3%; total arm, 5%; foot and lower leg, 6%; and total leg, 16% (Osterkamp, 1995). These percentages are derived largely from Caucasian individuals and may require some adjustment for other racial and ethnic groups. African Americans have proportionally longer lower extremities, and Asians have shorter extremities than Caucasians. The calculations are based on height, so preamputation values must be used for individuals with loss of both lower extremities. For paraplegic individuals, IBW is approximately 5% to 10% less than the calculated value, and for quadriplegic individuals, IBW is 10% to 15% less than calculated (Cox et al, 1985).

Body composition

The body composition—particularly the relative proportions of body fat and lean body mass (or fat-free mass) and the distribution of body fat—is much more relevant to health and fitness than the simple determination of the appropriateness of weight for height. Numerous methods are available for measuring body composition (Box 2-2).

Box 2-2   Methods of Assessing Body Composition

Anthropometric Measurements
- Height and weight
  Description: Weight is measured with a calibrated scale and height with a stadiometer.
    Advantages: Inexpensive; easy to perform; readily obtained; can be used for calculation of body mass index (BMI), which correlates well with other measures of body fatness.
    Disadvantage: No direct information about total body fat or regional fat distribution.
- Skinfold measurements
  Description: Skinfold(s) are measured with calipers at one or more sites, e.g., triceps (see Figure 2-2), subscapular, suprailiac, and midthigh.
    Advantages: Inexpensive, easy to perform, correlate well with size of subcutaneous fat deposits.
    Disadvantages: Substantial intraobserver and interobserver variation in measurements; skinfolds may be too large to measure with calipers in obese individuals; inaccurate when edema is present in the area measured; subcutaneous fat distribution may vary among races; an indicator of subcutaneous fat, which is less closely related to health risk than visceral fat.
- Waist circumference
  Description: The circumference is measured in a standing subject at the level of the iliac crest, at the end of normal expiration. The measuring tape must be parallel to the floor and snug, without compressing the skin.
    Advantages: Inexpensive; easy to perform; highly correlated with visceral fat, with waist circumferences of 102 cm (40 in) in men and 88 cm (35 in) in women indicating risk for the metabolic syndrome (see Chapter 5); may be more predictive of cardiovascular risk in some groups, such as Asian Americans, than BMI.
    Disadvantage: Visceral adiposity may vary among racial and ethnic groups.

Continued

Box 2-2   Methods of Assessing Body Composition—cont'd

Tissue Conductivity Techniques

■ Bioimpedance analysis (BIA)

Description: BIA requires passage of small electrical current, undetectable to the individual, between two electrodes placed on the body. Tissues rich in water (muscle and other lean tissues) are good electrical conductors, whereas fat is a poor conductor. BIA measures body water and from that estimates fat content.

Advantages: Relatively inexpensive, portable equipment; easy and fast to perform; reproducible; can measure intracellular and extracellular water compartments; segmental analysis allows estimation of muscle and fluid in segments of the body, e.g., trunk or extremity.

Disadvantages: Accuracy is affected by numerous factors that may be hard to control: changes in hydration, electrolyte concentrations, hematocrit, and skin temperature (fever or cold exposure), as well as recent eating, drinking, exercise, and position changes; inaccurate in cases of limb amputation or regional alterations of skeletal muscle, e.g., muscular dystrophy.

Comments: To decrease error, measurements should be taken after at least 4 hours of fasting and sedentary activity and 10 min after assuming a supine position. Do not use in individuals with a cardiac pacemaker or implantable defibrillator.

■ Total body electrical conductivity (TOBEC)

Description: The subject is surrounded by a low-level electromagnetic field in a detection chamber; the conductivity of hydrated tissues allows estimation of fat vs. fat-free mass (FFM).

Advantages: Easy and fast to perform; reproducible; accurate.

Disadvantages: Expensive equipment; not widely available; little information about regional fat distribution.

■ Near-infrared interactance

Description: A wand emitting near-infrared wavelengths of light is applied to the midpoint of the biceps in the dominant arm (midway between the antecubital fossa

Box 2-2   Methods of Assessing Body Composition—cont'd

and axilla), and FFM and fat mass are differentiated by the relative amounts of light reflected and absorbed (FFM reflects and fat absorbs the light).

Advantages: Relatively inexpensive, portable equipment; easy and fast to perform; reproducible.

Disadvantages: Accuracy is not as high as some of the other methods requiring instrumentation, and error may be greatest with very lean and very obese; few data for children under 5 years; little information about regional fat distribution.

Density Measurements

■ Hydrodensitometry or underwater weighing

Description: The subject exhales maximally and is weighed while submerged in water, and pulmonary residual volume is measured and deducted from the volume of water displaced. Fat mass and FFM are estimated from standard density measurements for fat and FFM derived from cadavers.

Advantages: Reproducible; easy to perform.

Disadvantages: Not suited to subjects who are unable or unwilling to be totally submerged in water; depends on accurate measurement of pulmonary reserve volume; provides no information about regional fat distribution.

■ Air displacement plethysmography (ADP; the "BOD POD")

Description: Displacement of air is measured while the person sits inside a small chamber; calculation is similar to that for hydrodensitometry.

Advantages: Reproducible, easy to perform, suited to individuals up to 227 kg (500 lb), applicable to children and infants (infants require special PEA POD equipment), no radiation exposure.

Disadvantages: Depends on accurate measurement of pulmonary reserve volume; subject must remain very still, with no change in breathing during test; provides no information about fat distribution.

Continued

Box 2-2   Methods of Assessing Body Composition—cont'd

Imaging Techniques

■ Dual energy x-ray absorptiometry (DEXA) or dual x-ray absorptiometry (DXA)

Description: Two x-ray beams with differing energies are passed through the body; their attenuation is used to estimate bone mineral density, fat mass, and lean body mass.

Advantages: Reproducible; easy to perform; provides a "multicompartment model," i.e., is able to separate the mass of bone from other FFM.

Disadvantages: Radiation exposure (very low); expensive equipment; requires trained radiology personnel to administer and interpret the scan; most current equipment is limited to use in individuals weighing 136 kg (300 lb) or less.

■ Computerized tomography (CT)

Description: Radiographic and computer analysis is used to determine the structure of internal organs.

Advantages: Provides a very accurate indication of regional body composition, e.g., visceral and subcutaneous abdominal fat.

Disadvantages: Radiation exposure (significant); expensive equipment; requires trained radiology personnel to administer and interpret the scan; infants and small children usually need sedation to remain still.

■ Magnetic resonance imaging (MRI)

Description: A powerful magnet is used to alter motion of atoms within the body; from these changes, computerized images of internal body tissues are produced.

Advantages: Provides an indication of regional body composition; enhanced technology has made it possible to measure fat stores within the muscle and the liver; no radiation exposure.

Disadvantages: Expensive equipment; requires trained personnel to administer and interpret the scan; subject must be completely still (infants and small children usually need sedation).

■ Ultrasonography

Description: A two-dimensional image of internal body structures is formed by use of ultrasonic frequencies.

Box 2-2   Methods of Assessing Body Composition—cont'd

Advantages: Equipment relatively widely available; no radiation exposure.

Disadvantages: Moderately expensive; requires skilled technicians to perform the tests.

Isotopic Techniques

■ Isotope dilution

Description: Two fluid samples (blood, saliva, or urine) are collected: one just before administration of a radioactive or stable (nonradioactive) isotope, to determine the natural background levels, and the second sample after waiting a sufficient amount of time for the isotope to equilibrate within the body. Typically the subject drinks water labeled with deuterium (^2H), tritium (^3H), or ^{18}O to label the body water pool; urine samples are collected for isotope analysis. Total body water is calculated, and from this fat mass and FFM are estimated.

Advantages: No radiation exposure if stable isotopes such as deuterium or ^{18}O are used; with the "double-labeled water" technique, water can be labeled with both deuterium and ^{18}O, allowing simultaneous measurement of body composition and energy expenditure in free-living individuals going about their daily activities.

Disadvantages: Moderately expensive; requires skilled technicians to analyze the samples; no measurement of regional body composition.

BMI, Body mass index; *FFM,* fat-free mass.

Not only total body fat but also regional distribution of fat is important in relation to long-term health. Abdominal fat is a predictor of cardiovascular risk, and abdominal fat exists in more than one depot, including the deep fat associated with the visceral organs (**visceral fat**) and the more superficial subcutaneous abdominal fat. Visceral fat is especially closely related to health risk. Only a limited number of the available methods (i.e., computerized tomography [CT] and magnetic resonance imaging)

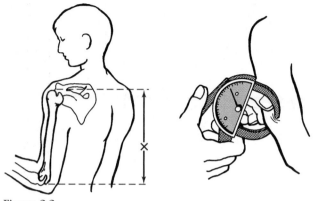

Figure 2-2
Triceps skinfold (TSF) measurements are performed at the midpoint of the upper arm.
(From Heimburger DC, Weinsier RL: *Handbook of clinical nutrition*, ed 3, St Louis, 1997, Mosby.)

assess visceral fat. CT and dual energy x-ray absorptiometry (DEXA) involve radiation exposure, albeit a very small amount with DEXA. This is a consideration in vulnerable populations, such as pregnant women and children, as well in performing repeated measurements in the same subject.

Biochemical or Laboratory Analyses

Good clinical judgment must be used in selecting laboratory analyses to be performed and interpreting test results. A thorough physical assessment and nutritional history can be as effective in identifying many cases of malnutrition as a battery of laboratory analyses.

Laboratory assessment of protein nutritional status is especially difficult (Table 2-1). Circulating proteins provide the simplest index of protein nutrition, but their serum or plasma concentrations rise and fall in sick or injured individuals for many reasons that have little to do with nutrition. The liver increases synthesis and release of **acute-phase reactants**, such as C-reactive protein, fibrinogen, serum amyloid A, and α_1-acid glycoprotein, in response to injury, trauma, inflammation, and infection. The same conditions can suppress circulating levels of albumin, transferrin, and prealbumin (reverse acute-phase reactants), since hepatic protein synthesis priorities are directed

Table 2-1   Laboratory Assessment of Protein Status

Protein Compartment and Test	Comments
Visceral proteins (serum or plasma proteins)	Synthesized in liver, decreased in liver disease; fall during the acute-phase response
Albumin	Long half-life (14-20 days) and thus relatively insensitive to nutrition change; lost in urine in nephrotic syndrome; "capillary leak" can cause loss from circulation in critical illness
Transferrin	Half-life 7-8 days; elevated in iron deficiency
Prealbumin (transthyretin)	Half-life 2-3 days
Retinol binding protein	Half-life 12-14 hr; elevated in renal failure
Somatic (muscle) proteins	Urinary excretion is an indicator of muscle mass
Creatinine excretion Expected 24-hr urinary excretion: 20 mg/kg body weight for children, 17 mg/kg for women, and 23 mg/kg for men	Requires accurate 24-hr urine collection; altered by renal failure; not a valid nutritional indicator in the presence of diseases affecting muscle
3-Methylhistidine (urine)	Specific indicator found only in muscle
Nitrogen balance Balance = [24-hr protein intake (g) × 0.16] − [24-hr urine urea nitrogen (g) + 4 g]*	Negative values occur when more nitrogen is lost than consumed (inadequate intake or catabolism); positive values are observed when more nitrogen is consumed than lost (e.g., nutritional repletion, growth, pregnancy) Requires accurate 24-hr urine collection and food intake records; altered by liver and renal failure

*Protein intake is multiplied by 0.16 because protein is approximately 16% nitrogen
4 g represents an estimate of daily fecal and skin losses, but this value can increase in the presence of severe diarrhea, fistula drainage, exudative losses, etc.

toward the acute-phase reaction. Fluid loss and fluid resuscitation also alter serum protein concentrations. A thorough physical assessment and diet/nutritional history provide more information about the presence of nutritional risk in acutely sick or injured individuals than measurement of circulating proteins does. However, serum protein measurements do correlate well with the patient's prognosis (and thus may help to identify patients at high risk for nutrition problems). Prealbumin's short half-life and small body pool make it one of the most sensitive visceral proteins for assessment of nutritional status. (**Sensitivity** is the probability that a test indicates a nutrient deficiency, given that the person actually does have a deficiency. **Specificity** is the probability that a test indicates no nutrient deficiency, given that the person does not have a deficiency.)

Table 2-2 lists representative tests used in nutrition assessment of selected minerals and vitamins. Reference values for nutrition-related laboratory tests are provided in Appendix F on Evolve. Blood, plasma, or serum concentrations are among the easiest values to obtain and the most commonly used tests for most vitamins and minerals. Nevertheless, with the exception of selenium, the circulating nutrient concentrations are unlikely to be sensitive or specific indicators of nutritional status. For many vitamins and minerals, homeostatic mechanisms maintain normal or near-normal circulating concentrations of the nutrient even though intake is inadequate and tissue stores are decreasing. However, alternative analyses are not always readily available. In many instances, measurements of tissue stores are poorly standardized (as in the case of hair and nail analyses) or difficult to apply on a wide basis. Functional tests (e.g., reduction in activity of an enzyme requiring a particular nutrient) are of great practical benefit, because they provide an indicator of a change in normal physiology and metabolism related to a nutritional deficit. To be most beneficial, functional indices must be specific for a deficiency of only one nutrient, a difficult criterion to meet. The most definitive indication of deficiency of many vitamins and minerals is the response to supplementation; for example, an increase in hemoglobin concentration within 1 month of initiating iron supplementation is consistent with the presence of iron deficiency.

Nutritional anemias

Nutritional anemias, resulting from deficiencies of iron, folate, vitamin B_{12} and other nutrients, are characterized by low hematocrit and hemoglobin concentrations. In order to distinguish between the types of anemia, judicious use of laboratory tests is essential (Figure 2-3). However, caution must be used in interpreting the tests. For example, the mean cell volume (MCV), a measure of the red blood cell size, is useful in differentiating the types of anemia, but it may be misleading for a number of reasons: (1) the MCV is normal in the early stages of virtually all anemias; (2) the reticulocyte, an immature form of the red blood cell, is larger than the mature cell, so that a marked increase in reticulocytes (e.g., following an acute hemorrhage) can elevate the MCV; and (3) combined deficiencies, as of iron and folate, may result in a normal MCV. Ferritin is an acute-phase reactant, and this can complicate the diagnosis of iron deficiency when inflammation is present. The serum transferrin receptor (sTfR) assay can help to identify iron deficiency when ferritin levels are high but iron saturation is low (Killip et al, 2007). Bone marrow aspiration may be necessary to determine whether marrow iron is depleted (i.e., in iron deficiency) or normal to high (as it may be in anemia of chronic disease) and to differentiate nutritional and nonnutritional (e.g., hemolytic anemias, leukemia) causes of macrocytic anemia.

Anemia of chronic disease is a complex disorder that occurs in a variety of conditions, including infection, inflammation, renal disease, and cancer. Contributing factors include suppression of bone marrow function by inflammatory cytokines, accelerated red blood cell breakdown with sequestration of iron in the reticuloendothelial system, and abnormalities in iron mobilization and delivery. Because of its prevalence among sick individuals, it is important to distinguish it from the nutritional anemias and recognize that it can occur concurrently with nutritional anemias.

If vitamin B_{12} deficiency is present, the cause (e.g., inadequate intake as in strict vegetarianism or inadequate absorption following ileal resection) must be determined. A subset of deficient individuals is lacking in intrinsic factor and have pernicious anemia. Intrinsic factor, secreted in the stomach, is required for vitamin B_{12} absorption. The presence of anti–intrinsic factor antibodies in the serum or an abnormal result on the Schilling test (an indicator of B_{12} absorption in the presence and absence of intrinsic factor) indicates intrinsic factor deficiency. Lifetime parenteral or intranasal vitamin B_{12} therapy is required in intrinsic factor deficiency or ileal resection, whereas low-dose oral therapy (2 to 3 mcg/day) will correct dietary inadequacy and large oral doses

Table 2-2   Laboratory Assessment of Selected Minerals and Vitamins

Nutrient	Tissue Concentrations	Indicators of Body Stores	Functional Indices Associated with Deficiency
Iron	Serum iron	Plasma or serum ferritin concentration* Serum transferrin saturation† Plasma-soluble serum transferrin receptor concentration (sTfR)	↓ Hgb, Hct, MCV (deficiency must be well advanced to be detected) ↑ Red cell distribution width (RDW) ↑ Erythrocyte protoporphyrin concentration
Calcium		Bone mineral density	
Zinc	Plasma zinc†	Red or white blood cell zinc Hair zinc White blood cell metallothionein (experimental, but promising results)	↓ Activity of zinc-dependent enzymes, such as alkaline phosphatase, copperzinc superoxide dismutase, lymphocyte 5′ -nucleotidase
Iodine	Urine iodine		↑ Thyroid-stimulating hormone ↓ Thyroxine (T$_4$) Thyroid gland enlargement (may also indicate tumor)
Selenium	Plasma selenium	Hair and nail selenium	↓ Plasma glutathione peroxidase activity

Copper	Plasma copper and ceruloplasmin (copper transport protein)	↓ Activity of copper-dependent enzymes, such as cytochrome-*c* oxidase in platelets and white blood cells
Folate	Serum or plasma folate Red cell folate	↑ Urinary excretion of FIGLU following an oral dose of histidine (may also be ↑ in vitamin B_{12} deficiency) Macrocytic anemia (↓Hct, ↓ Hgb, ↑ MCV; also a sign of B_{12} deficiency)
Vitamin A	Serum retinol Minimal dose response (measure baseline serum retinol and repeat measurement after small dose of vitamin A)	
Vitamin C (ascorbic acid)	Serum ascorbate Leukocyte ascorbate	
Vitamin K Vitamin B_{12}	Serum vitamin K Serum vitamin B_{12}	↑ Prothrombin time Macrocytic anemia (↓ Hct, ↓ Hgb, ↑ MCV; also seen in folate deficiency)
Vitamin E	Serum tocopherol	↑ Hemolysis (red cell peroxidation test)

FIGLU, Formiminoglutamate; *Hct*, hematocrit; *Hgb*, hemoglobin; *MCV*, mean (red blood) cell volume

*Increased by acute-phase reaction, ethanol intake, and hyperglycemia. Directly correlated with body mass index (BMI).

†Decreased during acute-phase reaction.

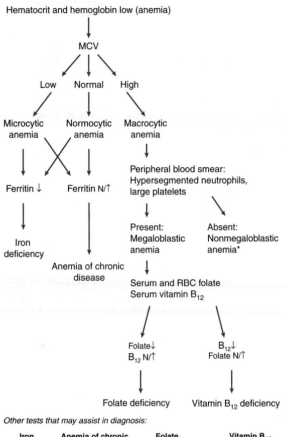

Hematocrit and hemoglobin low (anemia)

MCV

Low → Microcytic anemia

Normal → Normocytic anemia

High → Macrocytic anemia

Microcytic anemia → Ferritin ↓ → Iron deficiency

Normocytic anemia → Ferritin N/↑ → Anemia of chronic disease

Macrocytic anemia → Peripheral blood smear: Hypersegmented neutrophils, large platelets

Present: Megaloblastic anemia → Serum and RBC folate, Serum vitamin B_{12}

Absent: Nonmegaloblastic anemia*

Folate↓ B_{12} N/↑ → Folate deficiency

B_{12}↓ Folate N/↑ → Vitamin B_{12} deficiency

Other tests that may assist in diagnosis:

Iron deficiency	Anemia of chronic disease	Folate deficiency	Vitamin B_{12} deficiency
Serum iron↓	Serum iron↓	Serum homocysteine↑	Serum homocysteine↑
TIBC↑	TIBC↑	Methylmalonic acid (urine/serum) N	Methylmalonic acid (urine/serum)↑
Transferrin↑			
RDW↑			

Figure 2-3
Decision tree for laboratory tests differentiating among nutritional anemias. Anemia of chronic disease is not a nutritional anemia but is among the most common disorders in hospitalized and chronically ill patients and may coexist with nutritional anemias. ↓, Decreased; ↑, elevated; *MCV*, mean cell volume; *N*, normal; *RBC*, red blood cell; *RDW*, red blood cell distribution width; *TIBC*, total iron binding capacity. *Nonnutritional anemia; requires further evaluation.

(1000 mcg/day) may be sufficient to correct a deficiency caused by inadequate hydrochloric acid secretion. Vitamin B_{12} deficiency is associated with nerve damage that results in numerous neuropsychiatric symptoms, including abnormal gait, paresthesias, memory loss, disorientation, psychosis, spasticity, and visual loss (optic nerve atrophy). These symptoms may improve but are unlikely to be fully reversed with correction of the deficiency. Thus it is essential that B_{12} deficiency be diagnosed as early as possible and treated appropriately. High doses of folic acid can correct the anemia of vitamin B_{12} deficiency without correcting the nerve damage. Intake of folic acid from supplements and foods should be limited to 1 mg daily to reduce the risk of masking vitamin B_{12} deficiency. (Most over-the-counter folic acid supplements contain 0.4 mg in a daily dose, fortified cereals contain 0.1 mg folic acid per serving, and fortified flour and cornmeal provide 0.43 to 1.4 mg folic acid per pound [454 g].)

Clinical and Physical Assessment

Many nutrient deficiencies and excesses become apparent during careful physical assessment of the individual. Table 2-3 describes findings that may indicate malnutrition. In addition, the individual's medical record can provide some information needed for a thorough clinical assessment.

Diet or Nutritional History

Several methods can be used to obtain information about nutrient intake, depending on the depth and type of information needed.

24-hour recall

The individual is asked to recall everything consumed the previous day. If the previous day's intake was atypical for the person, a recent, more typical day may be substituted. A sample tool for collection of a 24-hour recall is shown in Figure 2-4. The advantage of this method is that it is easily and quickly done; however, the person being interviewed may not be able to recall intake accurately, and snacks, beverages, and supplements tend to be omitted. The interviewer must be trained in prompting and questioning the individual to obtain complete and accurate information. Serving sizes, in particular, may be reported incorrectly. Having available measuring cups, spoons, and dishes of different sizes may help the interviewee to describe serving sizes more accurately.

Text continued on p. 64.

Table 2-3   Signs That Suggest Nutrient Imbalance

Area of Concern	Possible Deficiency	Possible Excess
Hair		
Dull, dry, brittle	Pro	
Easily plucked (with no pain)	Pro	
Hair loss	Pro, Zn, biotin	Vit A
Flag sign (loss of hair pigment in strips around head)	Pro, Cu	
Head and Neck		
Bulging fontanel (infants)		Vit A
Headache		Vit A, D
Epistaxis (nosebleed)	Vit K	
Thyroid enlargement	Iodine	
Eyes		
Conjunctival and corneal xerosis (dryness)	Vit A	
Pale conjunctiva	Fe	
Blue sclerae	Fe	
Corneal vascularization	Vit B$_2$	

	Deficiency	Excess
Mouth		
Cheilosis or angular stomatitis (lesions at corners of mouth, see Figure 2-1)	Vit B$_2$	
Glossitis (red, sore tongue)	Niacin, folate, vit B$_{12}$, and other B vit	
Gingivitis (inflamed gums)	Vit C	
Hypogeusia, dysgeusia (poor sense of taste, distorted taste)	Zn	
Dental caries	Fluoride	
Mottling of teeth		Fluoride
Atrophy of papillae on tongue	Fe, B vit	
Skin		
Dry, scaly	Vit A, Zn, EFAs	Vit A
Follicular hyperkeratosis (resembles gooseflesh)	Vit A, EFAs, B vit	
Eczematous lesions	Zn	
Petechiae, ecchymoses	Vit C, K	
Nasolabial seborrhea (greasy, scaly areas between nose and lip)	Niacin, vit B$_{12}$, B$_6$	
Darkening and peeling of skin in areas exposed to sun	Niacin	
Poor wound healing	Pro, Zn, vit C	
Nails		
Spoon-shaped nails (see Figure 2-1)	Fe	
Brittle, fragile	Pro	

Continued

Table 2-3   Signs That Suggest Nutrient Imbalance—cont'd

Area of Concern	Possible Deficiency	Possible Excess
Heart		
Enlargement, tachycardia, failure	Vit B_1	
Small heart	Energy	
Sudden failure, death	Se	
Arrhythmia	Mg, K, Se	
Hypertension	Ca, K	
Abdomen		
Hepatomegaly	Pro	Vit A
Ascites	Pro	
Musculoskeletal Extremities		
Muscle wasting (especially temporal area)	Energy	
Edema	Pro, vit B_1	
Calf tenderness	Vit B_1 or C, biotin, Se	
Beading of ribs, or "rachitic rosary" (child)	Vit C, D	

Musculoskeletal Extremities

Bone and joint tenderness	Vit C, D, Ca, P
Knock-knee, bowed legs, fragile bones	Vit D, Ca, P, Cu

Neurologic

Paresthesias (pain and tingling or altered sensation in the extremities)	Vit B_1, B_6 B_{12}, biotin
Weakness	Vit C, B_1, B_6, B_{12}, energy
Ataxia, decreased position and vibratory senses	Vit B_1, B_{12}
Tremor	Mg
Decreased tendon reflexes	Vit B_1
Confabulation, disorientation	Vit B_1, B_{12}
Drowsiness, lethargy	Vit B_1
Depression	Vit B_1, biotin, B_{12} Vit A, D

Ca, Calcium; *Cu*, copper; *EFAs*, essential fatty acids; *Fe*, iron; *K*, potassium; *Mg*, magnesium; *Na*, sodium; *P*, phosphorus; *Pro*, protein; *Se*, selenium; *Vit*, vitamin(s); *Zn*, zinc.

The following questions may be used to elicit a 24-hour recall:
1. What time did you get up yesterday? _____
2. When was the first time you had anything to eat or drink? _____ (Avoid mentioning specific meals, e.g., "What did you have for breakfast?")
   What did you have? How much? _____ (For each food, ask for details if type or preparation method is unclear, e.g., was chicken fried or baked?; was milk whole, low-fat, or skim?)
3. When did you eat or drink something again? _____
   What did you have and how much? _____
   (Repeat question 3 until the individual has described the entire day.)
4. Did you eat or drink anything else? _____ (Review the day with the individual to see if any snacks have been omitted.)
5. Did you put anything else in your mouth and swallow it? _____ (Ask specifically about supplements: vitamin/mineral, health foods, herbal medications, etc.) Do you usually take any supplements or herbal medications that you did not take yesterday? _____
6. Was this day's intake different from usual? If so, in what way? _____
7. Do you eat differently on weekends than on weekdays? If so, in what way? _____

Figure 2-4
Tool for collection of a 24-hour recall.

Food frequency questionnaire

The health professional collects information regarding the number of times per day, week, or month the individual eats particular foods. A sample tool, focusing on cholesterol and saturated fat intake, is shown in Figure 2-5. When used with a 24-hour recall, the questionnaire can help validate the accuracy of the recall and provide a more complete picture of the individual's intake. If the goal of the nutritional history is to find out about intake of particular food components or nutrients (e.g., cholesterol and saturated fat), then the questionnaire can be designed to focus on those items. The food frequency method is economical in terms of time but provides limited information in comparison with some other methods that reveal time and circumstances of food intake, which may be helpful in identifying and changing poor eating habits (e.g., nighttime snacking during television viewing).

Mark the box showing how often you eat or drink each of the following:

	Daily	Several times a week	Once a week	Once or twice a month or less	Never
Whole milk	☐	☐	☐	☐	☐
Butter	☐	☐	☐	☐	☐
Cheese (regular)	☐	☐	☐	☐	☐
Cheese (low-fat)	☐	☐	☐	☐	☐
Cream	☐	☐	☐	☐	☐
Cream cheese	☐	☐	☐	☐	☐
Ice cream	☐	☐	☐	☐	☐
Eggs	☐	☐	☐	☐	☐
Liver	☐	☐	☐	☐	☐
Beef, pork, goat, or mutton/lamb	☐	☐	☐	☐	☐
Poultry	☐	☐	☐	☐	☐
Shellfish	☐	☐	☐	☐	☐
Salmon, tuna, sardines, or mackerel	☐	☐	☐	☐	☐
Other fish	☐	☐	☐	☐	☐
Lard	☐	☐	☐	☐	☐
Hydrogenated shortening	☐	☐	☐	☐	☐
Stick margarine	☐	☐	☐	☐	☐
Soft (tub or squeeze) margarine	☐	☐	☐	☐	☐
Corn, sunflower, or safflower oils	☐	☐	☐	☐	☐
Olive, peanut, or canola oils	☐	☐	☐	☐	☐
Pastries	☐	☐	☐	☐	☐
Gravies	☐	☐	☐	☐	☐
Walnuts or flax seed	☐	☐	☐	☐	☐
Cashews or macadamias	☐	☐	☐	☐	☐
Peanuts, mixed nuts, or peanut butter	☐	☐	☐	☐	☐

Figure 2-5
Food frequency questionnaire.

Food record

In keeping a food record, the individual records all the foods consumed, with portions weighed, measured, or estimated. Usually this is done for 3 days—1 weekend day and 2 weekdays. The food record provides more information than the 24-hour recall, particularly in quantifying the amounts eaten. Nevertheless, a food record relies heavily on the individual's cooperation. Also, food intake may be atypical during the recording period. In some cases the act of recording one's intake results in a change in eating patterns.

Food records are a valuable part of a program of weight control. Keeping food records on a regular basis increases the likelihood of success in weight loss and maintenance of weight loss.

Diet history

The individual is extensively interviewed to elicit detailed information about nutritional status, as well as general health, socioeconomic status, and cultural impact on nutrition. The diet history usually includes information similar to that collected by the 24-hour recall and food frequency questionnaire, as well as other information listed in Box 2-3. An accurate diet history requires an experienced interviewer, and it can be very time consuming. This method provides more information than either the 24-hour recall or the 3-day food record, however, and it can give an indication of food habits over several months or years. Table 2-4 illustrates diet history findings that may indicate nutritional deficits.

Evaluating nutrient intake

Computer databases can be used to calculate the amount of each nutrient in the diet. Numerous commercial databases are available. A free downloadable database can be found

Text continued on p. 70.

Box 2-3 Diet History

I. Socioeconomic data
 A. Income
  1. Adequate for food purchasing
  2. Eligibility for food stamps or other public assistance
 B. Ethnic or cultural background
  1. Influence of culture or religion on eating habits
  2. Educational level
II. Food preparation
 A. Problems in shopping for or preparing food
  1. Skill of person who shops and cooks
  2. Availability of market(s)
  3. Adequacy of facilities for cooking, food storage, and refrigeration
 B. Use of convenience foods

Box 2-3   Diet History—cont'd

III. Physical activity
    A. Occupation—type, number of hours per week, activity level
    B. Exercise—type and frequency
    C. Handicaps

IV. Appetite and perception of taste and smell—quality, any changes over the last 12 months

V. Allergies, intolerances, food avoidances, and special diets
    A. Foods avoided and reason
    B. Special diet—what kind, why followed, and who recommended it

VI. Oral health/swallowing
    A. Dentures; completeness of dentition
    B. Problems with chewing, swallowing, and salivation

VII. Gastrointestinal problems
    A. Heartburn, bloating, gas, diarrhea, vomiting, constipation — frequency of problems, any association with food intake or other occurrences
    B. Remedies used—laxatives, antacids

VIII. Medical or psychiatric illnesses
    A. Type of disease
    B. Type and duration of treatment

IX. Medications
    A. Vitamins, minerals, or other nutritional supplements—frequency, type, amount, and recommended or prescribed by whom
    B. Other medications, including over-the-counter and herbal—frequency, type, amount, and duration of use

X. Recent weight change
    A. Amount of loss or gain and over what period of time (most significant if during past year)
    B. Intentional or unintentional; if intentional, what method was used

XI. Usual food intake—description of a "typical" day's intake, or 24-hour recall with use of food frequency questionnaire

Table 2-4 Evaluation of Nutritional History

Area of Concern	History	Possible Deficiency
Inadequate intake	Alcohol abuse	Energy, pro, vit B$_1$, niacin, folate
	Avoidance of food groups	
	Fruits and vegetables	Vit A, C
	Breads and cereals	Vit B$_1$ and B$_2$, fiber
	Meat, eggs, dairy products	Vit B$_{12}$, pro, Fe, Zn
	Dairy products	Ca, vit D, vit B$_2$
	Constipation, hemorrhoids, diverticulosis	Fiber
	Poverty, disadvantaged environment	Various nutrients, especially pro and Fe
	Multiple food allergies	Depends on specific allergies
	Weight loss	Energy, other nutrients
Inadequate absorption	Drugs (especially antacids, cimetidine, anticonvulsants, cholestyramine, neomycin, antineoplastics, laxatives)	Various nutrients (see Appendix G on Evolve)
	Malabsorption (diarrhea, weight loss, steatorrhea)	Energy; vit A, D, E, K; pro; Ca; Mg; Zn
	Parasites	Fe
	Surgery	
	Gastrectomy	Vit B$_{12}$, Fe, folate
	Intestinal resection	Energy; vit A, D, E, K; Ca; Mg; Zn; vit B$_{12}$ if distal ileum

Impaired utilization	Drugs (especially antineoplastics, oral contraceptives, isoniazid, colchicines, corticosteroids)	Various nutrients (see Appendix G on Evolve)
	Inborn errors of metabolism	Depends on disorder
Increased losses	Diabetes	Zn, Cr
	Blood loss	Fe
	Diarrhea, fistula	Pro, Zn, fluid, electrolytes
	Draining abscesses or wounds	Pro, Zn
	Nephrotic syndrome	Pro, Zn
	Peritoneal dialysis or hemodialysis	Pro, water-soluble vit, Zn
Increased requirements	Fever	Energy, vit B_1
	Hyperthyroidism	Energy
	Physiologic demands (infancy, adolescence, pregnancy, lactation)	Fe, Ca; energy; other nutrients
	Surgery, trauma, burns, infection	Energy, pro, vit C, Zn
	Neoplasms (some types)	Energy, pro, other nutrients

Modified from Heimburger DC, Weinsier RL: *Handbook of clinical nutrition*, ed 3, St Louis, 1997, Mosby.
Ca, Calcium; *Cr*, chromium; *Fe*, iron; *Mg*, magnesium; *pro*, protein; *vit*, vitamin(s); *Zn*, zinc.

at http://www.nal.usda.gov/fnic/foodcomp. It also includes data about food components (e.g., **isoflavones** and flavenols) that can be difficult to find elsewhere. Once nutrient intake is calculated, it is then compared with some standard, usually the Dietary Reference Intakes (DRIs) (see Appendix A on Evolve). If an individual has an intake that meets the Recommended Dietary Allowance (RDA) or the Adequate Intake (AI) for a nutrient, the likelihood of dietary deficiency is low.

Some caveats should be noted in the use of any nutrient database. Diet analysis is limited by the accuracy of the food intake records, which depends on the skill and motivation of the record keeper. In addition, foods consumed may not have exactly the same nutrient composition as those in the database because of variations in growing and storage conditions, food processing, cooking procedures, and changes in fortification or formulation. Moreover, gaps exist in the food composition data in published tables and databases. Many foods have not been analyzed for all trace elements, for example. Despite these caveats, the databases are among the most useful and widespread methods for nutrition analysis. A free interactive "MyPyramid Tracker" program for consumers is available at www.cnpp.usda. gov/MyPyramidTracker.htm. Individuals enter their own food intake and physical activity data and receive an analysis of their diet and activity status as well as links to information about nutrition and physical activity.

Nutrition Screening

Health care providers rarely have the time to perform a complete nutrition assessment on every patient. It is most important that individuals who are nutritionally at risk or those who are malnourished be identified quickly; thorough assessment can then be performed on these individuals, and intervention can be planned as necessary. Nutrition screening of individuals consists of gathering some readily available subjective and objective information. Any of the following findings may indicate the presence of malnutrition or nutritional risk:

■ Unplanned loss of ≥10% of usual body weight within 6 months or ≥5% of usual body weight in 1 month; in infants (after the first week of life) and children, any weight loss (or failure to gain adequate weight) that causes deviation from

the child's usual percentile on standardized growth charts
(see www.cdc.gov/growthcharts)
- Body mass index (see Box 2-1) >25 or <18.5, or weight 10%
  greater than or less than ideal body weight; in infants and children,
  weight, length, or BMI less than the 10th percentile or greater than
  the 85th percentile (see Appendix D on Evolve)
- Presence of chronic disease
- Increased metabolic requirements (e.g., trauma, burns, systemic
  infection)
- Altered diet or diet schedules (e.g., recent surgery, serious illness, receiving total parenteral nutrition or tube feedings)
- Inadequate food intake (for adults, risk is greater if inadequate
  intake continues or is expected to continue for 7 days or more;
  infants and children are considered at risk with a shorter period
  of inadequate intake)

Estimating Nutrient Needs
Energy Needs

Energy expenditure can be divided into three components: (1) **basal
energy expenditure**, or energy required for basic life processes,
such as respiration, cardiac function, and maintenance of body temperature; (2) the thermic effect of food, or the energy required for
ingestion, digestion, absorption, and metabolism of nutrients from
food (generally a rather small contribution to energy expenditure);
and (3) physical activity. Basal (or resting) energy expenditure
(BEE) is determined largely by the amount of lean body mass
(LBM; also known as the fat-free mass). It can be measured by indirect calorimetry. This technique, which requires a metabolic cart,
is not available in all settings, and therefore various formulas are
used in estimation of energy needs.

Table 2-5 provides rough estimates of energy needs that
are sometimes used for a quick assessment of the adequacy of
energy intake. These estimates may not reflect accurately the
energy expenditure of a particular person. A number of more
detailed formulas are used in clinical practice in an effort to
derive more individualized estimates of energy expenditure.
Some common formulas are shown in Table 2-6. These formulas
yield basal or resting energy expenditure. Generally they are
multiplied by an activity factor to obtain an estimate of total
energy expenditure (Box 2-4). Alternative methods have been

Table 2-5   Estimates of Daily Energy Needs for Adults

Status/Activity Level	Kcal/kg	Kcal/lb
Obese	21	9.5
Sedentary or hospitalized	25-30	11-13.5
Moderately active (regular aerobic exercise plus routine activities)	30-35	13.5-16
Very active (manual laborer, athlete) or patient with major burns or trauma	40	18

Table 2-6   Selected Equations Used in Estimating Resting Energy Expenditure (kcal/day)

Age-Group	Males	Females
Harris-Benedict Equations		
Adults	$66 + 13.7(W) + 5(H) - 6.8(A)$	$655 + 9.6(W) + 1.7(H) - 4.7(A)$
Mifflin–St. Jeor		
Adults	$5 + 10(W) + 6.25(H) - 5(A)$	$-161 + 10(W) + 6.25(H) - 5(A)$
Owen		
Adults	$879 + (10.2 \times W)$	$795 + (7.18 \times W)$
World Health Organization		
0-3 yr	$(60.9 \times W) + 54$	$(61.0 \times W) + 51$
3-10 yr	$(22.7 \times W) + 495$	$(22.5 \times W) + 499$
10-18 yr	$(17.5 \times W) + 651$	$(12.2 \times W) + 746$
18-30 yr	$(15.3 \times W) + 679$	$(14.7 \times W) + 996$
30-60 yr	$(11.2 \times W) + 879$	$(8.7 \times W) + 829$
>60 yr	$(13.5 \times W) + 987$	$(10.5 \times W) + 596$

Modified from Harris JA, Benedict FG: Standard basal metabolism constants for physiologists and clinicians. In The Carnegie Institute of Washington: *A biometric study of basal metabolism in man, publication 279,* Philadelphia, 1919, JB Lippincott, p 223; Mifflin MD et al: A new predictive equation for resting energy expenditure in healthy individuals, *Am J Clin Nutr* 51:241, 1990; Owen OE: Resting metabolic requirements of men and women, *Mayo Clin Proc* 63:503, 1988; World Health Organization: *Energy and protein requirements. Report of a Joint FAO/WHO/UNU Expert Consultation,* Technical Report Series 724, Geneva, 1985, The Organization.
A, Age in years; *H,* height in cm (1 in = 2.54 cm); *W,* weight in kg (1 lb = 0.45 kg).

Box 2-4   Selected Equations Used in Estimation of Total Energy Expenditure

Equations Based on Basal or Resting Energy Expenditure

Used for both well and sick individuals

Multiply the basal or resting expenditure (see Table 2-6) by an activity factor to obtain an estimate of total energy expenditure:

Sedentary, obese, or hospitalized individual: 1.2 to 1.3

Active, nonhospitalized, normal-weight individual: 1.4 to 1.6

Example: A woman who has a sedentary job is 26 years old, 162.5 cm (5'4") tall, and 84 kg (185 lb).

BEE = 655 + 9.6(84) + 1.7 (162.5) − 4.7(26) = 1615 kcal/day

Estimated total energy expenditure = 1615 × 1.2 = 1938 kcal/day

Ireton-Jones Equations*

Developed in and used for sick hospitalized patients[†]

EEE(v) = 1784 − 11(A) + 5(W) + 244(S) + 239(T) + 804(B)

EEE(s) = 629 − 11(A) + 25(W) − 609(O)

A = age in years, EEE = estimated total energy expenditure in kcal/day, s = spontaneously breathing, S = sex (m = 1, f = 0), v = ventilator dependent, W = actual weight in kg. Diagnosis: B = burn, O = obesity (if present = 1, absent = 0), T = trauma.

Example: If the woman in the example above experienced respiratory failure and needed ventilatory support following drowning, her EEE would be as follows:

EEE(v) = 1784 − 11(26) + 5(84) + 244(0) + 239(0) + 804(0)
        = 1918 kcal/day

---

*Both Ireton-Jones equations can be applied to obese individuals, although obesity appears as a factor only in the equation for spontaneously breathing patients.

[†]Ireton-Jones C, Jones JD: Improved equations predicting energy expenditure in patients, the Ireton-Jones equations, *Nutr Clin Prac* 17:29, 2002.

proposed for calculation of total energy expenditure in ill patients (see Box 2-4).

The LBM is responsible for most of the energy expenditure. Obese people contain more of both fat and LBM than do normal-weight individuals, but LBM accounts for only about 25% of the excess weight in the obese. Elderly people have less LBM and a higher fat content, on average, than their younger counterparts. For this reason, estimates of energy needs for elderly persons should usually fall at the bottom end of the suggested range. Rather than drastically limiting their energy intake to maintain a desirable body weight, elderly people should be encouraged to exercise at a moderate intensity on a regular basis (e.g., walk as briskly as can be tolerated for 30 to 60 minutes almost every day). Regular exercise has two advantages: maintenance of LBM and increase in energy expenditure. With increased energy expenditure, and thus an increase in energy needs, it is easier for the elderly to obtain a diet adequate in vitamins, minerals, and other nutrients.

Protein Needs

Protein needs vary with the physiologic demands, degree of malnutrition (if present), and stressors. Estimated needs for growth in healthy children can be found in Appendix A on Evolve. For healthy adults or those undergoing elective surgery, 0.8 to 1 g/kg body weight is usually adequate. Athletes and individuals in catabolic states (sepsis, major trauma, and burns) may need as much as 1.2 to 2.0 g/kg daily. Individuals with liver or kidney failure may require lower protein intakes (see Chapters 11 and 16).

Assessing State of Hydration

The state of hydration is an important part of nutrition assessment. On one hand, fluid overload is a hazardous state that may compromise cardiorespiratory function. It is usually reflected in rapid weight gain (more than approximately 0.1 to 0.2 kg [¼ to ½ lb]/day in an adult over a period of several days). On the other hand, fluid deficits (**dehydration**) can become severe enough to cause shock and coma.

The three types of dehydration, which can be distinguished by the serum sodium level, are as follows:

1. *Hypertonic or hypernatremic*: Serum sodium >150 mEq/L. This occurs because loss of water is greater than loss of sodium.

Causes include inadequate water intake (e.g., institutionalized elderly individuals who may not feel or be able to express thirst, infants given improperly diluted powdered or concentrated formula, individuals with diarrhea and inadequate fluid intake) and osmotic diuresis (e.g., excessive urination in hyperglycemia).

2. *Isotonic*: Serum sodium 130 to 150 mEq/L. This is the most common form of dehydration; it occurs because of loss of balanced amounts of sodium and water. Causes include diarrhea, vomiting, and nasogastric suction with inadequate replacement of fluid and electrolytes.

3. *Hypotonic or hyponatremic*: Serum sodium <130 mEq/L. Sodium is lost in excess of water. Causes include viral gastroenteritis with rehydration with plain water, tea, or other low-sodium fluids; excessive sweating without fluid and electrolyte replacement; cystic fibrosis; and diuretic therapy.

Dehydration can be graded as mild, moderate, or severe. The amount of weight loss, along with clinical signs (Table 2-7), can be used to determine the severity of the fluid deficit.

Table 2-7   Judging Severity of Fluid Deficit

	Mild (3%-5%)	Moderate (6%-9%)	Severe (≥ 10%)
Blood pressure	N	N	N to ↓
Pulses	N	N to ↓	↓↓
Heart rate	N	↑	↑*
Skin turgor	N	↓ to ↓↓	↓↓ to ↓↓↓
Fontanel (infants)	N	Sunken	Sunken
Mucous membranes	Slightly dry	Dry	Dry
Eyes	N	Sunken	Deeply sunken
Capillary refill	N	Delayed	Delayed†
Mental status	N	N to ↓	N to ↓↓↓
Urine output	↓	↓↓‡	↓↓↓‡
Thirst	↑	↑↑	↑↑↑

N, Normal; ↓, slightly decreased; ↓↓, moderately decreased; ↓↓↓, severely decreased; ↑, slightly increased; ↑↑, moderately increased; ↑↑↑, severely increased.
*May become bradycardic in very severe dehydration.
†Skin cool and mottled.
‡<1 ml/kg/hr.

Structured Approaches to Nutrition Assessment, Intervention, and Evaluation
Nutrition Care Process

The registered dietitian is the professional prepared to address complex nutrition needs and education. The American Dietetic Association has developed a standardized **Nutrition Care Process** (NCP) to provide a framework for delivery of nutrition care to individuals, groups, or communities in order to facilitate the delivery of quality care by the nutrition professional, generate useful outcomes data, and demonstrate the value of professional nutrition care. The NCP has four steps: nutrition assessment, nutrition diagnosis, nutrition intervention, and nutrition monitoring and evaluation. Each step requires information gathering, critical thinking, and documentation. The nutrition assessment involves collection of data regarding nutritional adequacy, health status, and functional and behavioral status, as described earlier in this chapter. The nutrition diagnosis is the "identification and labeling that describes an actual occurrence, risk of, or potential for developing a nutritional problem" (Lacey and Pritchett, 2003). It is not the same as a medical diagnosis, which names a specific disease or pathology. Moreover, the nutrition diagnosis changes as the patient's, client's, or group's condition changes. Each nutrition diagnosis is clear, patient/client centered, and related to only one etiology. The nutrition diagnosis consists of three components, abbreviated as PES: the problem (P), or a description of the alterations in nutritional status; etiology (E), an identification of the cause or risk factors contributing to the problem; and signs/symptoms or defining characteristics (S) providing evidence that a nutrition-related problem exists. For example, a nutrition diagnosis for an obese individual who lost 25 kg but regained 22 kg could be: self-management deficit (P) related to lack of monitoring nutrient intake and physical activity (E) as evidenced by weight regain (S). An individual or group might have several nutrition diagnoses. Some standardized diagnoses have been developed (Hakel-Smith and Lewis, 2004), and others will be added as needs become evident. They are too numerous to list here but are available from the American Dietetic Association (ADA, 2006). The third step of the NCP, nutrition intervention, involves selecting, planning, and implementing appropriate actions to meet the needs associated with a specific diagnosis; above all, the intervention is individualized to the needs of the patient, client, or community. The final step of the NCP, nutrition monitoring and evaluation, allows the professional to determine what progress has been made and what outcomes have been achieved.

Nursing Process

Much like the nutrition care process, the nursing process relies on an assessment of the patient's or client's health status and teaching needs. Based on this assessment, an appropriate nursing diagnosis (or diagnoses) is assigned, individualized interventions are planned and implemented, and responses are monitored. The North American Nursing Diagnosis Association (NANDA) has developed, refined, and promoted a series of nursing diagnoses that can be divided into wellness issues, risk for problems, and actual problems (www. nanda.org). Examples of nursing diagnoses likely to be associated with nutritional health and problems include diagnoses related to the following:

1. Health perception–health management, e.g., health-seeking behaviors, risk for altered growth, delayed growth and development, ineffective health management

2. Nutrition-metabolism, e.g., effective breastfeeding; readiness for enhanced nutritional metabolic pattern; risk for imbalanced nutrition: more than body requirements, or imbalanced nutrition: more than body requirements; risk for imbalanced nutrition: less than body requirements, or imbalanced nutrition: less than body requirements; risk for aspiration; risk for imbalanced fluid volume; risk for constipation; risk for delayed surgical recovery; risk for impaired skin integrity; fluid volume deficit; fluid volume excess; ineffective breastfeeding; interrupted breastfeeding; ineffective infant feeding pattern; impaired swallowing; altered oral mucous membrane; impaired skin integrity; altered dentition

3. Elimination, e.g., risk for constipation; altered bowel elimination: constipation; altered bowel elimination: diarrhea

4. Activity-exercise, e.g., readiness for enhanced diversional activity pattern; readiness for enhanced activity-exercise pattern; diversional activity deficit; self-care deficit: feeding

5. Role relationship, e.g., risk for loneliness; risk for impaired parent/infant/child attachment; impaired parenting; social isolation

6. Self-perception/self-concept, e.g., risk for body image disturbance; disturbed body image; disturbed self-esteem
7. Coping–stress tolerance, e.g., risk for ineffective coping (individual, family, or community); caregiver role strain; ineffective individual coping; ineffective family coping

Conclusion

No single test or tool provides an adequate nutrition assessment. However, the use of a number of different anthropometric, laboratory, and dietary assessment techniques within structured frameworks such as the nutrition care and nursing processes ensures that nutrition problems can be detected and appropriately addressed.

REFERENCES

American Dietetic Association (ADA): *Nutrition diagnosis and intervention: standardized language for the nutrition care process,* Chicago, 2006, The Association.

Bogers RP et al: Association of overweight with increased risk of coronary heart disease partly independent of blood pressure and cholesterol levels, *Arch Intern Med* 167:1720, 2007.

Campillo B et al: Value of body mass index in the detection of severe malnutrition: influence of the pathology and changes in anthropometric parameters, *Clin Nutr* 23(4):551, 2004

Carvalho NF et al: Severe nutritional deficiencies in toddlers resulting from health food milk alternatives, *Pediatrics* 107(4):E46, 2001.

Cox SAR et al: Energy expenditure after spinal cord injury: an evaluation of stable, rehabilitating patients, *J Trauma* 25(5):419, 1985.

Dülger H et al: Pro-inflammatory cytokines in Turkish children with protein-energy malnutrition, *Mediators Inflamm* 11(6):363, 2002.

Fuhrman MP, Charney P, Mueller CM: Hepatic proteins and nutrition assessment, *J Am Diet Assoc* 104(8):1258, 2004.

Hakel-Smith N, Lewis NM: A standardized nutrition care process and language are essential components of a conceptual model to guide and document nutrition care and patient outcomes, *J Am Diet Assoc* 104: 1878, 2004.

Katz KA et al: Rice nightmare: kwashiorkor in 2 Philadelphia-area infants fed Rice Dream beverage, *J Am Acad Dermatol* 52(5 suppl 1):69, 2005.

Killip S, Bennett JM, Chambers MD: Iron deficiency anemia, *Am Fam Physician* 75(5):671, 2007.

Lacey K, Pritchett E: Nutrition Care process and model: ADA adopts road map to quality care and outcomes management, *J Am Diet Assoc* 103(8): 1061, 2003.

Liu T et al: Kwashiorkor in the United States: fad diets, perceived and true milk allergy, and nutritional ignorance, *Arch Dermatol* 137(5): 630, 2001.

Osterkamp LK: Current perspective on assessment of human body proportions of relevance to amputees, *J Am Dietet Assoc* 95(2):215, 1995.

Selected Bibliography

Alberda C, Graf A, McCargar L: Malnutrition: etiology, consequences, and assessment of a patient at risk, *Best Pract Res Clin Gastroenterol* 20(3):419, 2006.

Armstrong LE: Hydration assessment techniques, *Nutr Rev* 63(6 pt 2): S40, 2005.

Barbosa-Silva MC, Barros AJ: Indications and limitations of the use of subjective global assessment in clinical practice: an update, *Curr Opin Clin Nutr Metab Care* 9(3):263, 2006.

Boullata J et al: Accurate determination of energy needs in hospitalized patients, *J Am Diet Assoc* 107:393, 2007.

de Luis DA et al: Nutritional assessment: predictive variables at hospital admission related with length of stay, *Ann Nutr Metab* 50(4):394, 2006.

Hambidge M: Biomarkers of trace mineral intake and status, *J Nutr* 133:948S, 2003.

Kuhl J et al: Skin signs as the presenting manifestation of severe nutritional deficiency: report of 2 cases, *Arch Dermatol* 140(5):521, 2004.

Nassis GP et al: Methods for assessing body composition, cardiovascular and metabolic function in children and adolescents: implications for exercise studies, *Curr Opin Clin Nutr Metab Care* 9(5):560, 2006.

National Institutes of Health (NIH), National Heart, Lung, and Blood Institute (NHLBI), and North American Association for the Study of Obesity (NAASO): *The practical guide: identification, evaluation, and treatment of overweight and obesity in adults,* Washington, DC, 2000, NIH, NHLBI, and NAASO.

Niggemann B, Grüber C: Side-effects of complementary and alternative medicine, *Allergy* 58:707, 2003.

Raguso C, Dupertuis YM, Pichard C: The role of visceral proteins in the nutritional assessment of intensive care unit patients, *Curr Opin Clin Nutr Metab Care* 6:211, 2003.

U.S. Department of Agriculture, Agricultural Research Service: Composition of food raw, processed, prepared: USDA national nutrient database for standard reference, release 20. Available at www.nal.usda.gov/fnic/foodcomp/search. Accessed February 29, 2008.

PREGNANCY AND LACTATION

Pregnancy

Nutrition during pregnancy is important not only because it contributes to the health of the mother and her newborn but also because it establishes the nutritional foundations for a healthy adult life. Poor growth in utero, for example, increases the risk of heart disease and type 2 diabetes in later life.

Needs for most nutrients increase at least modestly during pregnancy (see Appendix A on Evolve). Nutritional deficiencies during pregnancy can have adverse effects on both the mother and her infant. Maternal diets are likely to be low in iron, zinc, calcium, magnesium, and folic acid (Giddens et al, 2000; Moran, 2007). Requirements for some important nutrients are described later in this chapter. Food sources of these nutrients are listed in Appendix B.

Objectives of nutrition care during pregnancy are for the woman to do the following: (1) recognize and alter any practices or findings that could interfere with optimal nutritional status and pregnancy outcome; (2) establish with the health care provider a goal for weight gain within the recommended range and achieve this goal with an appropriate rate of gain; and (3) cope with physiologic changes during pregnancy that interfere with optimal nutritional intake or comfort.

Assessment

A thorough nutrition assessment should be performed as described in Chapter 2 and should be carried out even before conception if possible. Box 3-1 highlights common or especially serious findings in pregnancy and lactation. If any maternal nutrition problems (e.g., poor eating habits; inappropriate weight for height; inadequate folate intake; or poor control of chronic maternal diseases such as hypertension, diabetes, or phenylketonuria) are apparent, they should be addressed before pregnancy or as soon

Text continued on p. 85.

Box 3-1   Assessment of Nutrition in Pregnancy and Lactation

Inadequate Energy Intake

History

Limited income; body image concerns; nausea and vomiting; lack of knowledge about optimal gain during pregnancy and nutrition needs during pregnancy and lactation; stress or fatigue; prepregnant BMI <19.8; poor obstetric history during previous pregnancies; smoking; substance abuse; adolescent pregnancy

Physical Examination

Pregnancy: failure to demonstrate adequate weight gain; lactation: poor milk production, inadequate gain by infant

Excessive Energy Intake

History

Emotional stress, indulgence, or boredom from interruption of job routine; decrease in activity because of awkwardness during pregnancy or interruption of job routine; prepregnant BMI >25

Physical Examination

Pregnancy: weight gain > recommended range; lactation: weight gain or maintenance of BMI >25

Inadequate Protein Intake

History

Limited income; vegan diet; nausea and vomiting during pregnancy; lack of knowledge about needs; fatigue (especially during lactation); frequent pregnancies (>3 within 2 years) or high parity; poor obstetric history during previous pregnancies (e.g., spontaneous abortion, delivery of an LBW infant); alcohol or illicit drug use; multiple gestation

Physical Examination

Edema (some lower-extremity edema is normal during pregnancy; look for edema in hands and periorbital area); changes in hair color and texture; hair loss

Continued

Box 3-1   Assessment of Nutrition in Pregnancy and Lactation—cont'd

Laboratory Analysis

Serum albumin <3.2 g/dl; prealbumin <10 mg/dl

Inadequate Vitamin Intake

Folate/Folic Acid

History

Failure to use a daily folic acid supplement and foods rich in folate; delivery of a previous infant with a neural tube defect; increased needs because of alcohol or drug abuse, smoking, or multiple gestation

Physical Examination

Pallor; glossitis

Laboratory Analysis

Hct <33%; ↑ MCV; ↓ serum and RBC folate

Vitamin B$_{12}$

History

Vegan diet with failure to use a supplement or foods fortified with vitamin B$_{12}$; ileal resection or disease; pernicious anemia

Physical Examination

Maternal findings: glossitis, pallor, ataxia; infant breastfed by vegan: delayed growth, pallor, glossitis, developmental delay

Laboratory Analysis

↓ Hct; ↑ MCV (in mother or infant); ↓ serum vitamin B$_{12}$ (in mother or infant)

Vitamin D

History

Failure to consume vitamin D–fortified milk because of strict vegetarianism, lactose intolerance, dislike of milk, or cultural practices; little exposure of skin to sunlight because of

Box 3-1   Assessment of Nutrition in Pregnancy
and Lactation—cont'd

residence in northern latitudes in winter or cultural prohibitions against exposing the body

Inadequate Mineral Intake

Iron

History

Failure to consume foods rich in iron because of vegan diet,
limited income, or dislike of these foods; frequent pregnancies or high parity with depletion of stores; adolescent with
increased needs for her growth as well as that of the fetus;
anemia during a previous pregnancy; pica; menorrhagia;
multiple gestation

Physical Examination

Pallor, especially of conjunctiva; blue sclerae; spoon-shaped nails

Laboratory Analysis

Hct <33%; Hgb <11 g/dl; ↓ MCV, serum ferritin, serum iron;
↑ free erythrocyte protoporphyrin (FEP)

Zinc

History

Use of supplement containing >30 mg iron (competition between zinc and iron for absorption); use of folic acid or
calcium supplement without zinc supplement; avoidance of
animal protein foods; frequent pregnancies or high parity
with depletion of stores; adolescent with increased needs for
her growth as well as that of the fetus; pica; alcoholism with
increased excretion

Physical Examination

Seborrheic dermatitis; alopecia; diarrhea; poor sense of taste;
distorted taste

Laboratory Analysis

↓ Serum zinc

Continued

Box 3-1   Assessment of Nutrition in Pregnancy and Lactation—cont'd

Calcium

History

Lactose intolerance; dislike of milk products; vegan diet or cultural food patterns that avoid milk; frequent pregnancies or high parity with depletion of stores; adolescent with increased needs for her growth as well as fetus

Potentially Harmful Substances (During Pregnancy)

Caffeine

History

Daily consumption of coffee, tea, and soft drinks (other than caffeine free), especially if more than the equivalent of 2 cups of coffee per day; use of over-the-counter cold or analgesic medications (not usually recommended during pregnancy; the woman should consult her health care provider before using)

Alcohol

History

Use of alcoholic beverages, especially if >1 oz/day or more than 3 or 4 times/wk

Cocaine/Other Drugs of Abuse

History

Use of illicit drugs, especially on a regular basis, during pregnancy

Laboratory Analysis

Positive urinary drug screen

BMI, Body mass index; *Hct,* hematocrit; *Hgb,* hemoglobin; *LBW,* low birth weight; *MCV,* mean corpuscular volume; *RBC,* red blood cell.

after conception as possible. Nutritional status should be reevaluated at each prenatal visit, bearing in mind that pregnancy alters the normal ranges for many laboratory tests commonly used in nutrition assessment (Box 3-2).

Nutrition Needs

Preconceptual weight, weight gain, and energy needs

Enlargement of maternal breasts, uterine tissue, blood volume, and energy (fat) stores, as well as development of the placenta, amniotic fluid, and fetus, contributes to maternal weight gain during pregnancy (Table 3-1). Appropriate weight gain does not necessarily equal good nutritional status, of course, but the amount of weight gain during pregnancy is closely related to pregnancy outcome. The mother's weight before pregnancy is another factor involved in

---

Box 3-2   Changes in Laboratory Values During Pregnancy

↓ Hematocrit
↓ Hemoglobin
↑ Lymphocyte count
↓ Serum albumin
↓ Serum ferritin
↑ Serum cholesterol
↓ Blood urea nitrogen
↓ Serum creatinine

Table 3-1   Components of Maternal Weight Gain at Term Gestation

Tissue	Pounds	Kilograms
Fetus	7.9	3.6
Placenta	1.1	0.5
Amniotic fluid	2.5	1.1
Increased uterus and breast tissue	4.0	1.8
Increased blood volume	4.4	2.0
Increased fat and other tissues	5.5	2.5
TOTAL	25.4	11.5

pregnancy outcome. Maternal and fetal risks are increased in the following cases:

1. *Underweight*: Women who are underweight before pregnancy are more likely to experience preterm labor and to deliver **low birthweight** (LBW; <2500 g [5.5 lb]) infants. LBW is the single greatest risk factor for the survival of the newborn.
2. *Overweight*: Women who are overweight before pregnancy are more likely to have hypertension and diabetes.
3. *Inadequate weight gain*: For normal-weight and underweight women, maternal weight gain is directly related to infant birth weight, and the risk of delivering an LBW infant is increased by inadequate gain.
4. *Excessive weight gain*: Overeating, multiple gestation, edema, and **pregnancy-induced hypertension** are some of the causes of greater-than-expected weight gain. There is increased risk of fetopelvic disproportion, operative delivery, birth trauma, and infant mortality with very high total weight gain, especially in short women (<157 cm [62 in]). Moreover, excessive fat stores tend to be retained after pregnancy, increasing the woman's likelihood of being overweight or obese.

Intervention and education
Optimal energy intake and weight gain. The optimum amount of weight gain during pregnancy is determined largely by the mother's weight before pregnancy. Recommendations have been developed for desirable ranges for total weight gain and rate of weight gain based on body mass index (BMI), an indicator of the appropriateness of weight for height. See Chapter 2 for the method of calculating BMI, or consult the chart inside the back cover of this book.

Current recommendations for total weight gain during pregnancy are as follows: underweight women (BMI <19.8), 12.5 to 18 kg (28 to 40 lb); normal-weight women (BMI 19.8 to 26), 11.5 to 16 kg (25 to 35 lb); overweight women (BMI 26 to 29), 7 to 11.5 kg (15 to 25 lb); and obese women (BMI >29), ≥6.8 kg (15 lb) (National Academy of Sciences, Institute of Medicine, 1992). Young adolescents (less than 2 years past menarche) are encouraged to make their weight gain goal the upper end of the recommended range for their BMI because their infants are smaller than those of adult women for any given amount of maternal gain. Weight gain recommendations for both adolescents and adults are currently undergoing study (NRC/IOM), 2007). After the pregnancy, many women have difficulty losing all the weight that they have gained. The effects that this excess weight may have on the long-term health of the mother have prompted some authorities to suggest that pregnancy weight gain recommendations should be reevaluated. Recommendations for weight gain are best made as part of a comprehensive plan encouraging optimal nutrition and regular physical activity (NRC/IOM, 2007).

Outcome of a twin pregnancy appears to be best if weight gain is approximately 16 to 20.5 kg (35 to 45 lb). Although there are insufficient data to make a conclusive recommendation, a gain of at least 22.7 kg (50 lb) in total, with a substantial gain in the first trimester, is suggested as the goal for triplet gestations (Luke, 2005).

Explanation of the components of weight gain in pregnancy (see Table 3-1) may help women to understand the importance of weight gain. On the other hand, excessive weight gain is associated with the development of diabetes and hypertension, an increased likelihood of Caesarean delivery, and overweight after pregnancy (Cedergren, 2007; NRC/IOM, 2007).

The pattern of weight gain is important in evaluating weight changes during pregnancy. Most women with singleton fetuses gain approximately 1.5 to 2 kg (3 to 5 lb) during the first trimester of pregnancy, when the fetus and the changes in maternal tissues are relatively small. Recommended weekly weight gains during the second and third trimesters are 0.5 kg (1.1 lb) for underweight women, 0.44 kg (1 lb) for normal-weight women, and 0.3 kg (0.66 lb) for overweight women. Gain of 1 kg (2.2 lb) or less per month in the second or third trimester by normal-weight women and 0.5 kg (1 lb) or less by obese women should be evaluated, as should a gain of 3 kg (6.6 lb) or more per month. In twin gestations the goal is a gain of approximately 0.75 kg (1.65 lb) per week during the second and third trimesters.

The Dietary Reference Intakes (DRIs) (Otten et al., 2006) suggest that during the second and third trimesters women 14 to 50 years of age should consume 340 and 452 kcal/day (respectively) more than their nonpregnant energy needs to promote an adequate gain (see Chapter 1 for discussion of DRIs.) The extra energy (kcal) needed daily is easily obtained by increasing intake of milk products by 1 or 2 servings per day and making small increases in intake of protein foods, fruits, and vegetables. There is little room in the diet for high-energy foods that are low in nutrients. Problems occur when women restrain their intake too much or, alternatively, eat excessively during pregnancy. Therefore it is especially important that pregnant women know their weight gain goal and understand how to follow a food plan to achieve it.

Healthful food plan. Nutrition needs for healthy pregnant women, except perhaps those for folic acid and iron, can be met through a varied diet of normal foods (e.g., the MyPyramid plan described in Chapter 1 or the Dietary Approaches to Stop Hypertension (DASH) diet described in Chapters 1 and 14). Adequate calcium is contained in 3 or 4 servings of milk, yogurt, cheese, or calcium-fortified juices or soy milk daily. A minimum of 6 or 7 servings of fruits and vegetables, 2 or 3 servings of meat or protein-rich substitutes (e.g., nuts or cooked dry beans), and 6 or 7 servings of whole and enriched grain products supplies the remainder of the needed nutrients. Prenatal vitamin-mineral supplements (Table 3-2) are

Table 3-2   Composition of a Representative Prenatal Multivitamin-Multimineral Supplement

Nutrient	Amount
Vitamin A	800 mcg
Vitamin D_3	10 mcg
Vitamin E	20 mg
Vitamin C (ascorbic acid)	120 mg
Folic acid	0.8 mg
Vitamin B_1 (thiamin)	3 mg
Vitamin B_2 (riboflavin)	3.4 mg
Vitamin B_6 (pyridoxine)	2 mg
Niacinamide	20 mg
Vitamin B_{12} (cyanocobalamin)	12 mcg
Biotin	30 mcg
Pantothenic acid	10 mg
Calcium	250 mg
Iodine	150 mcg
Iron	27 mg
Magnesium	100 mg
Copper	2 mg
Zinc	25 mg
Chromium	25 mcg
Molybdenum	25 mcg
Manganese	2 mg

commonly prescribed during pregnancy to ensure that intake of these nutrients is adequate.

Physical activity during pregnancy. Moderate physical activity is recommended in healthy women without obstetric conditions that would contraindicate such activity. No pregnant woman should participate in such activity without the guidance of her health care provider. Activities such as stationary or recumbent cycling, swimming, walking, and low-impact or water aerobics are recommended, and those such as skiing, water skiing, surfing, contact sports, scuba diving, and mountaineering at high altitudes are discouraged (ACOG, 2002). A moderate level of physical activity is one that would result in a heart rate (beats per minute) of approximately 140 to 155 in women younger than 20 years of age, 135 to 150 in women 20 to 29 years of age, 130 to 145 in women 30 to 39 years of age, and 125 to 140 in women older than 40 years. After the first trimester, women should avoid any exercises carried out lying on their backs, since this may impair the blood supply to the uterus. Pregnant women should also avoid exercising in especially hot, humid weather and should drink adequate water to replace losses during exercise.

Protein

An intake of 1.1 g/kg body weight/day, or a total of approximately 71 g of protein per day (25 g more than the nonpregnant recommendation), is recommended (Otten et al, 2006). This amount, which is easily provided by the average diet in the United States and Canada, is necessary for normal growth of the fetus, enlargement of the uterus and breasts, formation of blood cells and proteins as the blood volume expands, and production of amniotic fluid.

Intervention and education. The extra protein needed in addition to the prepregnant intake can be provided by approximately 1 cup (240 ml) of milk or soy milk and 2 oz (60 g) of meat or an equivalent protein food per day. There is no benefit in consuming protein in excess of the recommendations, and doing so increases the cost of the diet.

For low-income women who may have difficulty affording the additional protein foods and other nutrient-rich foods that are needed during pregnancy, the Special Supplemental Food Program for Women, Infants, and Children (WIC) provides vouchers for purchase of selected food items rich in protein, iron, and vitamin C. Low-income women may also be eligible for the food stamp program. When the woman's diet is found to be poor and there is little likelihood of its improving, or when other risk factors (adolescent pregnancy, maternal smoking, use of illicit drugs or alcohol, or multiple gestation) exist, vitamin-mineral supplementation is especially important (see the discussion that follows).

Vitamins and minerals
Folate (folic acid)

There is good evidence that a diet rich in folate (the food form of the vitamin) or folic acid (the form used in supplements or fortified foods) decreases the risk of giving birth to an infant with a neural tube defect. All women who have the potential to become pregnant are advised to consume 400 mcg of folic acid from supplements or fortified foods daily, in addition to the folate obtained from a varied diet (Otten et al., 2006). During pregnancy the recommendation for folic acid is increased to 600 mcg. It is needed for both maternal red blood cell production and the DNA synthesis entailed in fetal and placental growth.

Intervention and education. Folate intake is especially important during the periconceptual period, before pregnancy may even be suspected, and therefore good nutrition education is needed to ensure adequate intakes by nonpregnant teens and women in their childbearing years.

- A folic acid supplement is the best way to ensure that intake is adequate. Most over-the-counter multivitamins contain 400 mcg folic acid in a daily dose, and prenatal vitamins contain increased amounts (see Table 3-2).
- Fruit, juices, green vegetables, whole grains and enriched flour, and fortified cereals are reliable dietary sources.

Other vitamins

An increase in intake of vitamin C is recommended during pregnancy because of its many roles in metabolism, including its involvement in development of connective tissue. In addition, vitamin C improves iron absorption and facilitates activation of folate. Vitamin D plays an important role in calcium metabolism, and vitamin B_{12} is required for synthesis of nucleic acids, needed for the increased production of maternal red blood cells and growth of fetal tissue.

Intervention and education

- *Vitamin C*: A total of 85 mg is recommended for adult women during pregnancy, and a total of 80 mg is recommended for pregnant teens. Although vitamin C is contained in prenatal vitamin-mineral supplements, the recommended amounts can easily be achieved from a diet rich in foods such as citrus fruits, broccoli, green peppers, strawberries, and melons.
- *Vitamin D*: Regular exposure of the skin to sunlight or consumption of vitamin D–fortified milk and cereals generally provides sufficient amounts. A supplement of 5 mcg or 200 international units is suggested for strict vegetarians or other women with little intake of vitamin D–fortified milk, especially for women with little exposure of the skin to sunlight and those with very dark skin in northern latitudes.
- *Vitamin B_{12}*: This vitamin is found only in animal products, and therefore strict vegetarians need a supplement of at least 2.6 mcg daily unless they are consuming vitamin B_{12}–fortified food products. Women with pernicious anemia (inability to produce intrinsic factor, required for absorption of vitamin B_{12}) require parenteral or intranasal vitamin B_{12} for life, and those with disease of the ileum usually require similar therapy or very-high–dose oral supplements (1000 mcg daily).

Iron

The red blood cell mass expands by about 15% during pregnancy, which requires a substantial increase in the maternal content of iron. Iron is also needed for deposition of fetal stores, and inadequate maternal iron intake is linked with delivery of LBW infants (those less than 2500 g). The DRIs include a 50% increase in iron intake during pregnancy, from 18 to 27 mg daily. **Pica**, the consumption of substances usually considered nonfoods, could interfere with iron nutriture in two ways: (1) displacing nutritious foods in the diet and (2) interfering with absorption of iron and other nutrients from foods and nutritional supplements. Women who practice pica have been found to have significantly lower levels of hemoglobin, mean cell hemoglobin, and ferritin (a storage form of iron) than women who do not practice pica (López et al., 2007). Risk factors for pica during pregnancy include race (African American), living in a rural area, practicing pica during childhood, and having family members who practice pica. Ice or freezer frost, soil or clay, chalk, glue, cornstarch, and laundry starch are examples of substances consumed (Rose et al., 2000).

Intervention and education. A supplement of 30 mg of iron is recommended during the second and third trimesters of pregnancy (National Academy of Sciences, Institute of Medicine, 1992). Ferrous sulfate, 150 mg, provides 30 mg of elemental iron and is often prescribed because it is inexpensive and relatively well absorbed. Teaching points in relation to iron supplementation and iron nutrition include the following:

- Take the supplement between meals or at bedtime because certain food components interfere with iron absorption. These include phytates (in whole grains), oxalates (in deep green leafy vegetables), and tannins in tea and coffee.
- Take the supplement with liquids other than milk, coffee, and tea, which inhibit iron absorption.
- Take the supplement at bedtime if it causes gastrointestinal (GI) distress.
- Even with supplementation, include in the daily diet good sources of iron, such as meats and legumes, and vitamin C sources, which enhance iron absorption. Cooking foods in cast-iron cookware increases their iron content.
- Keep the supplement out of the reach of children.

Zinc

Zinc is needed for formation of new tissue. The DRI for zinc increases from 8 to 11 mg daily during pregnancy in women older than age 18 years and from 9 to 12 mg for pregnant adolescents.

Intervention and education

- Women need to consume reliable sources of zinc (e.g., shellfish, meats, and tofu and other products made from soybeans) daily. Whole grains, milk, cheese, and eggs contain smaller but important amounts of zinc.
- Vegetarians are especially apt to have marginal zinc status, both because meats and shellfish are some of the richest sources of zinc and because phytates and oxalates found in whole grains and

green leafy vegetables inhibit zinc absorption. For this reason they may need a zinc supplement (15 mg elemental zinc daily).

■ Absorption of zinc is inhibited by large intakes of iron and folic acid. Supplements of zinc (15 mg daily) and copper (2 mg daily) are recommended for women who require therapeutic doses of iron (more than 30 mg daily) to treat anemia (National Academy of Sciences, Institute of Medicine, 1992).

Calcium

Pregnant women are encouraged to consume at least 1000 mg of calcium per day, and pregnant adolescents are advised to consume 1300 mg (National Institute of Arthritis and Musculoskeletal and Skin Diseases, 2008). Both the maternal and the fetal skeletons require an ample supply of calcium.

Intervention and education. Women are encouraged to consume several good dietary sources of calcium daily:

■ Dairy products, particularly milk, buttermilk, yogurt, and cheese, are among the richest calcium sources available (Figure 3-1). Three or four daily servings meet most of the needs of pregnant women.

■ Sardines and other canned fish are excellent calcium sources if the bones are eaten.

■ Foods made with milk, such as pancakes, waffles, puddings, and cream soups, provide moderate amounts of calcium.

■ Most deep green leafy vegetables contain calcium; however, some of these vegetables, such as Swiss chard and spinach, are poor calcium sources because they contain oxalates that prevent absorption of the calcium.

■ A commercial lactase enzyme preparation can be used when consuming milk if the woman has lactose intolerance (cramping, bloating, and diarrhea following milk consumption, resulting from lack of lactase, the enzyme that digests lactose). Lactose-intolerant individuals usually tolerate yogurt and hard cheeses, which contain little lactose. Many individuals with lactose intolerance can tolerate milk as long as they drink only 0.5 to 1 cup at a time.

■ Calcium-fortified juices and calcium-fortified cereal products are good calcium sources.

■ A supplement of 600 mg daily is recommended for women under 25 years of age who consume less than 600 mg of

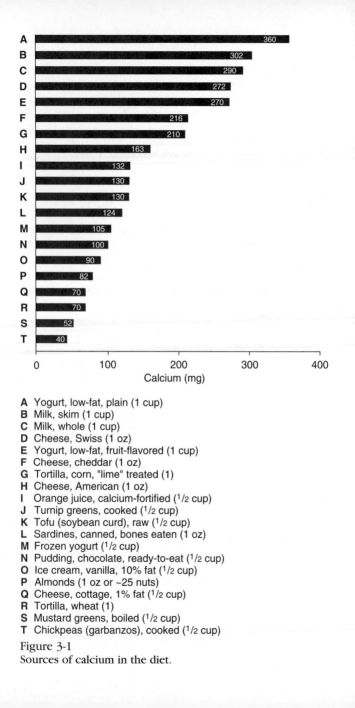

A Yogurt, low-fat, plain (1 cup)
B Milk, skim (1 cup)
C Milk, whole (1 cup)
D Cheese, Swiss (1 oz)
E Yogurt, low-fat, fruit-flavored (1 cup)
F Cheese, cheddar (1 oz)
G Tortilla, corn, "lime" treated (1)
H Cheese, American (1 oz)
I Orange juice, calcium-fortified ($1/2$ cup)
J Turnip greens, cooked ($1/2$ cup)
K Tofu (soybean curd), raw ($1/2$ cup)
L Sardines, canned, bones eaten (1 oz)
M Frozen yogurt ($1/2$ cup)
N Pudding, chocolate, ready-to-eat ($1/2$ cup)
O Ice cream, vanilla, 10% fat ($1/2$ cup)
P Almonds (1 oz or ~25 nuts)
Q Cheese, cottage, 1% fat ($1/2$ cup)
R Tortilla, wheat (1)
S Mustard greens, boiled ($1/2$ cup)
T Chickpeas (garbanzos), cooked ($1/2$ cup)

Figure 3-1
Sources of calcium in the diet.

calcium (two 8-oz glasses of milk) per day, because the bones of these women may still be increasing in density (National Academy of Sciences, Institute of Medicine, 1992). To maximize absorption of the supplement, it should be taken 1 to 2 hours before or after the iron supplement, and it should not be taken with bran or whole-grain cereals. Supplements containing unrefined oyster shell, bone meal, or dolomite should be avoided because they may include lead, mercury, or other toxic substances.

Harmful and Potentially Harmful Practices
Alcohol

Fetal alcohol syndrome (FAS) results from maternal alcohol intake during pregnancy. This disorder is characterized by some or all of the following features in the infant: microcephaly, prenatal and postnatal growth failure, mental retardation, facial abnormalities (Figure 3-2), cleft palate, skeletal-joint abnormalities, abnormal creases on the palms, cardiac defects, and behavioral abnormalities. There is no known safe level of alcohol intake during pregnancy and no safe time during pregnancy when alcohol can be consumed.

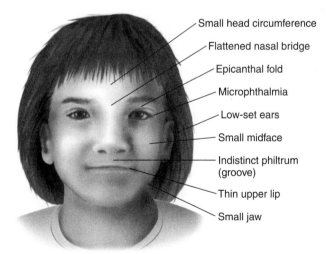

Figure 3-2
Abnormal findings of the head in fetal alcohol syndrome.

Regular (seven or more drinks/wk), heavy (two or more drinks/day), or binge (five or more drinks at a time) drinking is especially to be discouraged. Some children who do not develop all the characteristics of FAS are said to have alcohol-related birth defects (ARBDs) or alcohol-related neurodevelopmental disorder (ARND), depending on the disorders they display. ARBDs, such as facial anomalies, skeletal abnormalities, and damage to organ systems, most commonly occur because of drinking during the first trimester. Since the brain is forming throughout pregnancy, ARND may be caused by drinking at any time. Growth failure is commonly related to drinking during the last trimester. Hyperactive behavior, learning disabilities, developmental disabilities such as speech and language delays, and poor judgment and reasoning skills are signs of ARND. Difficulty in school and in maintaining employment, inappropriate sexual behavior, and violations of the law are problems likely to be exhibited by individuals with ARND.

Intervention and education. Avoiding alcohol altogether during pregnancy is the only known way to prevent FAS, ARBDs, and ARND. If the mother does not find this possible, she should be urged to limit her intake to no more than one drink at a time and not to drink every day. Every effort should be made to achieve abstinence from alcohol.

Other drugs of abuse

Increased risk of intrauterine growth restriction (IUGR) and preterm labor is associated with both marijuana and cocaine abuse. The risk of abruptio placentae is also increased by cocaine. Moreover, infants of mothers who abuse crack cocaine often display persistent learning and behavioral abnormalities. It is difficult to determine exactly what impact illicit drugs have on the nutritional status of the pregnant woman because drug abuse is often accompanied by abuse of other substances, such as alcohol or cigarettes, poverty, and poor education, all of which have detrimental influences on nutritional status.

Intervention and education. Vitamin and mineral supplements are recommended for women who abuse drugs, but supplements cannot be expected to correct the problems associated with drug use during pregnancy. Every effort should be made to convince the pregnant woman to stop using drugs.

Cigarette smoking

Infants of women who smoke during pregnancy have lower birth weights than infants of nonsmoking mothers. In addition, women who smoke have an increased risk of preterm delivery, perinatal mortality, placenta previa, and possibly spontaneous abortion. The mechanism by which smoking affects the fetus is not completely understood, but it is likely that it causes intrauterine hypoxia, perhaps through reduced placental blood flow. Also, smoking increases the metabolic rate and thus caloric needs. Weight gain and prepregnant weight tend to be lower in smokers than in nonsmokers, and the diets of smokers are reported to be poorer than those of nonsmokers. Women who smoke have decreased levels or increased needs for several nutrients, including vitamin C, folate, zinc, and iron. Women who stop smoking before pregnancy or early in pregnancy have been successful in increasing the birth weights of their infants.

Intervention and education. Vitamin and mineral supplementation of the woman who continues to smoke is advisable, but supplementation does not counteract the detrimental effects of smoking on the fetus. Smoking cessation should be the goal for all women who smoke.

Methyl mercury

Methyl mercury is a naturally occurring element and also an industrial pollutant that accumulates in some of the larger, long-lived fish and fish that eat other fish. The nervous system is especially susceptible to damage from mercury during fetal life, infancy, and early childhood.

Intervention and education. The U.S. Food and Drug Administration Center for Food Safety and Applied Nutrition (2007) advises pregnant women, those likely to become pregnant, and lactating women to do the following:

- Avoid shark, swordfish, king mackerel, and tilefish, but eat as much as 12 oz (360 g) of other ocean fish and farm-raised fish per week, as long as you eat a variety of types of fish, rather than a single type.
- Eat no more than 6 oz (180 g) albacore tuna weekly. Albacore (white) tuna contains higher amounts of mercury than canned light tuna.

- Choose seafood and fish such as shrimp, salmon, canned light tuna, pollock, and catfish. These commonly eaten fish are among those that are lowest in mercury content.
- Check local and state advisories about locally caught fish. If no advisory exists, consume up to 6 oz (180 g) of locally caught fish weekly, as long as no other fish is consumed during the week.

Listeria infection

The food-borne illness known as listeriosis can cause spontaneous abortion, stillbirth, and fetal infection. Pregnant women are about 20 times more likely than normal adults to contract listeriosis.

Intervention and education. To avoid listeriosis, pregnant women should not consume any of the following:

- Unpasteurized milk or items made with unpasteurized milk (e.g., cheeses) unless thoroughly cooked
- Undercooked or raw animal products, such as fish, shellfish, eggs, or meat
- Refrigerated smoked seafood, refrigerated pâtés or meat spreads, deli meats, cold cuts, or hot dogs (which can easily become contaminated after processing) unless they are thoroughly cooked
- Soft cheeses (Hard cheeses can be consumed.)
- Fresh fruits and vegetables before they are thoroughly washed

Caffeine and artificial sweeteners

The effect of caffeine intake on the fetus is not fully known. Moderate amounts of caffeine (approximately 300 mg, the amount contained in 500 ml [two 8-oz cups] or less daily) have not been found to be associated with either preterm birth or congenital defects (Browne, 2006; Bech et al., 2007).

Intervention and education

- *Caffeine*: Insufficient data are available to make a recommendation regarding caffeine use during pregnancy; however, until such data are available, it seems prudent to abstain from caffeine use or to limit daily intake to no more than 300 mg (equivalent to approximately two 8-oz cups [500 ml] of coffee). In addition to coffee, certain other foods, including tea and colas, can provide substantial amounts of caffeine (Table 3-3).

Table 3-3   Caffeine Content of Selected Beverages and Foods[*]

Beverage or Food	Caffeine (mg)
Coffees, 240-ml (8-oz) Servings	
Coffee, short (Starbucks)	250
Coffee, brewed, nongourmet	135
Orange cappuccino[†]	102
Coffee, instant	95
Café Vienna[†]	90
Mocha[‡] or Swiss mocha[†]	55-60
Café mocha, latte, or cappuccino (Starbucks)	35
Coffee, decaffeinated	5
Teas, 240-ml (8-oz) Servings Unless Otherwise Specified	
Bigelow Raspberry Royale	83
Tea leaf or bag; black, pekoe, or oolong	50
Snapple iced tea, all varieties, 480 ml (16 oz)	48
Nestea Pure Sweetened Iced Tea, 480 ml (16 oz)	34
Tea, green	30
Arizona iced tea, assorted varieties, 480 ml (16 oz)	15-30
Tea, instant	15
Tea, white	8-20
Tea, decaffeinated	<5
Tea, herbal or red	0
Soft Drinks, 360-ml (12-oz) Servings Unless Otherwise Specified	
Jolt	72
Mountain Dew	45
Coca-Cola, classic or diet; Pepsi, regular or diet; Dr. Pepper, regular or diet	29-39
Barq's Root Beer	18-23
7-Up or Diet 7-Up, A&W Root Beer, caffeine-free colas (all types, regular or diet), Minute Maid Orange Soda, Sierra Mist, Sprite or Diet Sprite	0
Red Bull energy drink, 250 ml (8.3 oz)	67
SoBe Adrenaline Rush, 250 ml (8.3 oz)	77
Others	
Ben & Jerry's No-Fat Coffee Fudge Frozen Yogurt, 1 cup	85

Continued

Table 3-3   Caffeine Content of Selected Beverages
and Foods*—cont'd

Beverage or Food	Caffeine (mg)
Others	
Coffee ice creams, 240 ml (1 cup)	30-60
Dannon coffee yogurt, 240 ml (1 cup)	45
Cappuccino or café au lait yogurts, 180-240 ml (6-8 oz)	<5
Chocolate bar, dark, bittersweet, or semisweet, 30 g (1 oz)	20
Chocolate bar, milk, 30 g (1 oz)	5
Cocoa, hot chocolate, or chocolate milk, 240 ml (8 oz)	5

From Center for Science in the Public Interest: Caffeine corner: products ranked by amount, *Nutrition Action Health Letter* (serial online). Available at http://www.cspinet.org/nah/caffeine/caffeine_corner.htm. Accessed March 30, 2007; McCusker RR et al: Caffeine content of decaffeinated coffee, *J Anal Toxicol* 30(8):611, 2006; McCusker RR, Goldberger BA, Cone EJ: Caffeine content of energy drinks, carbonated sodas, and other beverages, *J Anal Toxicol* 30(2):112, 2006; McCusker RR, Goldberger BA, Cone EJ: Caffeine content of specialty coffees, *J Anal Toxicol* 27(7):520, 2003.
*Many over-the-counter and some prescription medications contain higher levels of caffeine than these beverages and foods. Consult the product label or a pharmacist about the caffeine content of drugs.
†General Foods International Coffee.
‡Maxwell House Cappuccino.

▪ *Artificial sweeteners*: Four artificial sweeteners—saccharin, aspartame, acesulfame potassium, and sucralose—are approved by the Food and Drug Administration for use in the United States, including consumption during pregnancy. Aspartame (NutraSweet) has not been found to have adverse effects on the normal mother or fetus, but its use should be avoided by pregnant women homozygous for phenylketonuria (PKU).

Pregnancy Complications with Nutritional Implications
Nausea and vomiting

Nausea and vomiting, or "morning sickness," is common during the first trimester of pregnancy. "Morning sickness" is a misnomer because the symptoms can occur at any time of the day. Although annoying, nausea and vomiting are rarely severe and prolonged enough to impair nutritional status. Severe nausea and vomiting that may continue throughout pregnancy occur in about 3.5/1000 births.

Known as **hyperemesis gravidarum**, this condition is associated with electrolyte imbalance, dehydration, weight loss, and ketonemia.

Intervention and education. Suggestions for coping with morning sickness are as follows:

- Eat small, frequent meals; hunger can worsen nausea.
- Avoid fluids for 1 to 2 hours before and after meals.
- Consume plain, starchy foods (crackers, dry toast, melba toast, rice, pasta or noodles, plain boiled or baked potatoes, unsweetened cooked or ready-to-eat cereals) during times of nausea because they are easily digested and unlikely to cause nausea. Spicy foods can worsen nausea.
- Decrease intake of fats and fried foods. Fat delays gastric emptying and can increase nausea.
- Minimize exposure to strong food odors. Avoid cooking foods with strong odors during times of nausea, maintain adequate ventilation in the kitchen, and use lids on pots during cooking.
- Avoid brushing teeth immediately after eating because this causes some individuals to gag.
- Try salty foods (e.g., potato chips and pretzels) or tart foods (e.g., lemonade), which are tolerated well by some women with nausea.
- Sniff the cut edge of a lemon.
- Try consuming ginger or using P6 acupressure; there is evidence that both may be effective (Helmreich et al., 2006).

The woman suffering from hyperemesis gravidarum with weight loss may require parenteral or enteral nutrition support to restore fluid and electrolyte balance and maintain an adequate nutrient supply for the mother and fetus. When vomiting has diminished, small amounts of low-fat, easily digested starches, skinless poultry, and lean meats are reintroduced orally, with the diet gradually advanced as tolerated. Occasionally, nausea and vomiting will be so severe and prolonged that the woman requires prolonged enteral tube feeding or parenteral nutrition (see Chapters 8 and 9).

Constipation

Constipation is most common during the last half of pregnancy. Contributing factors include decreased GI motility resulting from increased progesterone levels, increased pressure on the GI tract by the bulky uterus, effects of iron supplementation, and decreased physical activity.

Intervention and education

- Maintain a dietary fiber intake of at least 28 g/day (see Appendix C on Evolve).
- Consume 35 to 50 ml fluid/kg body weight daily to ensure that adequate fluid is available to form soft, bulky stools.
- Obtain aerobic exercise (e.g., walk briskly) daily or almost daily to improve muscle tone and stimulate bowel motility.

Preeclampsia

Preeclampsia, a form of hypertension that occurs in pregnancy, is associated with proteinuria and usually with excessive edema. The cause is unknown, but possibilities include improper trophoblast invasion of the uterus, immunologic problems, cardiovascular mal-adaptation to pregnancy, genetic tendencies, and nutritional imbalances or deficiencies. Obesity increases the risk of preeclampsia (Dixit and Girling, 2008).

Intervention and education. If possible, obese women should reduce their weight before pregnancy. Diets that are adequate in vitamins and minerals and rich in long chain omega-3 fatty acids seem to be associated with the lowest incidence of preeclampsia (Hösli et al., 2007). Therefore diet instruction should focus on intake of a wide range of foods from all groups, regular consumption of omega-3 sources such as fish, flax, and walnuts, and possibly the use of a multivitamin-mineral supplement. The DASH diet (see Chapter 14) is a healthful guide that can be used. This diet pattern emphasizes intake of fruits and vegetables, low-fat dairy products, and whole grain and enriched grain products.

Diabetes

For the diabetic woman who becomes pregnant or the woman who develops **gestational diabetes mellitus (GDM;** diabetes that is first evident during pregnancy), the goal is to maintain normoglycemia during pregnancy. Women with a high risk of GDM (marked obesity, history of GDM during a previous pregnancy, glucose in the urine, or a strong family history of diabetes) should undergo glucose testing as soon as they enter prenatal care. If they are found not to have GDM initially, they should be retested between 24 and 28 weeks of gestation. Women of average risk should have testing undertaken at 24 to 28 weeks of gestation. Women at low risk of GDM (those meeting all of the following criteria: less than 25 years, normal weight before pregnancy, member of an ethnic group with low prevalence of GDM, no known diabetes in first-degree relatives, no history of abnormal glucose tolerance, and no history of poor obstetric outcome) require no glucose testing. The diagnosis of GDM is made by abnormal results on an oral glucose tolerance test (American Diabetes Association, 2004). GDM in some women can be controlled by dietary measures (medical nutritional therapy) alone; for those who cannot, insulin is the pharmacologic agent most commonly used.

For women with insulin-dependent diabetes before pregnancy, insulin requirements usually decline during early pregnancy but increase during the second trimester and remain high until delivery. Poor control of blood glucose levels during pregnancy is associated with an increased number of congenital malformations and fetal deaths. In fact, it is important for diabetic women to achieve good control before conception; an increased risk of preeclampsia and of producing infants with malformations is present for those who do not (American Diabetes Association, 2004).

Intervention and education. The diet for diabetes in pregnancy is discussed in Chapter 17.

- Tight control of blood glucose reduces the risk of congenital deformities of the fetus. Insulin-dependent women receive several daily injections or continuous infusions with an insulin pump.
- Self-monitoring of blood glucose, usually several times daily, is associated with better control than periodic monitoring by the health care provider.
- Moderate physical activity should be a part of treatment for women without physical or obstetric contraindications to exercise.
- For obese women, a moderate energy restriction (≈ 25 kcal/kg per day) has been shown to reduce hyperglycemia and hypertriglyceridemia without increasing urine ketone excretion. Restriction of carbohydrate to about 35% to 40% of total energy improves maternal and fetal outcomes (American Diabetes Association, 2004).

Maternal phenylketonuria

Individuals with PKU, an inborn error in the metabolism of the amino acid phenylalanine to tyrosine, appear to have better neurologic and mental function if they maintain a low phenylalanine diet for life. However, those women who have relaxed their dietary control need intensive counseling to return to the diet and achieve target blood phenylalanine concentrations before conception. If conception occurs before control is achieved, every effort should be made to achieve good control by 8 weeks of gestation. Pregnant women with PKU in poor control are at risk of delivering infants with defects that include low birth weight, microcephaly, and congenital heart disease. Although maternal blood phenylalanine concentrations of 120 to 360 μmol/L are desirable, it is difficult to achieve such stringent control. Adequate protein intake and weight gain reduce the incidence of delivering infants with microcephaly and congenital heart defects (Matalon et al., 2003), but the diet must be carefully planned. Special low-protein foods are included, and much of the protein comes from a low phenylalanine formula (medical food). Education and follow-up by a dietitian skilled in working with individuals with PKU are essential (Maillot et al., 2007).

Lactation

Human milk is an ideal food for the infant, and both the American Academy of Pediatrics (AAP, 2005) and the American College of Obstetrics and Gynecology (ACOG, 2007) recommend that infants receive breast milk as their sole source of nutrition for the first 6 months of life whenever possible. The advantages of breastfeeding are summarized in Box 3-3. Even if breastfeeding does not continue for 6 months, or the infant receives formula and infant foods in addition to breast milk, breastfeeding can be beneficial for both mother and child. For the infant, colostrum provides immunologic advantages, and for the mother, breastfeeding speeds involution of the uterus and stimulates weight loss.

The objectives of nutrition care in lactation are for the woman to (1) maintain an adequate diet to replenish stores that were diminished during pregnancy and produce sufficient milk for growth of the infant, (2) lose the weight gained during pregnancy, (3) avoid nutrition practices that could harm the infant, and (4) establish a successful breastfeeding relationship with her infant.

Box 3-3   Advantages of Breastfeeding

Infant Benefits

- Reduced risk of diarrheal diseases, respiratory diseases, bacterial meningitis, and otitis media. Human milk contains a variety of antiinfective factors and immune cells—such as IgA, IgM, IgG, B and T lymphocytes, neutrophils, macrophages, complement, and lactoferrin—not found in infant formula. In addition, human milk appears to contain immunomodulation factors that stimulate the infant to produce interferon and other agents of immunity.
- Reduced risk of overfeeding.
- Ease of digestion. Lactalbumin protein in human milk forms a soft, easily digested curd in the infant's stomach. Lipase enzyme in human milk improves the digestion of milk fat.
- Improved absorption of zinc and iron, compared with absorption from formula.
- Potential for enhanced cognitive development. Infants fed human milk have been found to have higher scores on intelligence tests at school age than those fed formula. These findings may be related to the fact that human milk is rich in certain long-chain polyunsaturated fatty acids believed to be needed for neurologic development. These fatty acids are especially important for preterm infants, who are more immature neurologically than term infants.

Maternal Benefits

- Less postpartum bleeding and more rapid uterine involution. Oxytocin levels are increased in the breastfeeding mother.
- Convenience (once lactation is established).
- Economy.
- More rapid postpartum weight loss.
- Increased child spacing because of delayed resumption of ovulation. Note that this does not mean that breastfeeding is a reliable method of contraception.
- Reduced risk of ovarian and premenopausal breast cancer.
- Improved bone mineralization in the postpartum period, with a reduced risk of postmenopausal hip fractures.

Mutual Benefit

- Promotion of mother-infant bonding.

Assessment

Assessment is summarized in Box 3-1.

Nutritional Requirements

Energy

The DRI for energy intake during the first 6 months of lactation is set at 330 kcal/day more than nonpregnant needs, and during the second 6 months it is 400 kcal/day more than nonpregnant needs. During the first 6 months of lactation, the DRI is calculated to be approximately 170 kcal/day less than needed to meet the mother's needs. Therefore consuming the DRI would result in continuing weight loss, helping the woman to return to her prepregnant weight more rapidly than women who do not breastfeed. During the second 6 months, the mother's weight is assumed to be stable, but the DRI is increased only slightly because milk intake by the older infant is reduced as more and more foods are added to the infant's diet.

Intervention and education. The increased energy needs should be met by use of additional milk products and small increases in meat and meat substitutes, fruits and vegetables, and whole-grain or enriched breads and cereals. Fatigue and the demands of the infant on the woman's time may interfere with food preparation. Commercially prepared foods such as low-salt and low-fat frozen meals may be helpful during the early postpartum period.

The MyPyramid Plan for Pregnancy and Breastfeeding (www.mypyramid.gov) or DASH plan (see Chapter 1), with inclusion of approximately 3 servings of milk, yogurt, or cheese, is appropriate during lactation. A variety of foods from all food groups should be consumed.

It is important to exercise regularly after the birth of the baby to promote weight control, reshape the figure, and foster a feeling of health and well-being. The lactating woman can participate in any activity she enjoys. It is essential that she have adequate fluid intake during and after exercise to replace losses in perspiration and to avoid interfering with milk production. After very heavy exercise, lactic acid may accumulate in the milk and cause the infant to reject the following feeding. This condition is usually temporary, with the infant nursing well at the next feeding.

Protein

Recommendations for protein during lactation are the same as during pregnancy (1.1 g/kg/day, or approximately 71 g/day). This amount is easily obtained in the U.S. diet; women often consume this much protein or more even before becoming pregnant.

Intervention and education. Protein intake is usually adequate if women consume approximately 3 servings of milk, yogurt, or cheese; 6 to 7 ounce equivalents of meat and beans; and and 6 to 10 servings of grains (depending on energy needs) daily.

Vitamins, minerals, and fluid

Vitamin B_{12}, calcium, and fluid are of special concern during lactation. Most normal adults have long-lasting stores of vitamin B_{12}, but approximately two thirds of lactating women who have followed strict vegetarian (vegan) diets for several years are lacking in reserves of this vitamin, and their milk contains little or no vitamin B_{12}. Megaloblastic (macrocytic) anemia, poor growth, and neurologic abnormalities have occurred in infants breastfed by such mothers (Centers for Disease Control and Prevention, 2003). The DRI for calcium during lactation remains the same as during pregnancy (1000 mg/day for adult women and 1300 mg/day for teens).

Intervention and education

- *Vitamin B_{12}*: Vegan mothers need a supplement (at least 2 to 3 mcg of vitamin B_{12}) or daily consumption of sufficient food sources fortified with vitamin B_{12} (e.g., at least 2 or 3 servings of vitamin B_{12}–fortified soy milk).
- *Calcium*: For women who do not drink milk, other good sources of calcium are listed in Figure 3-1. The use of milk in cooking (e.g., in mashed potatoes, grain products, and soups) can greatly increase milk intake. If the woman's diet appears likely to be inadequate, a daily calcium supplement is advisable.
- *Fluid*: To produce adequate milk, women need 35 to 50 ml of fluid/kg of body weight per day (16 to 23 ml/lb/day) plus an additional 500 to 1000 ml.
  - Water, milk, tea, decaffeinated coffee, soft drinks, fruit juices, and ices can be used to meet fluid needs.

- If energy intake is likely to be excessive, then emphasis should be placed on skim milk and calorie-free beverages. Women may perceive 100% fruit juices as healthful drinks, but these contain about 60 kcal in 120 ml and are a significant source of energy if used to quench thirst.

Diabetes

Breastfeeding may have a positive effect on blood glucose control in women with diabetes. Women with type 2 diabetes are likely to be overweight or obese, and breastfeeding is especially likely to benefit these women because it stimulates weight loss. Successful breastfeeding is associated with a kcal prescription of at least 31 kcal/kg of maternal weight (14 kcal/lb). Women with diabetes should be carefully monitored for mastitis because it is more common in diabetic than in nondiabetic women.

Potential Contraindications and Concerns About Breastfeeding

In a few circumstances, mothers should not be encouraged to breastfeed. These include the following:

- Classic galactosemia (galactose 1-phosphate uridyltransferase deficiency, or congenital inability to metabolize galactose) in the newborn.
- Serious maternal infections that pose a threat to the infant, such as active untreated tuberculosis. Women with human T-lymphotrophic virus type I or II infection should not breastfeed. In the United States and other industrialized nations, women positive for the human immunodeficiency virus (HIV) are advised not to breastfeed because the virus is present in milk. In developing countries, however, the antiinfective properties of human milk, which protect the infant from many diarrheal and respiratory infections associated with high mortality, may outweigh the risk of transmission of HIV posed by breastfeeding. Women in developing countries should be advised not to add complementary foods while breastfeeding, because that has been associated with higher rates of HIV infection in the infant than formula feeding (AAP, 2005).
- Maternal need for certain drugs secreted in milk that may have deleterious effects on the infant (for an extensive list of such drugs, see Lawrence and Lawrence, 1999).
- Maternal disinclination to breastfeed.

Certain medical conditions are compatible with breastfeeding as long as there is careful supervision by the health care provider:

- *Phenylketonuria (PKU) in the infant*: Human milk is relatively low in phenylalanine, and many infants with PKU can be totally or partially breastfed if their phenylalanine levels are closely monitored.
- *Severe "breast milk jaundice"*: Jaundice is more common in the first few days of life in breastfed than formula-fed infants, and it occurs most often when breastfeeding is delayed or inadequate, i.e., "nonfeeding" jaundice. Prevention is the key to management of nonfeeding jaundice (de Almeida and Draque, 2007). Policies that encourage breastfeeding, such as placing the infant at the breast in the delivery room and rooming in, improve breastfeeding success. Mothers should be encouraged to breastfeed 8 to 12 times a day initially. The adequacy of breastfeeding needs to be evaluated in the first 24 to 48 hours after birth; this includes latching on to the breast, effectiveness of suckling, and emptying of the breasts. Breastfeeding should be re-evaluated within 2 to 3 days after hospital discharge. Human milk contains an inhibitor of bilirubin conjugation and excretion. and therefore in some cases of severe hyperbilirubinemia, pediatricians may recommend temporary interruption of breastfeeding. After 12 to 24 hours of formula feeding, bilirubin usually declines, and breastfeeding can continue. The mother should be reassured that her milk is not bad for the infant and instructed to pump her breasts during the interruption of breastfeeding to maintain her milk supply.
- *Hepatitis B*: Carriers of hepatitis B may breastfeed as long as their infants have received hepatitis B immune globulin at birth and hepatitis B vaccine before hospital discharge.

Some specific foods and lifestyle practices may have negative effects on the success of lactation or the health of the infant:

- *Alcohol and drugs of abuse*: Maternal alcohol intake during lactation can impair the mother's milk ejection reflex. In addition, alcohol and other drugs appear in breast milk. If a woman chooses to drink alcohol during lactation, she should limit it to an occasional, single, small drink and avoid breastfeeding for 2 hours afterward (AAP, 2005). Drugs of abuse, including amphetamines, cocaine, heroin, marijuana, and phencyclidine hydrochloride (angel dust), should be avoided during lactation.

- *Coffee and caffeine*: Only 1% of the caffeine consumed by the mother is passed into her milk, but infants are unable to metabolize and excrete caffeine as effectively as adults. Some infants of mothers who consume caffeine have been noted to have irritability and insomnia, and mothers who note these symptoms would be well advised to limit to 300 mg daily their intake of caffeine from coffee, tea, chocolate, soft drinks, and over-the-counter drugs (Lawrence and Lawrence, 1999).
- *Smoking*: Smoking should be avoided. Nicotine appears in milk, but the major risk to the infant is from "passive smoking"— exposure to tobacco pollutants within the home environment. This increases the risk of asthma and other respiratory diseases.
- *Antigens in foods*: Where there is a family history of atopic disease (an allergy, probably hereditary, characterized by symptoms such as asthma, hay fever, or hives produced on exposure to a particular antigen), evidence suggests that lactating mothers who avoid antigenic foods reduce the risk of atopy in their infants (Kramer and Kakuma, 2006). Some common antigenic foods include peanuts, tree nuts, cow milk, eggs, and shellfish.
- *Methyl mercury in fish:* Avoid shark, swordfish, king mackerel, and tilefish, but eat as much as 12 oz (360 g) of other ocean fish and farm-raised fish per week, as long as a variety of types of fish is consumed, rather than a single type. Eat no more than 6 oz (180 g) albacore tuna weekly. Albacore (white) tuna contains higher amounts of mercury than canned light tuna. Choose seafood and fish such as shrimp, salmon, canned light tuna, pollock, and catfish. These commonly eaten fish are among those that are lowest in mercury content. Check local and state advisories about locally caught fish. If no advisory exists, consume up to 6 oz (180 g) of locally caught fish weekly, as long as no other fish is consumed during the week (U.S. FDA/CFSAN, 2008).

Lactating women are sometimes advised to avoid "gas-forming" foods, such as onions, cabbage, legumes, chocolate, and spicy foods. There is little basis for these prohibitions. Very rarely a mother will note that some food she consumes causes a rash, diarrhea, or irritability in her infant on a consistent basis. Elimination of this food from her diet readily corrects this problem.

Establishing Successful Breastfeeding

Many actions by health care providers can enhance the likelihood of successful breastfeeding. Early and sustained contact between the infant and mother (e.g., the opportunity to breastfeed within the first hour of life and to room in with the infant in the hospital) is an important measure. The infant should not be given supplements of water, glucose solutions, or formula unless the infant's medical condition makes supplementation necessary. A supportive layperson who has breastfed successfully can be a valuable resource for new breastfeeding mothers. In general, supplements and pacifiers should be used only after lactation is established, if at all. When juices, formula, and solid foods are introduced, the mother's milk production declines, and these foods and fluids are generally unnecessary until at least 6 months of age. Growth spurts occur during infancy, and the infant may seem continually hungry at these times. The mother can be reassured that this is normal and that her milk is sufficient; more frequent feedings will increase her milk supply so that the infant's needs are met.

For the infant, some signs of successful breastfeeding include a moist tongue and good hydration, weight gain of 15 to 30 g/day after the milk comes in, at least three or four bowel movements and four to six urinations daily after the third day of life, and rhythmic sucking with audible swallowing during breastfeeding. Signs of success in the mother include milk "coming in" by 72 hours after delivery (the breasts feel full and warm, and milk may leak), comfortable feedings, and letdown of milk, evidenced by the infant's swallows, leaking of milk, and softening of the breasts after feeding.

Conclusion

The intrauterine environment apparently has lifelong effects on the health of the offspring. Insulin resistance, diabetes, hypertension, coronary heart disease, chronic renal failure, breast cancer, and osteoporosis are just some of the diseases that are suggested to have their origins during fetal life (Martin-Gronert and Ozanne, 2006). Optimal weight gain and nutrient intake during pregnancy play an important role in programming the infant for a low risk of chronic disease (Buckley et al., 2005; Martin-Gronert and Ozanne, 2006).

REFERENCES

ACOG Committee on Obstetric Practice: Committee Opinion No.267: Exercise during pregnancy and the postpartum period, *Obstet Gynecol* 99(1):171, 2002.

American Academy of Pediatrics (AAP): Breastfeeding and the use of human milk, *Pediatrics* 115:496, 2005.

American College of Obstetricians and Gynecologists (ACOG) Committee Opinion No. 361: Breastfeeding: maternal and infant aspects, *Obstet Gynecol* 109(2 Pt 1):479, 2007.

American Diabetes Association: Gestational diabetes mellitus, *Diabetes Care* 27(Suppl 1):88, 2004.

Bech BH et al: Effect of reducing caffeine intake on birth weight and length of gestation: randomised controlled trial, *BMJ* 334(7590):409, 2007.

Browne ML: Maternal exposure to caffeine and risk of congenital anomalies: a systematic review, *Epidemiology* 17(3):324, 2006.

Buckley AJ, Jaquiery AL, Harding JE: Nutritional programming of adult disease, *Cell Tissue Res* 322(1):73, 2005.

Cedergren MI: Optimal gestational weight gain for body mass index categories, *Obstet Gynecol* 110(4):759, 2007.

Centers for Disease Control and Prevention: Neurologic impairment in children associated with maternal dietary deficiency of cobalamin—Georgia, 2001, *JAMA* 289:979, 2003.

de Almeida MFB, Draque CM: Neonatal jaundice and breastfeeding, *NeoReviews* 8:e282, 2007.

Dixit A, Girling JC: Obesity and preeclampsia, *J Obstet Gynaecol* 28(1):14, 2008.

Giddens JB et al: Pregnant adolescent and adult women have similarly low intakes of selected nutrients, *J Am Dietet Assoc* 100(11):1334, 2000.

Helmreich RJ, Shiao SY, Dune LS: Meta-analysis of acustimulation effects on nausea and vomiting in pregnant women, *Explore (NY)* 2(5):412, 2006.

Hösli I et al: Role of omega 3-fatty acids and multivitamins in gestation, *J Perinatal Med* 35 (Suppl 1):S19, 2007.

Kramer MS, Kakuma R: Maternal dietary antigen avoidance during pregnancy or lactation, or both, for preventing or treating atopic disease in the child, *Cochrane Database Syst Rev* 3:CD000133, 2006.

Lawrence RA, Lawrence RM: *Breastfeeding: a guide for the medical profession*, ed 5, 1999, St Louis, 1999, Mosby.

López LB, Langini SH, Pita de Portela ML: Maternal iron status and neonatal outcomes in women with pica during pregnancy, *Int J Gynaecol Obstet* 98(2):151, 2007.

Luke B: Nutrition and multiple gestation, *Semin Perinatol* 29(5):349, 2005.

Maillot F et al: A practical approach to maternal phenylketonuria management, *J Inherit Metab Dis* 30(2):198, 2007.

Martin-Gronert MS, Ozanne SE: Maternal nutrition during pregnancy and health of the offspring, *Biochem Soc Trans* 34(pt 5):779, 2006.

Matalon KM, Acosta P, Azen C: Role of nutrition in pregnancy with phenylketonuria and birth defects, *Pediatrics* 112:1534, 2003.

Moran VH: A systematic review of dietary assessments of pregnant adolescents in industrialized countries, *Br J Nutr* 97(3):411, 2007.

National Academy of Sciences, Institute of Medicine: *Nutrition during pregnancy and lactation*, Washington, DC, 1992, National Academies Press.

National Institute of Arthritis and Musculoskeletal and Skin Diseases: Pregnancy and bone health. Available at http://www.niams.nih.gov/ Health_Info/Bone/Bone_Health/Pregnancy/default.asp. Accessed March 7, 2008.

National Research Council, Institute of Medicine (NRC/IOM): *Influence of pregnancy weight on maternal and child health.* Washington, DC, 2007, National Academy Press.

Otten JJ, Hellwig JP, Meyers LD, editors: *Dietary Reference Intakes: the essential guide to nutrient requirements*, Washington, DC, 2006, National Academies Press.

Rose EA, Porcerelli JH, Neale AV: Pica: common but commonly missed, *J Am Board Fam Pract* 13(5):353, 2000.

U.S. Food and Drug Administration Center for Food Safety and Applied Nutrition (U.S. FDA/CFSAN): Fresh and frozen seafood: selecting and serving it safely. Available at http://www.cfsan.fda.gov/~lrd/seafsafe. html. Accessed March 15, 2008.

INFANCY, CHILDHOOD, AND ADOLESCENCE

During infancy, childhood, and adolescence, adequate nutrition is essential for the promotion of growth and the establishment of a framework for lasting health. Growth is the simplest and most basic parameter for evaluation of nutritional status in children.

Evaluating Growth

Adequate nutrition is reflected in a child's progress on standardized growth charts depicting height/length for age, weight for age, weight for stature, head circumference for age (up to 36 months of age), and body mass index for age. Gender- and age-specific charts are available for children from birth through 20 years (see Appendix D on Evolve).

Each child establishes an individual growth pattern and should follow this pattern consistently. Children should be evaluated for nutritional or medical disorders when one of the following occurs:

- They are consistently below the 5th or above the 95th percentile for any growth parameter. Some normal children fall outside the boundaries of the 5th and 95th percentile markings, but all children outside these boundaries should be evaluated to be sure that their growth patterns are reasonable for them (e.g., consistent with the size of their parents and other family members).
- They fail to stay within one percentile marking of their previous growth parameter (e.g., weight has been at 75th percentile marking and it then declines below the 50th percentile).
- Weight and height (or length) are inconsistent with each other (e.g., weight is at the 90th percentile, but height is at the 25th percentile).

Infancy

Goals of nutrition care are to assist the infant to consume an adequate diet for optimal growth and development; to avoid practices that may contribute to obesity, poor dentition, or other health problems; and to begin to develop good food habits. A thorough nutrition assessment should be performed as described in Chapter 2. Box 4-1 highlights common or especially serious findings in the infant.

Nutrition for Normal Growth and Development

Overfeeding is more likely than underfeeding, but parents frequently worry about whether they are feeding their infants enough, especially if the infants are breastfed. Infants who are gaining weight steadily and are wetting at least six to eight diapers per day are usually taking in enough milk.

Human milk feedings

The American Academy of Pediatrics (AAP, 2005) recommends that infants should receive breast milk unless there is a specific contraindication. Hospitals should implement policies to foster breastfeeding, including rooming-in and avoiding offering breast-fed infants water, glucose water, or formula.

Human milk is ideally suited to meet the needs of the term infant (see Box 3-3). The composition of human milk changes over the first few weeks of lactation. **Colostrum**, the milk produced for about the first 3 to 5 days, is yellowish, rich in immunoglobulins and lymphocytes, and higher in protein than mature human milk. Mature human milk is produced after about 10 to 14 days. It appears watery and may be bluish; it has more lactose and lipid than does colostrum. Transitional milk, produced in the period between colostrum and mature milk production, has some features of each type of milk.

Intervention and education. The following information should be included when instructing the breastfeeding mother:

■ Initially the baby should be breastfed 8 to 12 times daily. The breast should be offered whenever the infant shows signs of hunger, such as increased alertness, rooting, or mouthing. Crying is a late sign of hunger (AAP, 2005).

Box 4-1   Assessment in Growth and Development

Inadequate Energy or Protein Intake

History

Poverty; chronic illness or frequent acute illnesses; altered parent-infant relationship manifested by failure to feed infant adequately; fear of becoming obese; obsession with thinness (older children and adolescents); inadequately planned vegetarian diet

Physical Examination

Length, height, or weight <5th percentile, or >10% decrease in these parameters; edema, ascites; hair changes: alopecia, loss of pigmentation (flag sign), altered texture; muscle wasting; TSF <5th percentile for age; signs of self-induced vomiting: tooth erosion, gastric bleeding, weak and flabby muscles, poor skin turgor, abrasions on dorsal side of fingers

Laboratory Analysis

↓ Serum albumin, transferrin, and prealbumin; ↓ serum potassium (from self-induced vomiting)

Excessive Energy Intake

History

Overfeeding; sedentary lifestyle: frequent and prolonged television viewing/electronic gaming, lack of regular physical activity; one or both parents overweight or obese

Physical Examination

BMI >85th percentile; TSF >85th percentile for age

Inadequate Mineral Intake

Iron

History

Poverty; dislike of iron-containing foods; vegetarianism; increased needs, especially in an infant 4 to 12 months of age or adolescent female); excessive milk consumption by toddler; infant receiving cow milk before 12 months of age; infant born preterm with poor stores

Box 4-1   Assessment in Growth and Development—cont'd

Physical Examination

Pallor; blue sclerae; spoon-shaped nails; diminished learning ability

Laboratory Analysis

↓ Hgb, Hct, MCV, serum iron, serum ferritin; ↑ free erythrocyte protoporphyrin (FEP)

Zinc

History

Poverty; dislike of zinc-containing foods; vegetarianism (large intake of grains and vegetables containing phytates and oxalates that impede absorption); abnormal losses (severe or prolonged diarrhea); infant born preterm with poor stores

Physical Examination

Seborrheic dermatitis; anorexia; diarrhea; alopecia; poor growth

Laboratory Analysis

↓ Serum zinc

Calcium (Ca)

History

Failure to consume milk products, calcium-fortified soy milk or formula, or a calcium supplement daily because of food preferences, vegetarianism, dieting, or frequent reliance on fast foods

Inadequate Vitamin Intake

A

History

Failure to consume vitamin A (liver; deep green, leafy or deep yellow vegetables) at least every other day; frequent reliance on fast foods

Continued

Box 4-1   Assessment in Growth and Development—cont'd

Physical Examination

Dry skin, mucous membranes, or cornea; follicular hyperkeratosis (resembles gooseflesh); poor growth, susceptibility to
infection

Laboratory Analysis

↓ Serum retinol

B_{12}

History

Child or adolescent following vegan diet without a supplement
or use of fortified soy milk; ileal resection or disease; infant
breastfed by vegan mother

Physical Examination

Pallor; glossitis; neurologic abnormalities (altered sensation,
altered sense of balance); confusion, depression

Laboratory Analysis

↓ Serum vitamin B_{12}, Hct; ↑ MCV

BMI, Body mass index; *Hct,* hematocrit; *Hgb,* hemoglobin; *MCV,* mean corpuscular
volume; *TSF,* triceps skinfold.

- Make sure that the infant "latches on" well. The infant's mouth
  should cover as much of the areola (the dark area around the
  nipple) as possible and never cover just the nipple (Figure 4-1).
  If the infant is grasping only the nipple or nursing is painful to
  the mother, then she should insert her finger between the breast
  and the infant's mouth to break the seal and then reposition the
  infant's mouth before beginning again. Improper grasp of the
  nipple makes nipples sore and can lead to cracking.
- Feed the infant from both breasts at each feeding. Begin each
  feeding with the breast the infant ended with at the last feeding to
  ensure that the breast is drained at least every other feeding. Emptying the breasts encourages milk production. If twins are being
  breastfed, feed each baby on alternate breasts every other feeding.
  One baby is likely to be a more vigorous feeder than the other.

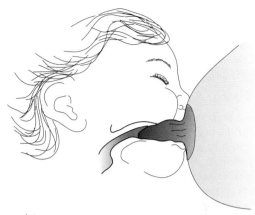

Figure 4-1
Infant properly latched on at the breast. Note that most of the areola is in the infant's mouth.

- Exposing the nipple to the air helps to heal it if it becomes sore or cracked (e.g., leave flaps of nursing bra down for a few minutes after feedings). Begin with brief feedings (<5 minutes per breast) to avoid nipple soreness, but progress to 15 to 20 minutes per breast. Milk fat is usually released only after 10 to 20 minutes of suckling, and the infant needs the fat to grow properly and to be satisfied between feedings.
- Avoid offering bottle feedings until the mother's milk supply is established, or preferably until 4 to 6 weeks after birth. After that time it may be possible to give a bottle so that the mother can be away from the infant. Many mothers who return to work outside the home continue to breastfeed for months, either by pumping their breasts during breaks at work or by adjusting to partial breastfeeding (e.g., only two or three feedings per day). Ideally pacifiers should not be used until after lactation is well established.
- Use different infant positions (e.g., cradle hold across the mother's body; lying beside the mother; and football hold with the infant's head in the mother's hand, nursing from the breast on the same side of the body as that hand) to drain different portions of the breast and decrease the risk of clogging the milk ducts. Clogging causes discomfort and may lead to mastitis or

breast infection. If signs of clogging (redness, enlargement, and pain in a portion of the breast) occur, then the mother should nurse more frequently, beginning on the affected side. The baby is hungrier at the beginning of the feeding and will nurse more effectively, helping to relieve the clogging.

Formula feeding

Infants who are not breastfed should receive iron-fortified infant formula for the first year (AAP, 2004). Infants given cow milk before 12 months of age are likely to develop iron deficiency anemia. Cow milk, whether whole, low-fat (1% or 2% fat), or skim, can cause gastrointestinal (GI) blood loss in infants. Also, cow milk is extremely low in iron and has excessive amounts of protein, calcium, phosphorus, and sodium for infants; excreting the unneeded nitrogen and minerals can place stress on the kidneys by increasing the renal solute load. It is especially important that skim milk not be used. Skim milk lacks essential fatty acids that are needed for optimal growth and maintenance of skin integrity.

Commercial formulas closely resemble human milk. Standard formulas and human milk contain about 20 kcal/oz (66 kcal/100 ml). Commercial formulas contain higher levels of protein and most minerals than human milk to compensate for less complete absorption and utilization. The formulas are manufactured with or without added iron. The low-iron formulas are virtually iron free, as is cow milk. Anemia is common in infants receiving low-iron formulas. For infants who are not breastfed, use of iron-fortified formulas for the first year of life provides a reliable source of dietary iron. Commercial formulas are available in three forms: ready-to-feed, concentrate (to be diluted with an equal volume of water), and powder. The three forms are the same in nutritional value (except for fluoride), and the concentrate or powdered forms are almost always less expensive than ready-to-feed.

Intervention and education. When teaching the parents of a formula-fed infant, the following information is appropriate:

▪ Hold the infant closely during feedings. Never prop a bottle or leave an infant unattended during feeding, both for safety reasons and because feedings are an important time for nurturing.

■ Be attuned to the infant's degree of hunger. Never encourage the infant to take more at a feeding than he or she seems to want. Table 4-1 gives general guidelines as to the amount of formula to feed, but the individual infant may have different needs.

■ Burp the infant regularly during feeding, every 0.5 to 1 oz initially and less often as the infant grows.

Recommended supplements

The AAP Committee on Nutrition has made the following recommendations (AAP, 2004):

■ *Vitamin D*: All breastfed infants should receive 5 mcg (200 international units) daily.
■ *Vitamin B_{12}*: Approximately 0.3 to 0.5 mcg daily is needed for breastfed infants of vegan mothers.
■ *Iron*: 10 mg daily is recommended for breastfed infants older than 6 months if they do not consume food sources of dietary iron (e.g., iron-fortified infant cereal) daily.
■ *Fluoride*: 0.25 mg daily is needed for infants over 6 months of age who are fed human milk, ready-to-feed formula, or formula reconstituted with water containing less than 0.3 parts per million (ppm) fluoride. No fluoride supplementation is recommended before 6 months of age.

Table 4-1   Approximate Daily Amount of 20 kcal/oz Formula Needed by Infants Younger Than 6 Months

Infant Weight			
lb	kg	Caloric Need	Ounces (ml) of Formula Needed
3	6.6	324	16.2 (486)
4	8.8	432	21.6 (648)
5	11.0	540	27.0 (810)
6	13.2	648	32.4 (972)

Solid foods

The AAP recommends that solid foods be started between 4 and 6 months of age in developed countries (AAP, 2004). Solid foods are not recommended before that time because of the following:

- The tongue extrusion reflex, which tends to push solid foods out of the mouth, does not fade until the infant is about 4 months of age.
- Production of pancreatic amylase, an important enzyme for digestion of starches in infant foods, is low before 4 to 6 months.
- Infants can maintain good head control at 4 months of age and can sit fairly well by 6 months of age. Thus they are better prepared than younger infants to participate in the feeding process; for example, an infant can turn the head away from the spoon to indicate that he or she is full.
- Exclusive breastfeeding for 4 to 6 months decreases the chance that infant at high risk of atopic disease will develop allergies (Greer et al., 2008).
- Early introduction of solid food has no effect on sleep patterns. Many parents introduce solid foods early, erroneously believing that this will cause the infant to sleep through the night.
- Solid foods can inhibit absorption of iron and other nutrients from human milk.
- The duration of breastfeeding tends to be shorter for infants who receive solid foods earlier (AAP, 2005).

Intervention and education. When introducing solid foods, the parents should follow these guidelines:

- Begin with foods that provide needed nutrients. For breastfed infants, this means good sources of iron, zinc, protein, and energy. Pureed meats are especially good sources of these nutrients. Other nutritious choices include iron-fortified infant cereals, vegetables, and fruits.
- Introduce only one new food every 3 to 5 days, and observe the infant for hypersensitivity reactions after each food. If a reaction is thought to have occurred, then stop that food for several weeks and try again later. If the same thing occurs after the second or third trial, then the infant is probably sensitive to this

food. Use single-grain cereals until it is clear that the infant tolerates all grains contained in mixed cereals.

- Wait until the infant is at least 12 months old to introduce egg white and shellfish, which are among the foods most likely to cause allergy. Avoid nuts and nut butters in infancy because of their potential for being allergens, as well as the choking hazard they pose.
- Begin with about 1 tsp at a time, and advance the amount as the infant seems ready.
- Offer solid foods at the beginning of feedings while the infant is hungry.
- Thin foods with formula or expressed breast milk initially to help the infant make the transition from human milk or formula to foods with thicker consistencies.
- Feed the infant with a spoon. Adding foods to formula in a bottle deprives the infant of a chance to learn feeding skills. Infants with certain medical disorders are exceptions to this rule. Thickening the formula with infant cereal may help to control gastroesophageal reflux, for example.
- Never feed the infant from the jar. If any food is left over, amylase enzyme in the saliva will digest starches in the food, making it watery. Also, bacteria from the mouth contaminate the food and might cause spoilage.
- Avoid serving desserts regularly; these are usually low in nutrients and establish a desire for sweets.
- Consider the developmental state of the infant in choosing foods. For instance, between 7 and 9 months of age the infant's purposeful grasp improves and he or she picks objects up and moves them to the mouth. This is an ideal time to offer finger foods such as toast, zwieback, dry cereals, and cheese slices.

Some parents may wish to prepare food at home for the infant. When preparing infant foods at home:

- Use fresh or frozen fruits, vegetables, and meats without added salt.
- Cook foods in as little water as possible, and do not overcook; this preparation preserves the vitamin content.
- Add no sugar or salt. Infants have a well-developed sense of taste and do not require flavor enhancers. The infant receives enough sodium from unsalted foods, and routine use of sugar

and salt causes the infant to develop a taste for these unnecessary food additives.

■ Puree foods in a blender or food grinder initially; chop or mash foods once the infant has more teeth and can chew lumpier foods.

■ Freeze prepared foods in ice trays for later use; the appropriate number of cubes can be used each time for an infant-sized serving.

Minimizing the risk of obesity

To minimize the risk of obesity, parents can do the following:

■ Reduce formula and milk intake as infants consume more solids.

■ Recognize and respond to cues that the infant has reached satiety. Satiety cues from a younger infant include withdrawing from the nipple, falling asleep, closing the lips tightly, and turning the head away. Cues from an older infant include closing the lips tightly, shaking the head "no," playing with or throwing utensils or food, and handing the cup or bottle back to the parent.

■ Never insist that the infant finish a bottle, dish, or jar of food. Before 6 months, an average serving size is about 2 to 5 tablespoons, and after 6 months, it is approximately one-half to one jar of baby food. Infants' needs vary widely, however, and an individual infant may not need an average serving.

Promoting dental health

Nursing bottle caries is a form of tooth decay resulting from prolonged contact of sugar-containing fluids (milk, juice, fruit drinks) with developing teeth. Although it usually occurs in bottle-fed infants, it can also occur in breastfed infants. To reduce the risk of caries, these guidelines should be followed:

■ If infants are put to bed with a bottle, then it should contain only water so that exposure of the teeth to sweet fluids is minimized. When infants are put to bed with a bottle, they suck on it periodically and keep the mouth full of fluid.

■ Avoid giving the infant a bottle or breastfeeding whenever the infant cries. Learn to distinguish cries of hunger from cries for other needs, and feed only in response to hunger.

- Infants less than 6 months of age should not be introduced to fruit juice, since it is not required to meet their nutrition needs. Fruit juice should be given only in a cup, not a bottle. Infants over 6 months of age should receive no more than 4 to 6 oz (120 to 180 ml) of juice daily because excessive intake of juice and other sugary beverages is associated with increased numbers of dental caries (AAP, 2004).
- Fruit drinks, even those that contain some fruit juice, are not equivalent to fruit juice and should not be included in the infant diet.

Feeding safety

Infants are at special risk for certain types of food-borne infections and for choking. Infant food safety practices include the following:

- Infants less than 1 year of age should not consume honey. *Clostridium botulinum* spores in honey can cause infant botulism. Symptoms range from constipation through progressive weakness and diminished reflexes to sudden death. In contrast, botulism in older persons is almost always caused by consuming the toxin released by the bacteria in spoiled food, not by consuming spores.
- When infants are given fruit juice, it should be pasteurized.
- Infants should not receive hot dogs, grapes, hard foods such as raw carrot, or any other food that is likely to cause choking and block the airway.

Nutritional Problems in Infancy

Acute gastroenteritis

Acute episodes of diarrhea and vomiting, usually associated with viral illness, are common during infancy and early childhood. These illnesses damage the intestinal mucosa and diminish the absorptive surface.

Intervention and education. The Centers for Disease Control and Prevention (CDC) (King et al., 2003) has made specific recommendations regarding management of acute gastroenteritis in children in the United States, based on the presence and degree of dehydration, and these are summarized below. The degree of dehydration can be determined using the criteria in Table 2-7. Treatment takes place in two stages. In the rehydration stage, fluid deficits are replaced over a period of approximately 3 to 4 hours and a state of adequate hydration is achieved. This is followed by the maintenance stage, where maintenance fluid and energy are provided. Nutrition should not be restricted. Breastfeeding should continue throughout therapy, even during rehydration, and bottle-feeding should resume as soon as the rehydration stage is over. The majority of bottle-fed infants tolerate lactose-containing full-strength formulas, although infants with severe malnutrition, diarrhea, or enteropathy (disease of the GI tract) may benefit from a lactose-free formula.

Children receiving semisolid or solid foods should continue to receive their usual diet during episodes of diarrhea. Carbonated soft drinks, fruit juice, fruit drinks, gelatin desserts, and other liquids and foods high in simple sugars should be avoided because they can cause osmotic diarrhea. It is often recommended that fat be restricted, but there does not appear to be much clinical evidence that this reduces diarrhea.

Children with diarrhea but minimal or no dehydration. Children with diarrhea but minimal or no dehydration should continue to receive an age-appropriate diet with increased fluids to replace losses. A commercial oral rehydration solution (ORS) is preferred for fluid replacement (Table 4-2). Most children with little or no dehydration can be treated at home.

- If the child is hospitalized, soiled diapers can be weighed, with the estimated weight of the dry diaper deducted, and 1 ml fluid administered for every gram of stool output.
- To replace ongoing losses in children at home, parents can be instructed to give 10 ml of ORS per kilogram body weight for each watery stool or 2 ml/kg body weight for each episode of emesis. As an alternative, children weighing less than 10 kg can be given 60 to 120 ml ORS for each episode of vomiting or diarrheal stool, and those weighing more than 10 kg can be given 120 to 240 ml.
- Some children object to the salty taste of ORS. The solutions may be better accepted if frozen into ice pops. Some of the commercial solutions are flavored to improve their acceptance.

Children with more significant dehydration

- *Mild to moderate dehydration*: Fluid deficits should be replaced quickly, over 2 to 4 hours, using 50 to 100 ml fluid per kilogram of usual body weight plus additional fluid as needed to replace

Table 4-2   Appropriate and Inappropriate Solutions for Oral Rehydration (Composition per Liter)

Composition	Rehydration Solutions*	Solutions Inappropriate for Oral Rehydration		
		Cola	Apple Juice	Chicken Broth	Sports Drink
CHO (g)	13.5-30	700	690	0	58
Na (mmol)	50-75	2	3	250	20
K (mmol)	20-25	0	32	8	3
Citrate (mmol)	10-34	11	0	0	3
Chloride (mmol)	45-65	2	0	0	0
Osm (mOsm/kg)	170-245	570-750	730	500	280-340

CHO, Carbohydrate; *K*, potassium; *Na*, sodium; *Osm*, osmolality.

*Carbohydrate–electrolyte solutions that are commercially available (e.g., Pedialyte [Ross], Enfalyte [Mead Johnson], Rehydralyte [Ross], WHO/UNICEF oral rehydration salt packets [http://rehydrate.org/solutions/packaged.htm]).

ongoing losses. Ongoing losses are replaced as described for children with minimal or no dehydration. A commercial ORS (see Table 4-2) is the preferred fluid. Use of an ORS is less expensive than intravenous treatment and is associated with fewer complications. Very small amounts of ORS (e.g., 5 ml every 10 to 15 minutes) should be administered initially, with the volume increased as tolerated. If vomiting prevents oral rehydration, or the infant/child is unable or unwilling to consume sufficient fluid, the ORS can be administered continuously through a nasogastric (NG) tube. NG rehydration has been successful even in the presence of vomiting. After rehydration many children can undergo maintenance ORS therapy at home, if the parents are carefully instructed in administration of ORS, signs of dehydration, and findings to report to the health care provider and if they have the ability to return to the health care facility if needed.

■ *Severe dehydration*: Severe dehydration is a medical emergency requiring immediate rehydration. Lactated Ringer's (LR) solution, normal saline, or a similar isotonic solution should be given intravenously (20 ml/kg body weight for previously healthy infants and small children; 10 ml/kg in frail or malnourished infants, where sepsis might be confused with dehydration) until pulse, perfusion, and mental status return to normal. Monitor the patient closely for edema of the eyelids and extremities, signs of overhydration. Once the mental status has returned to normal, maintenance fluid therapy can be given as described for infants with minimal or no dehydration, using ORS or IV fluids.

Other treatment measures. No medication is required for treatment of most acute diarrheal illnesses but may be warranted in cases where the disease does not respond to supportive therapy. Nonspecific antidiarrheal agents such as the adsorbents (e.g., kaolin-pectin) and antimotility drugs (e.g., loperamide) have been used, but their efficacy is unproven. The underlying problem in most cases is increased secretion of fluid and electrolytes by intestinal crypt cells.

Prebiotics (food ingredients that stimulate the growth or activity of nonpathogenic bacteria such as bifidobacteria and lactobacilli in the colon, e.g., oligofructose) and **probiotics** (live microorganisms such as lactobacilli, bifidobacteria, or the nonpathogenic yeast *Saccharomyces boulardii*) may alter intestinal microflora in a beneficial manner and reduce the duration of diarrheal diseases. No specific recommendations for the therapeutic use of these agents can be made at this time. The oligosaccharides found in human milk are prebiotics, however, and acute diarrhea is less prevalent among breastfed infants, providing an excellent reason for promotion of breastfeeding.

Diarrhea can result from malabsorption of sorbitol and fructose in fruit juices (AAP, 2004). If diarrhea is chronic, rather than acute, then the child's intake of fruit juices should be evaluated.

Food hypersensitivity

In infants and small children, symptoms of **food hypersensitivity** or allergy (an immunologic reaction to ingestion of a food or food additive) can include anaphylaxis, failure to thrive, vomiting, abdominal pain, diarrhea, rhinitis, sinusitis, otitis media, cough, wheezing, rash, urticaria, and atopic dermatitis (AAP, 2004). Egg white, cow milk, peanuts, nuts from trees, and shellfish are among the most allergenic foods for children.

Intervention and education. If a mother is breastfeeding an infant who is at high risk for food hypersensitivity (e.g., an infant with a family history of allergies), it may be necessary for her to avoid these foods with high allergenic potential during lactation. There is no need for a mother breastfeeding an infant at low risk of allergy to avoid any specific foods unless it becomes evident that her infant is displaying allergic symptoms. If the infant is formula fed and displays an allergy to cow milk, there is a high likelihood that the infant will also be allergic to soy. Protein hydrolysate formulas (in which the protein is broken down so that no large protein molecules are present to stimulate an allergic response) are often used for infants with allergic symptoms. About 85% of children with milk allergy outgrow it by their fourth year of life (AAP, 2004). Reintroduction of milk or any other suspected allergen into the diet should be done in a setting where epinephrine, intravenous fluids, and respiratory support are available.

Failure to thrive

Failure to thrive describes the infant who does not regain his or her birth weight by 3 weeks of age or the infant who exhibits continuous weight loss or failure to gain weight at the appropriate rate (see Appendix D on Evolve). This condition results from an inadequate food supply or illness in the infant. *Organic* failure to thrive is a condition in which a physiologic reason for the infant's failure to thrive is apparent. Insufficient milk production by the breastfeeding mother and cystic fibrosis in the infant are two examples of this condition. When no physical cause is apparent, the infant has inorganic failure to thrive. Impairments in the parent-child relationship, knowledge deficits in the parent or caregiver, and inadequate parenting skills are some reasons for inorganic failure to thrive. Assessments of these social, psychologic, and emotional issues and an individualized plan of care are essential to address inorganic failure to thrive adequately.

Toddlers and Preschoolers

As the child leaves infancy, the growth rate slows, but nutrition needs remain high. The goals of nutrition care are to foster development of good eating habits that will ensure adequate nutrient intake and minimize the risk of obesity and other health problems. Nutrition assessment is summarized in Box 4-1.

Nutrition for Normal Growth and Development
Developing good eating habits

Children need to consume a variety of foods from all food groups. Chronic diseases such as heart disease and type 2 diabetes are likely to have their start in childhood, and thus it is essential that healthy eating habits be established early to provide a basis for lasting health.

Intervention and education. Parental food habits strongly influence those of children, so parents may need to make an effort to eat a balanced and varied diet and avoid voicing distaste for any foods. Young children begin to develop food likes and dislikes (Box 4-2). Parents should continue to encourage their children to eat a variety of foods while respecting children's preferences as much as possible. Children sometimes refuse foods simply because they are unfamiliar with them, but parents should not take this refusal to be permanent. Children's opinions of particular foods improve after they are served those foods repeatedly. **Food jags**, during which children consume only one or two foods for several days, are common. Parents should avoid making an issue of food jags because

---

Box 4-2   Food Preferences of Young Children

Likes

- Crisp, raw vegetables
- Foods that can be served and eaten without help, such as finger foods (sandwiches cut into strips or shapes, raw fruit or vegetables cut into small pieces, cheese cubes) and milk and other beverages that can be poured from a child-sized pitcher
- Foods served lukewarm
- Single foods that have a characteristic color and texture; preferably, different foods should not even touch each other on the plate

Dislikes

- Strong-flavored vegetables such as cabbage and Brussels sprouts; overcooked vegetables
- Highly spiced foods
- Large servings of beverages or foods
- Foods served at temperature extremes
- Combination foods (e.g., mixed vegetables) where flavors mingle and textures become similar; exceptions: pizza, spaghetti, macaroni and cheese

---

this disapproval can put parents into the position of struggling with the child for control of the child's behavior. Parents should provide a variety of nutritious foods at each meal, and they should not allow the child to eat only sweets. Food jags are not usually harmful; intake over a period of several weeks balances out.

Young children want to feed themselves and need to learn the necessary skills. Although the process is messy, it should be encouraged. Overemphasis on neatness creates stress at mealtimes and could interfere with the development of good eating habits.

Nutrient dense foods that are not high in saturated fat or cholesterol such as low-fat dairy products, whole grains, vegetables, and lean meats should be encouraged and *trans* fatty acids should be avoided as much as possible. Fish, especially oily fish such as salmon, broiled or baked, should be eaten frequently. For children 1 to 2 years, 2% milk can be used; after 2 years, skim milk is preferable (Gidding et al., 2005).

Fiber helps to reduce the risk of heart disease and improves bowel function. Children 1 to 3 years of age should consume 19 g of fiber daily, and those 4 to 8 years of age need 25 g daily (Food and Nutrition Board, Institute of Medicine, 2005). Good fiber sources—whole grains, fruits, and vegetables—should be an important part of the child's diet. Appendix C on Evolve lists rich sources of fiber.

Energy intake and risk of obesity

A simple rule of thumb states that energy needs in early childhood are approximately 1000 kcal plus 100 kcal per year of life. That is, a 3-year-old needs about 1300 kcal/day. A more careful estimate, using body weight as well as height and activity level for older preschoolers and school-aged children, is advocated by the Food and Nutrition Board (2005). For children 13 to 16 months of age, estimated energy requirements (EERs) are as follows: $(89 \times$ weight in kg $- 100) + 20$ kcal. The EER for boys 3 to 8 years of age is calculated by the formula: $88.5 - (61.9 \times$ age in years$) +$ PA $\times (26.7 \times$ weight in kg $+ 903 \times$ height in meters$) + 20$ kcal; and the formula for EER for girls of the same age is as follows: $135.3 - (30.8 \times$ age in years$) +$ PA $\times (10 \times$ weight in kg $+ 934 \times$ height in meters$) + 20$ kcal. PA is determined by the level of physical activity. The PA is equal to 1 if the child is sedentary. For low active children the PA is 1.13 for boys and 1.16 for girls. For active children the PA is 1.26 for boys and 1.31 for girls. For very active children the PA is 1.42 for boys and 1.56 for girls.

Intervention and education. Parents may be concerned about what they perceive to be poor food intake by toddlers and preschoolers. They need to be reminded that the growth rate is slowing, and children's appetites will reflect this change. Needs for protein, vitamins, and minerals remain high; however, there is little room for "empty calories" from high-fat or high-sugar foods. Some steps that parents can take to reduce the risk of obesity are as follows:

- Avoid overwhelming the child with servings that are too large. More can be served if the child is still hungry after the initial serving.
- Keep fruits or vegetables available, include them in every meal, and offer them as snacks. Children learn to control their own energy intake when parents provide healthful foods but let the children determine the amount that they will consume. Fresh,

frozen, or canned fruits and raw vegetables make better snacks than chips, cookies, or candy.

■ Choose no-fat or low-fat dairy and whole-grain products, as well as lean meats and poultry, because energy needs are too low to allow for consumption of many high-fat foods.

■ Limit intake of fruit juice to no more than 4 to 6 fl oz (120 to 180 ml)/day for children 1 to 6 years of age. Whole fruits, a good source of fiber, should make up the remainder of the fruit servings. Water is the preferred beverage if children are thirsty.

■ Limit the amount of time that children are involved in sedentary activities, such as watching television and using a computer or electronic game, to no more than 1 to 2 hours daily (Gidding et al., 2005).

■ Encourage at least 1 hour of vigorous physical activity daily, and model a physically active lifestyle for their children (Gidding et al., 2005).

Mineral intake

The highest incidence of iron deficiency in the United States is found in children under age 5 years. Children at special risk include Mexican Americans, Native Americans, the poor, and those who consume 1 quart or more of milk per day (CDC, 2002). Milk, which is low in iron, may take the place of iron-rich foods in the diet. Iron deficiency is associated with decreased attentiveness, narrow attention span, and impaired problem-solving ability.

The recommended calcium intake for children 1 to 3 years old is 500 mg/day, and for children 4 to 8 years of age it is 800 mg/day. Development of bones and teeth depends on adequate calcium intake. Further, the habit of consuming a diet rich in calcium is important for the prevention of osteoporosis in later life. Milk and cheese are the richest calcium sources in the diets of most young children. Juices, fruit drinks, and other beverages should not be allowed to replace milk in the diet.

Intervention and education. To ensure an adequate intake of iron, children should do the following:

■ Eat at least 4 or 5 oz equivalents of meat, poultry, fish, or legumes and 5 oz of enriched or whole-grain breads and cereals daily, depending on level of physical activity (Figure 4-2). Deep green, leafy vegetables can also supply some iron.

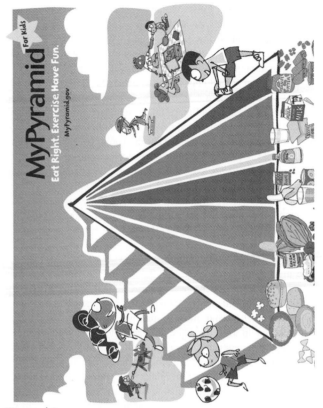

Figure 4-2
Food guide pyramid for young children.
(From USDA Center for Nutrition Policy and Promotion.)

- Avoid excessive milk intake (i.e., 1 L or more daily), since milk provides little or no iron and can displace iron-containing foods in the diet.
- Consume good vitamin C sources daily to improve iron absorption.

To ensure adequate intake of calcium, parents should encourage children to follow these guidelines:

- Consume approximately 2 cups (240 ml) of milk or yogurt daily unless the child is lactose intolerant, a condition that is

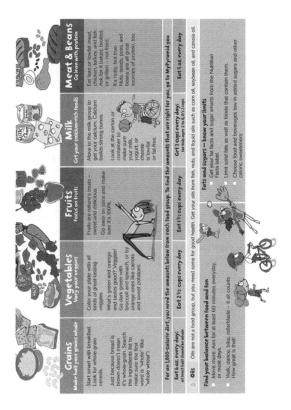

Grains Make half your grains whole	Vegetables Vary your veggies	Fruits Focus on fruits	Milk Get your calcium-rich foods	Meat & Beans Go lean with protein
Start smart with breakfast. Look for whole-grain cereals. Just because bread is brown doesn't mean it's whole-grain. Search the ingredients list to make sure the first word is "whole" (like "whole wheat").	Color your plate with all kinds of great-tasting veggies. What's green and orange and tastes good? Veggies! Go dark green with broccoli and spinach, or try orange ones like carrots and sweet potatoes.	Fruits are nature's treats—sweet and delicious. Go easy on juice and make sure it's 100%.	Move to the milk group to get your calcium. Calcium builds strong bones. Look at the carton to make sure your milk, yogurt, or cheese is lowfat or fat-free.	Eat lean or lowfat meat, chicken, turkey, and fish. Ask for it baked, broiled, or grilled — not fried. It's nutty but true. Nuts, seeds, peas, and beans are all great sources of protein, too.

For an 1,800-calorie diet, you need the amounts below from each food group. To find the amounts that are right for you, go to MyPyramid.gov.

Eat 6 oz. every day; at least half should be whole	Eat 2½ cups every day	Eat 1½ cups every day	Get 3 cups every day; for kids ages 2 to 8, it's 2 cups	Eat 5 oz. every day

Oils Oils are not a food group, but you need some for good health. Get your oils from fish, nuts, and liquid oils such as corn oil, soybean oil, and canola oil.

Fats and sugars — know your limits
- Get your fat facts and sugar smarts from the Nutrition Facts label.
- Limit solid fats as well as foods that contain them.
- Choose food and beverages low in added sugars and other caloric sweeteners.

Find your balance between food and fun
- Move more. Aim for at least 60 minutes everyday, or most days.
- Walk, dance, bike, rollerblade - it all counts. How great is that!

less common in children than in adults. There is no significant difference in the absorption of calcium from chocolate milk and unflavored milk, so chocolate milk can be used if the child prefers it. Yogurt can be consumed often as a snack or part of a meal.

- Limit intake of soft drinks, which are empty of nutrients other than energy and displace milk and other nutritious foods in the diet.
- Eat cheese often. Parents can offer cheese for snacks, use cheese in main dishes such as macaroni and cheese, or use cheese sauce over vegetables. Low-fat or "part skim" versions of some cheeses help to reduce children's fat intake, which is often excessive.

Promoting dental health

Good dental health is promoted by encouraging the child to consume a diet adequate in calcium and phosphorus. Two cups of milk daily provide the calcium and phosphorus needed. Avoid offering sticky carbohydrates such as chewy candies, cookies, and pastries, which cling to the teeth. Develop the habit of regular brushing as soon as the child has teeth, and begin flossing as soon as teeth touch each other.

Fluoride makes the teeth more resistant to caries; therefore the American Dental Association (ADA) and the AAP (2004) recommend providing some children with fluoride supplements. If the local water supply contains less than 0.3 ppm of fluoride, then the recommended daily supplement of fluoride is 0.25 mg before age 3 years, 0.5 mg between ages 3 and 6 years, and 1 mg from 6 to 16 years. If the water supply provides 0.3 to 0.6 ppm of fluoride, then the recommended dosage for fluoride supplementation is 0 to 3 years of age, none; 3 to 6 years, 0.25 mg; and 6 to 16 years, 0.5 mg. No supplement is routinely recommended for children of any age whose water supply provides greater than 0.6 ppm of fluoride.

Feeding safety

All juices served to children should be pasteurized to reduce the risk of food-borne infection. Another safety concern is that most deaths resulting from asphyxiation by food occur in children under age 3 years. To help prevent asphyxiation, these guidelines should be followed:

- Provide adult supervision for very young children while they eat.
- For children under age 3 years, avoid foods such as hot dogs, hard candy, caramels, jelly beans, gum drops, nuts or peanuts, grapes, popcorn, and raw carrots, which are difficult to chew or swallow and are an appropriate size to block the airway. If the parent chooses to give the child foods that are likely to be aspirated, the parent should modify these foods to make them less likely to obstruct the airway. Grapes can be quartered, carrots cooked, and meat cut into very small pieces. Hot dogs can be cut lengthwise into four strips.
- Insist that children sit down while they eat and keep eating times as calm as possible. A child who is laughing or extremely excited could aspirate food.

School-Age Children

The goals of nutritional care are to develop sound eating habits that minimize the risk of obesity and other health problems while providing adequate amounts of all nutrients and fiber. Specifically, teaching should include choosing a balanced diet and encouraging physical activity.

Assessment is summarized in Box 4-1.

Nutrition for Normal Growth and Development
Healthful food and lifestyle choices

Peers, teachers, and other significant adults begin to influence food choices during the school years, and home influences decline. As children grow older and have more money to spend, they consume more snacks and meals outside the home. Vending machines and fast-food restaurants offer foods that are likely to be high in fat, salt, and sugar and low in vitamins and minerals. Eating habits with long-lasting effects are set during childhood. Dietary intake can influence the incidence of chronic health problems, such as obesity, heart disease, cancer, and osteoporosis. A survey of U.S. adolescents (Larson et al., 2007) found that they consumed less than the recommended amounts of fruits and vegetables and that their intake of fruits and vegetables declined from early to late adolescence. Approximately 18% of children 6 to 19 years of age in the United States are overweight or obese, a substantial increase over the previous estimates (National Center for Health Statistics, 2008). Similarly, about 29% of Canadian teens are estimated to be overweight or obese (Shields, 2006). Overweight and obesity are linked to a poor diet, particularly a lack of fruits and vegetables, and a more sedentary lifestyle that may include, for example, excessive television viewing and use of electronic games and computers (Shields, 2006). An alarming increase in cases of insulin resistance and type 2 diabetes (disorders commonly associated with overweight and obesity) has occurred in children and teens. Evidence of cardiovascular disease is also present among children and teens (Steinberger and Daniels, 2003). Thus lifestyle changes to prevent overweight and promote physical activity are a high priority in child health.

Intervention and education. Children need to consume a wide variety of fruits, vegetables, whole grains, dairy products, legumes, fish, poultry, and lean meat. Their diets should be moderate in fat, high in calcium, and adequate but not excessive in energy. In addition, children need daily physical activity. The following guidelines help to achieve these goals:

- Parents can encourage children to eat a nutritious diet by involvement and example. It may take as many as 10 tries to convince a child to include a new food in his or her diet, but it is worth the effort to encourage children to eat a wide variety of foods. Establish a rule that all family members eat at least one meal together daily, if at all possible. This rule not only encourages family interaction, but also makes it easier to control the amount of sodium, sugar, and unhealthful fats, and cholesterol in the diet.
- Emphasis should be placed on making healthy food choices rather than on foods to avoid. Nutritious foods, including ample amounts of fruits, fresh vegetables, low-fat dairy products, and whole grains, should be provided for meals and snacks. The family must avoid relying regularly on fast-food meals, which tend to be high in energy, fat, and sodium and low in milk products, vegetables, and fruits. Low-fat cooking methods (grilling, baking, stir-frying) are preferred over deep-frying.
- Involve children in obtaining or preparing food. Children can be involved in gardening if the family grows some vegetables, in choosing food at the market with adult guidance, and in age-appropriate cooking and food preparation tasks. This involvement gives children a personal stake in the family meals and is a good way to introduce elementary nutrition.
- Make nutritious snacks available at all times to discourage the consumption of high-energy, low-nutrient foods. Good choices for snacks include fresh or dried fruits; raw vegetables; yogurt; air-popped or other low-fat popcorn; cheese, especially low-fat varieties; cottage cheese with raisins or other fruits; unsalted, dry-roasted seeds or nuts; bran or oat muffins; fruit juice frozen into pops; and peanuts or peanut butter (in moderation because of the high fat content).
- Prepare foods attractively, because meals with "eye appeal" are more likely to be enticing to youngsters. Choose appealing color combinations for foods served in a meal, and be sure that vegetables are not overcooked, to avoid causing their colors and textures to deteriorate. Bread for sandwiches can be cut with cookie cutters into inviting shapes, and pancakes can be poured

in the shape of the child's initials or other fun shapes. If vegetable intake is a problem, try incorporating vegetables into other foods, e.g., bake carrot or zucchini muffins, or add finely grated vegetables to meatballs or meatloaf.

■ Ensure that children participate almost daily in physical activity that involves use of large muscle groups—either team sports or individual aerobic exercises. Parent example and involvement are especially important, and parents should plan enjoyable family activities that involve physical activity. Opportunities to obtain activity during the school day are also essential, and all schools should have trained physical education teachers (National Center for Chronic Disease Prevention and Health Promotion, 2008). After-school care programs should provide opportunities for vigorous physical play. Youth sports and recreation programs are additional ways to obtain physical activity. The American Heart Association recommends at least 60 minutes of moderate to vigorous physical activity every day for children and adolescents (Steinberger and Daniels, 2003). Excessive sedentary activity (more than 2 hours daily of television watching or electronic gaming) should be avoided (AAP, 2003).

The child's social, emotional, and family environment may contribute as much as the nutritional and physical environment to the problem of overweight. The mother who has always struggled with maintaining weight at a stable level may put undue pressure on her child to stay slim, for example. The child's self-esteem and sense of independence can suffer as a result. Ultimately, this attitude may contribute to development of eating disorders. Parents need help from the health care team when they are too rigid in trying to control the child's behaviors or too disorganized to provide children with the structure and support they need to maintain a healthy body weight. Children benefit from counseling and modeling of behaviors that help them to improve their self-esteem and self-reliance.

Attention-Deficit/Hyperactivity Disorder

Attention-deficit/hyperactivity disorder (ADHD) is characterized by focusing on irrelevant stimuli, impulsive behavior, overactivity (not in all children), inconsistency, and lack of persistence. The Feingold diet has been recommended as a treatment for ADHD. It excludes foods containing salicylates, compounds that cross-react with salicylates, artificial flavors, colors, and preservatives. Controlled studies have not provided clear-cut evidence that this diet is effective (Rojas and Chan, 2005). Positive effects from the diet may be a result of the placebo effect or of the fact that it takes pressure off the child (placing the blame for behavior on the diet, rather than on the child). Unfortunately, some of the supposed salicylate-containing foods, such as oranges, peaches, grapes, raisins, apples, berries, and cherries, are nutritious and are commonly enjoyed by children. A modified Feingold diet, restricting only food additives, allows a more varied diet. There should be no objection if family members want to follow such a diet, unless they substitute the diet for medication or counseling needed by the child or family or unless emphasis on the diet promotes behavioral problems by forcing the child to be "different" from peers.

Sugar has also been proposed as a cause of ADHD, but there is little solid evidence for this (Rojas and Chan, 2005). Studies done so far indicate that parents expect their children to be hyperactive after consuming large amounts of sugar-containing foods, and this parental expectation may explain why children sometimes have behavioral problems after high sugar intake. Also, sugar intake tends to be high at parties and on holidays, when children are usually excited; the children's excitement over the event itself can confuse parents into thinking that sugar is causing the problem.

Adolescence

The goal of nutrition care is to help adolescents learn to make wise food choices that provide the necessary nutrients while maintaining a desirable body weight and a healthy lifestyle. Nutrition assessment of the adolescent is summarized in Box 4-1.

Nutrition for Normal Growth and Development

Healthy food and lifestyle choices

Energy needs for adolescent growth are high. Despite these needs, many adolescents do not consume an adequate diet. In a recent survey in the United States, less than 3% of teenagers consumed the current recommended number of servings of fruits and vegetables (Guenther et al., 2006). Snacks furnish about 40% of energy in adolescent diets. Although snacking is not bad in itself, traditional snack foods such as chips, cookies, and soft drinks are low in nutrients and high in energy. Adolescents rely heavily on fast-food restaurants, which have limited menus and serve foods that, for the most part, are high in energy (kcal), fat, and sodium and limited in fruit and vegetable options.

Intervention and education
Fat and cholesterol. To reduce fat and cholesterol intake, these guidelines should be followed:

- Limit use of fried foods to 1 serving per day or less.
- Choose poultry, fish, or grain and legume main dishes often, and reduce the use of red meat. When meats are consumed, choose lean meats rather than high fat choices such as cold cuts, hot dogs, and regular hamburger meat.
- Use dairy products made with skim milk whenever possible. Chapter 14 provides additional information for limiting fat and cholesterol intake.
- Fiber has a cholesterol-lowering effect. Girls 9 to 18 years old should consume 26 g of fiber daily. The recommendation is 31 g for boys 9 to13 years of age and 38 g for boys between the ages of 14 and 18 years (Food and Nutrition Board, Institute of Medicine, 2005). To increase fiber intake, choose abundant servings of fruits and vegetables daily and select whole-grain products.

Mineral intake. Lack of calcium and iron is particularly common among teenage girls. Bone growth requires an increase in calcium intake, with a Dietary Reference Intake (DRI) of 1300 mg/day. Growth and onset of menstruation necessitate an increase in iron needs; the Recommended Dietary Allowance (RDA) for adolescent girls is 15 mg/day. Fast foods and traditional snack foods tend to be low in calcium and iron. Also, girls concerned about their weight often consider dairy products, which are rich sources of calcium, to be too fattening to include in their diets. To ensure adequate vitamin and mineral intake, these guidelines should be followed:

- Consume at least 3 servings of milk or milk products daily (especially important for adolescent girls). Skim milk and yogurt, cheese, and cottage cheese made of skim milk are low in energy and may be acceptable to dieting teens. For those who do not use milk products, calcium-fortified juice and cereals are reliable calcium sources, and tortillas, pancakes, and other grain products made with milk or calcium provide additional calcium (see Figure 3-1).

- Use a daily supplement if the diet is low in milk products or other good sources of calcium. Calcium citrate is a well-absorbed form of calcium. Calcium carbonate, a common antacid, is 40% calcium. To improve absorption, it should be taken with foods but preferably not with bran or whole grains.
- Eat lean meat, poultry, fish, legumes, enriched or whole grains, or deep green, leafy vegetables daily to receive dietary iron (see Appendix B on Evolve). Even if adolescent girls use a variety of these foods daily, they may still have an inadequate or marginal iron intake. A daily supplement (15 mg) may be needed. This amount is available in many over-the-counter multivitamin-multimineral supplements. Avoid taking such supplements with milk, coffee, or tea to improve iron absorption.

Effective weight control. Overweight, obesity, and the associated disorders, including type 2 diabetes and cardiovascular disease, occur at epidemic proportions even among youth in North America and much of the developed world. To avoid excessive energy intake, these guidelines should be followed:

- Limit fat intake.
- Choose high-fiber foods (see Appendix C on Evolve) because they are bulky and require more chewing than low-fiber, refined foods. The person feels full after eating less energy. Whole grains, legumes, and crisp salads without excessive additions such as dressing, eggs, meat, and bacon are nutritious, low-energy foods.
- Obtain approximately 60 minutes of moderate exercise most days of the week. Some teens wish to participate in team sports, which can be encouraged. Others need to choose individual activities that they will continue on a long-term basis. Parents continue to be significant role models for teenagers, and it is important that the parents be physically active on a regular basis and that they plan family activities that include physical exercise. In addition, physical activity needs to be a part of the school day for adolescents, and opportunities for exercise can also be obtained through extracurricular sports and youth recreation programs (National Center for Health Statistics, 2008).

Chapter 5 shows how to calculate the target heart rate for cardiovascular fitness and includes recommendations for becoming and remaining physically fit. Excessive sedentary leisure activity (more than 2 hours daily), especially "screen" time, should be discouraged.

■ Make sure that snacks are nutritious and low in energy, because they are such an important part of the adolescent's diet. Some examples are fresh or dried fruits; fresh vegetables with a dip made of low-fat yogurt and herbs; no-fat or very low-fat microwave popcorn; bagels (plain or with low-fat or fat-free cream cheese or other low-fat topping); fruit ices; and yogurt, cottage cheese, or cheese made with skim milk.

■ Limit fruit juice consumption to 8 to 12 oz (240 to 360 ml) daily. It is easy to overconsume energy in this liquid form, and many juices (e.g., apple) are relatively low in nutrient density. This limit does not apply to whole fruits, which contribute a range of nutrients, as well as dietary fiber and nutraceutical components. Consume sugar-containing soft drinks and sport drinks infrequently; water is the best beverage for quenching thirst.

■ Teens have such busy schedules that convenience is an overwhelming concern for them. Thus parents need to ensure that nutritious snacks and convenience foods are readily available at home, and schools need to keep vending machines and snack bars stocked with fruits, yogurt, low-fat granola bars, and other healthful, low-fat items.

■ Include a healthful breakfast in the day's meal pattern. Teens that regularly skipped breakfast had higher BMIs than those that usually ate breakfast (Timlin MT et al., 2008). Whole grains are an especially important part of healthful breakfasts.

Inappropriate weight control practices

Fad diets are popular among teens but are more likely to promote transient water loss than lasting changes in eating habits. In fact, dieting often leads to development of poor eating habits, such as binge eating and skipping breakfast, that contribute to weight gain (van den Berg et al., 2007). Magazines aimed at adolescent girls focus on physical appearance, with thinness given extreme importance. The cultural emphasis on a slim figure contributes to the prevalence of anorexia nervosa and bulimia (see Chapter 19), eating disorders that usually develop during the teen years.

Intervention and education. Because teens are so interested in weight-reduction diets, they need to be taught to recognize a safe and effective eating plan. Fad diets promise and often deliver quick results, but much of the weight loss is fluid and lean body mass, rather than fat. A good plan meets the criteria outlined in Box 7-2.

Eating disorders often appear during adolescence. Magazines and television programming focused on adolescents place a priority on appearance. Adolescents who are seriously committed to certain sports or recreational activities—such as gymnastics, figure skating, wrestling, or ballet—may feel compelled to maintain unrealistically low body weights. Primary prevention of eating disorders should be the goal. Some topics to include in a primary prevention program are as follows: (1) normal physiologic, social, and psychologic changes during puberty, the normal changes in fat deposition, and the diversity that occurs among individuals; (2) general nutrition, meal skipping, and other eating habits; (3) physical activity—its importance and appropriate levels; (4) weight control—realistic and safe methods of weight control, realistic goals for weight, myths and fads about dieting, the physiologic and psychologic effects of food restriction and chronic dieting; (5) body image issues and how to determine one's appropriate body weight; (6) autonomy and self-esteem; (7) impact of nutritional habits on athletic performance; and (8) information about anorexia and bulimia. If parents observe their children to be dieting inappropriately, they need to intervene early. The prognosis is much better if intervention occurs early in the course of the illness. See Chapter 19 for a more detailed discussion.

Vegetarianism

The teen years are a time of experimentation, which may take the form of adopting vegetarianism. There are many types of vegetarians (see Chapter 1). Unless carefully planned, vegetarian diets may be nutritionally inadequate.

Plant sources of protein include legumes (soybeans; peanuts; beans such as pinto, navy, northern, or kidney; and peas such as blackeye and crowder), grains, nuts and seeds, and vegetables other than legumes. Plant sources of protein differ from animal sources such as meat, milk, and eggs in that most plant sources are not **complete proteins**. A complete protein is one that contains all the **essential amino acids (EAAs)** in sufficient amounts and in proportion to one another so that it can support growth and maintenance of tissues. EAAs are those that cannot be synthesized in the body in the amounts needed for the building of tissues and therefore must be provided by the diet. Most plant proteins are low in one or more EAAs and are therefore **incomplete proteins**. Fortunately, the amino acid patterns of the different plant protein sources vary. For example, most grains are low in the amino acid lysine but contain moderate amounts of methionine, and conversely most legumes are relatively low in methionine but contain moderate amounts of lysine. Consuming proteins from a variety of plant sources on a daily basis is the best way to ensure that the diet includes adequate amounts of all amino acids. Use of milk products also helps to ensure that the diet has high-quality protein sources, and adolescents should be encouraged to include milk, cheese, and yogurt in their diets.

Intervention and education. A vegetarian food guide has been developed for use as a teaching tool in diet planning (Messina et al., 2003). To ensure that nutritional intake is adequate, the adolescent vegetarian needs to be aware of the following:

■ Consuming a wide variety of grains, legumes, nuts, and seeds allows the vegetarian to obtain adequate amounts of all amino acids. A diet including eggs and dairy products ensures that the vegetarian has complete protein in the diet, but an adequate diet (with the exception of vitamin B_{12}) without animal products is possible with careful planning.
■ Whole grains; legumes; and deep green, leafy vegetables contain iron and zinc. Additional iron can be obtained from dried fruits, molasses, soy sauce, and use of iron cookware. Iron from plant sources is better absorbed if it is consumed with a vitamin C–containing food, such as citrus fruit. Coffee and tea inhibit iron absorption; thus it is best not to consume these beverages with meals.
■ Vegetarians who avoid dairy products often have difficulty consuming enough calcium. Further, plant foods are usually lower in zinc and iron than animal products, and phytate (in whole grains) and oxalate (in chocolate, green leafy vegetables, and rhubarb) form complexes with minerals and inhibit their absorption. Calcium-fortified juice, cereals, tofu, and soy milk can be valuable sources of calcium for vegetarians who do not use dairy products. Adolescent girls, in particular, may benefit from daily use of dairy products or a calcium supplement. Dairy products are among the richest dietary sources of calcium, and lactose in

dairy products stimulates calcium absorption. See Figure 3-1 or Appendix B on Evolve for other good sources of calcium.

■ Vitamin B_{12}–containing products must be consumed several times per week. Eggs, dairy products, and all other animal products contain vitamin B_{12}. Some soy milk and nutritional yeast is fortified with vitamin B_{12} (consult the label). If no dietary vitamin B_{12} sources are used, then the individual will need a vitamin B_{12} supplement (2 to 3 mcg/day), which can be obtained in a daily multivitamin.

■ Although the vegetarian diet can be a healthful one, as demonstrated in Table 4-3, interest in such a diet can also signal an eating disorder in an adolescent. The diets of adolescent vegetarians need to be carefully assessed to determine that they are associated with healthful eating patterns.

Table 4-3   Sample Vegetarian Diet Plan

Foods Eaten	Number of Servings from MyPyramid
Breakfast	
4 oz calcium-fortified orange juice	½ cup fruit
1 cup whole-grain oat cereal	1 oz eq grain
1 small peach, sliced	½ cup fruit
1 cup fortified soy milk*	1 cup milk
Lunch	
1 veggie burger on a bun	2 oz eq meat and beans, 2 oz eq grain
2 slices tomato, 1 slice onion, and 1 large lettuce leaf	½ cup vegetable
1 small apple	1 cup fruit
Dinner	
1½ cups whole wheat spaghetti	3 oz eq grain
1 cup sauce (tomato and textured vegetable [soy] protein)	2 oz eq meat and beans, ½ cup vegetable
2 cups mixed raw greens with ½ oz sunflower seeds and vinaigrette dressing	1 cup vegetable, 1 oz eq meat and beans
½ cup broccoli florets	½ cup vegetable
1 cup soy milk	1 milk

Table 4-3   Sample Vegetarian Diet Plan—cont'd

Foods Eaten	Number of Servings from MyPyramid
Snack	
1 cup fortified soy yogurt*	1 cup milk
Total Servings	6 oz eq grain
	2½ cups vegetables
	2 cups fruit
	5 oz eq meat and beans
	3 cups milk

Oz eq, Ounce equivalents.
*Calcium and vitamin B_{12} fortified.

Conclusion

Although nutritional status is impacted by countless health and developmental issues in growing children, one of the most worrisome problems is the increasing prevalence of overweight and obesity among children. The increase in body weight has led to a marked increase in chronic health problems among young people, such as type 2 diabetes, hypertension, and hyperlipidemia that are normally thought of as adult diseases (Lobstein and Jackson-Leach, 2006). No one factor is responsible for the increase in childhood obesity; the causes lie with changes in the family, community, and society as a whole (Anderson and Butcher, 2006). Thus all these social units must come together as a whole to encourage healthy food choices, decrease screen time (computers, video games, television), and increase time spent in physical activity.

REFERENCES

American Academy of Pediatrics (AAP), Committee on Nutrition: *Pediatric nutrition handbook*, ed 5, Elk Grove Village, Ill, 2004, The Academy.

American Academy of Pediatrics (AAP), Committee on Nutrition: Prevention of pediatric overweight and obesity, *Pediatrics* 112:424, 2003.

American Academy of Pediatrics (AAP), Section on Breastfeeding: Breastfeeding and the use of human milk, *Pediatrics* 115:496, 2005.

Anderson PM, Butcher KE: Childhood obesity: trends and potential causes, *Future Child* 16(1):19, 2006.

Centers for Disease Control and Prevention (CDC): Iron deficiency –
United States, 1999–2000. *MMWR Morb Mortal Wkly Rep* 51:897, 2002.

Food and Nutrition Board, Institute of Medicine: *Dietary reference intakes
for energy, carbohydrate, fiber, fat, fatty acids, cholesterol, protein, and
amino acids*, Washington, DC, 2005, National Academies Press.

Gidding SS et al: Dietary Recommendations for Children and Adolescents: A Guide for Practitioners: Consensus Statement From the
American Heart Association, *Circulation* 112(13):2061, 2005.

Greer FR et al: Effects of early nutritional interventions on the development
of atopic disease in infants and children. *Pediatrics* 121(1):183, 2008.

Guenther PM et al: Most Americans eat much less than recommended
amounts of fruits and vegetables, *J Am Diet Assoc* 106:1371, 2006.

King CK et al: Managing acute gastroenteritis among children: oral rehydration, maintenance, and nutritional therapy, *MMWR Recomm Rep*
52(RR-16):1, 2003.

Larson NI et al: Trends in adolescent fruit and vegetable consumption,
1999-2004: Project EAT, *Am J Prev Med* 32:147, 2007.

Lobstein T, Jackson-Leach R: Estimated burden of paediatric obesity and
co-morbidities in Europe. 2. Numbers of children with indicators of
obesity-related disease, *Int J Pediatr Obes* 1(1):33, 2006.

Messina V, Melina V, Mangels AR: A new food guide for North American
vegetarians, *J Am Diet Assoc* 103:771, 2003.

National Center for Chronic Disease Prevention and Health Promotion
(NCCDPHP): Promoting better health for young people through physical activity and sports: a report to the President. Available at http://
www.cdc.gov/healthyyouth/physicalactivity/promoting_health/#
CalltoAction. Accessed March 8, 2008.

National Center for Health Statistics (NCHS): Prevalence of overweight
among children and adolescents: United States, 2003-2004. Available
at http://www.cdc.gov/nchs/products/pubs/pubd/hestats/overweight/
overwght_child_03.htm. Accessed February 17, 2008.

Rojas NL, Chan E: Old and new controversies in the alternative treatment
of attention-deficit hyperactivity disorder, *Ment Retard Dev Disabil Res
Rev* 11:116, 2005.

Shields M: Overweight and obesity among children and youth, *Health
Rep* 17(3):27, 2006.

Steinberger J, Daniels SR: Obesity, insulin resistance, diabetes, and cardiovascular risk in children, *Circulation* 107(10):1448, 2003.

Timlin MT et al: Breakfast eating and weight change in a 5-year prospective
analysis of adolescents: Project EAT (Eating Among Teens), *Pediatrics*
121(3):e638, 2008.

van den Berg P et al: Is dieting advice from magazines helpful or harmful?
Five-year associations with weight-control behaviors and psychological
outcomes in adolescents, *Pediatrics* 119(1):e30, 2007.

ADULTHOOD AND AGING

A nutritious diet and regular physical activity are major factors contributing to fitness and health in the adult years. Habits that promote healthy lifestyle choices should be developed early and maintained throughout life.

Nutrition Assessment in the Adult Years

The goal of nutrition intervention in adulthood is maintenance of good health and well-being and reduction of the risk of chronic and debilitating diseases. A thorough nutrition assessment should be performed as described in Chapter 2. Box 5-1 highlights common or especially serious findings of adults.

Health Promotion

Nutrition and lifestyle practices among many adults are poor. In particular, approximately half of North American adults do not obtain the recommended amount of physical activity (Centers for Disease Control and Prevention [CDC], 2007). Women are less active than men, and Hispanics, Native Americans, and African Americans are more sedentary than Caucasians. Sedentary habits begin to develop early in life, with activity levels decreasing in adolescence, particularly among girls. Surveys of food intake are equally concerning, indicating that fewer than 30% of adults consume at least five servings of vegetables and fruits daily (Kruger et al., 2007).

Overweight/Obesity and a Sedentary Lifestyle

Overweight and obesity are prevalent in the United States and Canada. For convenience, overweight is generally defined as a body mass index (BMI) of 25 to 29.9, and obesity is defined as a BMI of 30 or greater (CDC, 2008b). Based on this definition, the CDC estimates that two thirds of U.S. adults are either overweight

Box 5-1   Assessment in Early and Middle Adulthood

Overweight and Overnutrition

History

Sedentary lifestyle; excessive energy intake

Physical Examination

Weight >120% of desirable or BMI >25; waist circumference >102 cm (men) or >88 cm (women); TSF>95th percentile; hypertension; acanthosis nigricans*

Laboratory Analysis (Plasma)

↑ Triglycerides, ↑ LDL cholesterol, ↓ HDL cholesterol, ↑ glucose

Inadequate Fiber Intake

History

Frequent use of processed foods; low intake of fruits and vegetables, whole grains, and legumes; constipation, diverticulosis

Inadequate Antioxidant Intake

History

Poor intake of fruits and vegetables

Medications

History

Supplement usage, medications (prescribed or over the counter)

BMI, Body mass index; *HDL,* high-density lipoprotein; *LDL,* low-density lipoprotein; *TSF,* triceps skinfold.
*Darkening of the skin, especially over the elbows, knees, neck, and groin; associated with insulin resistance (but not a highly specific or sensitive indicator).

or obese, and one third are obese (National Center for Health Statistics, 2008). About 60% of all Canadian adults are overweight or obese and 23% are obese (Tjepkema, 2006). Obesity and overweight are risk factors for numerous chronic illnesses including cardiovascular disease; hypertension; type 2 diabetes; and certain types of cancers, including breast (postmenopausal), colorectal, endometrial, renal cell, and gallbladder cancers.

About 47 million adults in the United States (almost 25% of the adult population) and growing numbers around the world have a disorder known as the **metabolic syndrome.** This disorder is characterized by obesity, particularly in the upper body; hypertension; abnormal serum lipids; and **insulin resistance** (impaired responsiveness of the tissues to insulin, evidenced by elevated fasting glucose). The National Heart, Lung and Blood Institute (NHLBI) and the American Heart Association (AHA) have jointly published criteria for diagnosing the metabolic syndrome (Grundy et al., 2005), and the International Diabetes Federation (IDF) has published separate criteria (Alberti et al., 2006). Both sets of criteria include the presence of three of the following five findings:

- *Increased waist circumference.* For non–Asian Americans, the NHLBI/AHA guidelines specify a waist circumference ≥102 cm (≥40 in) in men or ≥88 cm (≥34 in) in women. For Asian Americans the NHLBI/AHA criteria suggest a lower waist circumference cut point (≥90 cm [≥35 in] in men and ≥80 cm [≥31 in] in women). The IDF defines an increased waist circumference as one that is ≥94 cm (≥37 in) in men or ≥80 cm (≥31 in) in women, and the IDF criteria mandate that an increased waist circumference (plus two other findings listed below) be present for a diagnosis of metabolic syndrome.
- *High triglycerides.* Both sets of guidelines define this as serum triglyceride concentrations ≥150 mg/dl (≥1.7 mmol/L) or use of a medication for high triglycerides.
- *Low high-density lipoprotein cholesterol (HDL-C).* This is defined as HDL-C ≤40 mg/dl (≤1.03 mmol/L) in men or ≤50 mg/dl (≤1.3 mmol/L) in women or the use of a drug to raise HDL-C.
- *Elevated blood pressure.* A systolic pressure ≥130 mm Hg, a diastolic pressure ≥85 mm Hg, and/or receiving treatment for hypertension is defined as elevated blood pressure.
- *Elevated fasting blood glucose.* A fasting blood glucose measurement ≥110 mg/dl, drug treatment for hyperglycemia, or a previous diagnosis of type 2 diabetes meets this criterion.

The metabolic syndrome is likely to be a precursor to cardiovascular disease and type 2 diabetes. Since overweight/obesity and a sedentary lifestyle are major contributing factors to the metabolic syndrome, these factors are key targets in efforts to prevent and correct the syndrome.

Intervention and education

Maintaining a healthy weight. The content in this chapter focuses primarily on prevention of developing overweight and obesity. Although there is some overlap with Chapter 7, that chapter deals in more detail with weight loss measures for individuals who are overweight or obese. The first step in maintaining a healthy weight is for the individual to recognize what that is. A healthy weight range for the individual is generally a weight for height that results in a BMI of 18.5 to 24.9 (see Chapter 2 or the chart on the inside the back cover for methods of determining the BMI). Although some healthy individuals have weights that cause them to fall outside that range, health risks are statistically greater for those outside the range.

Healthy eating habits. A weight-maintaining diet includes a wide variety of foods, especially those rich in fruits and vegetables and moderate in fat.

- Whole grains, e.g., whole-wheat, oat, and rye breads; whole-grain pasta; brown rice; oatmeal; and whole-grain breakfast cereals, are preferable to refined products. Fiber from whole grains, along with that from fruits and vegetables, not only provides bulk that helps the individual feel full but also has beneficial effects on serum cholesterol levels and bowel function.
- Fat is needed in the diet to supply essential fatty acids, but, more important for individuals trying to control their weight, it helps to promote satiety. Oils rich in monounsaturated fats (olive, canola, safflower, peanut) and polyunsaturated fats (sunflower, corn) are especially good choices because of their beneficial effects on serum cholesterol. Peanuts; tree nuts such as walnuts, pecans, pistachios, and almonds; and seeds such as sunflower, sesame, and pumpkin are good sources of monounsaturated and polyunsaturated fats and can be used in moderate amounts as cholesterol-free replacements for some of the meat servings in the diet. A moderate intake of fat (25% to 35% of energy intake) is part of a prudent diet (Lichtenstein et al., 2006).
- Lean meat, fish, and poultry can be part of a healthful diet, but portion sizes are best limited to about 4 oz (120 g), about the size of a deck of cards. Red meats and processed meats such as smoked sausages and cold cuts are associated with an increased risk of cancer. A recent recommendation is to consume no more

than 500 g (18 oz) of red meat weekly, with very little processed meat in the diet (World Cancer Research Fund, American Institute for Cancer Research, 2007).

■ Broiling, grilling, steaming, and sautéing in small amounts of oil or with the use of nonstick cookware and vegetable cooking spray are low-fat cooking methods preferable to frying.

■ Food labels should be read carefully. "Low-fat" items (e.g., cottage cheese, milk, cold cuts, frozen meals and entrees) can be helpful in controlling fat and energy intake, but "low fat" does not always mean that an item provides substantially less energy than its higher-fat alternative. For example, 2 tablespoons of low-fat peanut butter provide 166 kcal, whereas 2 tablespoons of regular peanut butter contain 188 kcal; three low-fat Oreo cookies contain 150 kcal, whereas three regular cookies provide 160 kcal; and two low-fat fig cookies provide 100 kcal, whereas two regular cookies provide 111 kcal.

■ Healthful foods such as fresh fruits or vegetables (pared and cut into appropriate eating sizes if possible), low-fat dairy products, and nuts and seeds should be kept readily available as alternatives to less healthful snack choices, such as chips and cookies. Sugary drinks such as fruit drinks and regular soft drinks should be avoided, and foods of high energy density (approximately 225 to 275 kcal/100 g food) should be limited (World Cancer Research Fund, American Institute for Cancer Research, 2007).

■ Eating out can be a special challenge to the individual trying to control body weight. Teaching tips include the following:

   ■ At fast-food or quick-serve restaurants, use the nutrition information available in the restaurant and on the websites for the chain in making the wisest food choices. Avoid the temptation to "super size" items. Choose small sandwiches and do not add cheese or bacon. Select salads with low-fat dressing or grilled chicken or fish rather than burgers or fried fish.

   ■ At full-service restaurants, the customer can ask about food preparation methods before ordering if there is any question about the fat or energy content of an item and request sauces and salad dressings to be served "on the side" so that the patron can determine how much to use. Serving sizes are likely to be large, so meals can be shared with a companion or part of the meal can be taken home for later consumption.

- Psychologic and emotional skills can help avoid overeating. Teaching tips include the following:
    - Eat only when hungry. Learn to recognize cues for eating that have nothing to do with hunger (e.g., situations such as watching television or movies, seeing commercials about food, emotional stresses, boredom), and avoid eating in response to those cues. Chewing sugar-free gum helps some individuals cope with the need to eat when not hungry.
    - Eat slowly to allow the body to recognize satiety before overeating has already occurred. Avoid eating "on the run" because it is easy to overeat while focusing on matters other than eating.
    - Keep a record of all food eaten to recognize the actual amounts consumed as well as times when overeating is likely. The individual may not find it necessary to do this always, but it can be helpful to do it for a few days whenever weight gain occurs to identify unhealthful eating practices and provide a basis for planning changes.
    - Avoid skipping meals. In particular, eating breakfast every day is associated with lower BMI among adults and also a reduced chance of regaining weight after a substantial weight loss (Timlin and Pereira, 2007).
- Moderate intake of alcohol is associated with a reduced risk of cardiovascular disease, but alcohol intake at any level appears to increase the risk of cancer. If alcohol is consumed, it should be limited to two drinks per day for men and one for women. Pregnant women and children should avoid alcohol altogether (World Cancer Research Fund, American Institute for Cancer Research, 2007).

Physical fitness. Regular physical activity throughout life is an extremely valuable tool for health maintenance. It not only helps to maintain muscle mass and decrease fat accumulation but also reduces the tendency to gain weight as the metabolic rate declines with age.

- *Changes in incidental activity can improve fitness and stimulate energy expenditure.* A few examples include the following: park further from the door to increase the walking needed to get into a building, take the elevator rather than the stairs whenever practical, and walk or bicycle rather than driving when running errands close to home or work.

- *Optimal exercise duration.* Moderate intensity activity for 30 minutes on 5 or more days per week, or a minimum of 20 minutes of vigorous intensity at least 3 days per week, reduces the risk of cardiovascular disease and diabetes (CDC, 2008a), but it is unlikely to be sufficient to prevent overweight in adults as they age. About 60 minutes of daily activity of at least moderate intensity is believed to be necessary for avoiding weight gain, and 60 to 90 min may be necessary for maintaining weight loss (USDHHS and USDA, 2005).

- *Exercise intensity.* Intensity of exercise can be judged in various ways (CDC, 2008a):

  - *The talk test.* A person should be able to sing while performing light activity and carry on a conversation comfortably while engaged in moderate activity. Exercise is vigorous if the person is too winded or breathless to talk comfortably.

  - *Target heart rate.* For moderate-intensity exercise, a person's heart rate should be between 50% and 70% of the maximum (HR_{max}). HR_{max} can be estimated as 220 minus the age in years. For example, for a 40-year-old, HR_{max} would be 180 beats/min. To determine the target heart rate, $180 \times 0.5 = 90$ beats/min, and $180 \times 0.7 = 126$ beats/min. Thus the target heart rate for moderate intensity exercise at 40 years of age is 90 to 126 beats/min. For vigorous intensity exercise the target heart rate should be 70% to 85% of the HR_{max}. For the 40-year-old, the target heart rate for vigorous intensity exercise would be 126 to 153 beats/min.

  - *Perceived exertion (Borg scale).* The Borg scale is based on the individual's perception of how much exertion he or she is doing. The person's perception of increase in heart rate, work of breathing, sweating, and muscle fatigue may give a good indication of the actual heart rate. On this scale a rating of 6 means no exertion at all, and a rating of 20 indicates maximal exertion. A rating of 7.5 is very light activity, 11 is light, 13 is somewhat hard, and 15 is hard. Moderate-intensity exercise would be rated at approximately 12 to 14 on the scale.

  - **Metabolic equivalent (MET) level.** Activities are rated according to the relative energy (oxygen) use required. One MET is the energy required while sitting quietly—for example, while reading a book. The harder the body works, the higher the MET rating for the activity (Table 5-1). The same activity may be categorized as light, moderate, or vigorous

Table 5-1   Level of Intensity of Selected Physical Activities

Light Activity* <3 METs† (<3.5 kcal/min)	Moderate Activity* 3-6 METs† (3.5-7 kcal/min)	Vigorous Activity* >6 METs† (>7 kcal/min)
Walking casually, less than 3 miles per hour (mph)	Walking at a moderate or brisk pace, 3-4.5 mph on a level surface	Race walking or aerobic walking, 5 mph or faster
		Jogging or running
		Wheeling your own wheelchair
		Backpacking
	Walking with crutches; Roller-skating or in-line skating at a leisurely pace	Roller-skating or in-line skating at a brisk pace
		Mountain or rock climbing
Bicycling <5 mph	Bicycling 5-9 mph with few hills	Bicycling >10 mph or on steep uphill terrain
Stationary cycling with light effort	Stationary cycling with moderate effort	Stationary cycling with vigorous effort
Stretching exercises—slow warm-up	Yoga	Karate, judo, tae kwon do, jujitsu
	Gymnastics	Jumping rope
	Using a stair climber machine or a rowing machine at a light to moderate pace	Using a stair climber machine or rowing machine at a fast pace

Aerobic dancing—stretching and slow warm-up period	Aerobic dancing—high impact	Aerobic dancing—high impact
Swimming—floating	Water aerobics	Step aerobics
	Swimming—recreational	Swimming—steady-paced laps
	Water-skiing	Water polo
	Snorkeling	Scuba diving
	Surfing, body or board	Downhill skiing—racing or with vigorous effort
	Downhill skiing—with light effort	Cross-country skiing
	Ice skating at a leisurely pace (≤9 mph)	Sledding
		Playing ice hockey
Gardening and yard work: pruning, weeding while sitting or kneeling, or slowly walking and seeding a lawn	Gardening and yard work: raking the lawn, bagging grass or leaves, digging, hoeing, shoveling <10 lb/min	Gardening and yard work: heavy or rapid shoveling (>10 lb/min), carrying heavy loads
		Felling trees, carrying large logs, swinging an ax, hand-splitting logs, or climbing and trimming trees

Continued

Table 5-1   Level of Intensity of Selected Physical Activities—cont'd

Light Activity* <3 METs[†] (<3.5 kcal/min)	Moderate Activity* 3-6 METs[†] (3.5-7 kcal/min)	Vigorous Activity* >6 METs[†] (>7 kcal/min)
Using a riding mower	Planting trees, trimming shrubs and trees, hauling branches Pushing a power lawn mower or tiller	Pushing a nonmotorized lawn mower

From U.S. Department of Health and Human Services, Public Health Service, Centers for Disease Control and Prevention, National Center for Chronic Disease Prevention and Health Promotion, Division of Nutrition and Physical Activity: *Promoting physical activity: a guide for community action,* Champaign, Ill, 1999, Human Kinetics.

*For an average person, defined as 70 kg, or 154 lb. The activity intensity levels in this chart are most applicable to men aged 30 to 50 yr and women aged 20 to 40 yr. Intensity is a subjective classification. For older individuals the classification of activity intensity might be higher. For example, what is moderate intensity to a 40-year-old man might be vigorous for a man in his 70s.

[†]The ratio of exercise metabolic rate. One MET is defined as the energy expenditure for sitting quietly, which, for the average adult, approximates to 3.5 ml of oxygen uptake per kilogram body weight per minute, or approximately 1.2 kcal/min for a 70-kg individual. A 3-MET activity requires 3 times the metabolic energy expenditure of sitting quietly.

intensity, depending on the effort put into it. In addition, at different ages, the same activity may have different intensities. A moderate activity for a woman in her 30s might be vigorous for a woman in her 60s.

- *Type of physical activity.* Almost any activity that can be performed vigorously enough to raise the heart rate to reach the target level and keep it elevated can provide aerobic benefit. Physical activity is more likely to be maintained if it is an enjoyable activity for the individual, easy to access on a daily basis, easy to fit into the daily schedule, financially reasonable, and low in negative consequences (injury, negative peer pressure, etc.). Walking and gardening are two of the most popular physical activities among adults, and they should be encouraged to perform them regularly and vigorously enough to obtain moderate intensity exercise. Wearing a pedometer and ensuring that one takes at least 10,000 steps per day are ways of incorporating physical activity into the daily routine.

- *Resistance and flexibility training.* For a well-rounded exercise program, resistance and flexibility training should be performed at least 2 or 3 days per week. Resistance training consists of at least 8 to 12 repetitions (10 to 15 for elderly or very frail individuals) of 8 to 10 different exercises that condition the major muscle groups (e.g., weight training). Flexibility training stretches the major muscle groups. In the frail elderly, resistance and balance training should precede aerobic training to ensure that aerobic exercise can be done without increased risk of injury.

Oxidative Stresses

"Free radicals" are electrically charged particles formed as the natural by-product of normal cell processes. Exposure to various environmental factors, including tobacco smoke and radiation, can lead to increases in free radical formation. In humans the most common form of free radicals is oxygen. The oxygen radical causes damage to the DNA and other cellular molecules by binding to electrons on those molecules (thereby oxidizing the molecules). Over time, such damage may become irreversible and lead to disease, including cancer. **Carotenes** or **carotenoids** (vitamin A precursors) and vitamins E and C have **antioxidant** properties, meaning that they interact with free radicals to protect cell molecules. In addition, the mineral selenium is part of antioxidant enzymes. Several clinical trials have examined whether diets rich in antioxidant nutrients might decrease the risk of certain types of cancers. Although some trials have shown promising results, others have not. Beta-carotene, vitamin A, and vitamin E supplements may increase mortality from some cancers, while further study of selenium and vitamin C supplements is needed (Bjelakovic et al., 2007).

Another disorder related to oxidative damage is age-related macular degeneration. This problem, an irreversible cause of visual loss in middle-aged and elderly individuals, appears to be less common in people with higher circulating levels of carotenoids. Two carotenoids, lutein and zeaxanthin, are found in especially high concentrations in the macula of the retina, where they protect it from damaging blue light.

Intervention and education. Antioxidants are abundant in fruits and vegetables, as well as in some nuts and other food sources. No study has ever found fruit and vegetable intake to be harmful, and many epidemiologic studies have shown cancer and other disease rates to be lower in individuals with the highest fruit and vegetable intakes. Therefore there is good reason to recommend that all individuals consume more than five servings of fruits and vegetables daily. Emphasis should be on consuming a wide variety of fruits and vegetables, to increase the types of nutrients and antioxidants obtained. Specific antioxidants and good sources include the following:

- *Beta-carotene*: deep yellow vegetables and fruits such as carrots, pumpkin, and mango; deep green, leafy vegetables
- *Lycopene (a carotenoid)*: tomatoes, watermelon, guavas, pink grapefruit, apricots (Most of the lycopene in the American diet comes from tomatoes.)
- *Lutein and zeaxanthin*: deep green, leafy vegetables; corn and yellow cornmeal, broccoli, Brussels sprouts, green beans, green peas, summer squash (yellow or zucchini), persimmons
- *Selenium*: grains, meats, Brazil nuts
- *Vitamin C*: many fruits and vegetables, especially citrus fruits, strawberries, melons, broccoli, cauliflower, Brussels sprouts
- *Vitamin E*: oils; nuts, especially almonds; broccoli; cauliflower; spinach; mangoes
- *Anthrocyanins, polyphenols, and flavonoids (nonnutrient antioxidants, so these are **functional foods** in terms of their antioxidant role)*: blueberries, blackberries, cherries, cranberries, strawberries, raspberries, red cabbage, red sweet potatoes

Bone Density

Peak bone mass is achieved by approximately age 35 years in women and a few years later in men. It is especially important to have a diet rich in calcium and adequate in vitamin D to achieve the maximum possible bone density and reduce the risk of later fractures.

Intervention and education. A diet rich in calcium (at least 1000 mg daily) and adequate in vitamin D (at least 10 mcg daily for adults under age 70 years and 15 mcg for those over age 70 years) enhances bone mass. In addition, very thin adults usually have lower bone mass than those with greater BMI. Caucasian, Asian, Hispanic, and Native American women appear to be at higher risk of developing osteoporosis than African-American women (Pothiwala et al., 2006).

- Consume 3 servings of low-fat dairy products daily, in addition to leafy green vegetables and foods made with milk.
- Consume adequate amounts of magnesium daily, approximately 320 mg for women and 420 mg for men. Intake of magnesium from supplements should total no more than 350 mg daily, but this limit does not apply to food intake (Otten et al., 2006). Good sources of magnesium include deep green, leafy vegetables, nuts, seeds, whole grains, fish, and chocolate (approximately 75 to 100 mg per serving). Legumes (dry beans and peas) and potatoes provide about 60 to 75 mg per cup (240 ml).
- Participate in weight-bearing exercise, such as walking, running, or aerobic dance, daily.
- Avoid smoking, and drink alcohol moderately, if at all.
- If weight loss is needed, focus on lifestyle changes such as making healthy food choices and increasing activity, rather than overly restricting intake. Develop a realistic view of body weight and strive for a healthy weight, rather than an excessively low weight.

The Aging Adult

All the nutrition needs of younger adults, discussed earlier, also apply to the elderly. However, the physiologic and psychologic changes of aging create unique needs and concerns affecting nutritional status. Use of multiple medications, missing teeth or poorly fitting dentures, chronic illnesses, loss of muscle mass and physical function, role changes, and depression or other psychologic problems predispose older adults to nutrition problems (Feldblum et al., 2007; Labossiere and Bernard, 2008) (Table 5-2). Assessment of nutrition in the aging population is summarized in Box 5-2. Obtaining accurate values for height in the elderly can be problematic, because loss of vertebral mineralization and volume in intervertebral disks results in loss of height and because ill individuals may not be able to stand for measurement. Long bones, however, do not shorten with age. Knee height (length from sole of foot to anterior thigh with both ankle and knee bent at 90-degree angle) can be used to estimate height. A number of different investigators have developed equations to estimate total height from knee height for individuals from different ethnic and racial groups (e.g., Bunout et al., 2007; Chumlea et al., 1998; Van Lier et al., 2007).

Chronic and Acute Illnesses

Malnutrition is unfortunately a common finding among the elderly, and acute or chronic disease processes are often contributing factors. Disease processes may interfere with food intake or increase nutritional requirements, require modified diets that are unappealing to the individual, or require drug therapy that influences nutritional status (see Appendix G on Evolve). Coronary heart disease and type 2 (formerly referred to as non–insulin-dependent) diabetes are two nutrition-related chronic diseases that become increasingly prevalent with aging. Diet modifications used in treatment of these disorders are described in Chapters 14 and 17.

Declines in cognitive function are of great concern among seniors, and numerous investigations have been undertaken to determine whether nutrition intervention can improve cognitive ability or delay declines in functioning. Thus far, no specific nutrients, including vitamin E and other antioxidants, have proven effective in averting or delaying dementia (Gray et al., 2008).

Intervention and education
Guidelines for choosing a healthful diet. The elderly can be encouraged to choose a variety of foods from all food groups daily, including grains (especially whole grains); fruits and vegetables; lean meats, poultry, and fish or meat substitutes; and low-fat dairy products. Food is the preferred source of nutrients in the elderly, just as

Text continued on p. 167.

Table 5-2 Nutritional Implications of Changes Related to Aging

Change	Nutritional Implications
Physiologic Changes and Impairments of Physical Function	
Decreased muscle mass (sarcopenia) and increased percentage of body fat	Decline in basal metabolic rate of about 2% per decade after age 30 yr; daily energy need declines; potential for weight gain and obesity
Decreased skin capacity for cholecalciferol (vitamin D) synthesis; decreased renal activation of cholecalciferol; decreased responsiveness of the gut to stimulation of vitamin D	Impaired absorption of calcium, contributing to osteoporosis
Diminished sense of taste and smell	Disinterest in food; anorexia; some individuals salt or sugar their food heavily to compensate for loss of taste; may eat spoiled food
Poor vision, especially in dim light	Difficulty preparing food
Impaired dentition	Difficulty eating; food choices limited (raw or crisp fruits and vegetables and high-fiber grains often avoided; softer, low-fiber foods, which are frequently higher in energy, are substituted); can contribute to constipation, weight loss, or weight gain

Continued

Table 5-2   Nutritional Implications of Changes Related to Aging—cont'd

Change	Nutritional Implications
Physiologic Changes and Impairments of Physical Function—cont'd	
Decreased secretion of hydrochloric acid (needed for absorption of vitamin B_{12}), pepsin (protein digestive enzyme), and bile (needed for fat absorption)	Potential for impaired absorption of calcium, iron, zinc, protein, fat, fat-soluble vitamins, vitamin B_{12}
Arthritis and impaired mobility	Difficulty opening food packages and preparing food
Psychosocial Changes	
Fixed income	Potential for difficulty affording food or being unwilling to spend money on food, particularly foods perceived as expensive, e.g., milk, meats, fruits, vegetables, which are important sources of calcium, riboflavin, protein, iron, zinc, vitamins C and A, and fiber
Lack of socialization; loneliness	Apathy about meals; poor intake; potential for alcohol abuse
Vulnerability to advertising and food fads related to alleviation of the effects and discomforts of aging	Wasting of limited income on diet or health aids with dubious value; potential for toxic intakes of nutrients, particularly vitamins A and D
Confusion, memory loss	Potential for forgetting to eat or forgetting what has been eaten (and therefore consuming an unbalanced diet)

Box 5-2   Assessment in Aging

Underweight and Undernutrition

History

Loss of 4.5 kg (10 lb) or more in the last 6 months; fixed income; inadequate money for food; usually eats alone; loss of spouse or friends; difficulty chewing or swallowing; pain in mouth, teeth, or gums; poor appetite; follows a modified diet; regular use of medications, particularly those that impair appetite, e.g., digoxin, especially if three or more drugs are used; presence of chronic disease; avoidance of or inadequate intake from one or more food groups or eats inadequate servings; consumption of more than 1 alcoholic drink per day (woman) or more than 2 drinks per day (man); difficulty getting to market or transporting purchases home; lack of food preparation skills; lack of facilities for food storage or preparation; difficulty feeding self

Physical Examination

BMI <18.5; low level of body fat, TSF <5th percentile; muscle wasting; edema; glossitis, angular stomatitis

Laboratory Analysis

↓ Serum albumin, transferrin, prealbumin

Overweight/Obesity

History

Gain of 4.5 kg (10 lb) or more in the last 6 months; excessive intakes, especially of fat, snack items, and sweets; increase in intake of energy-dense refined foods because of difficulty chewing high-fiber foods; little physical activity; loss of muscle mass with resulting decrease in energy expenditure

Physical Examination

BMI >25; TSF >95th percentile

Continued

Box 5-2   Assessment in Aging—cont'd

Potential for Fluid Deficit

History

Altered mental status (confusion or coma) with inability to feel or express thirst; decreased thirst sensation with aging; vomiting, diarrhea, febrile illness, or extremely hot weather

Physical Examination

Poor skin turgor; dry sticky mucous membranes; rapid weight loss over 1 to 2 weeks; oliguria; lethargy, hypotension

Laboratory Analysis

↑ Hct, BUN, serum sodium

Inadequate Calcium and Vitamin D Intake

History

Avoids milk because of lactose intolerance, difficulty carrying milk home from the market, knowledge deficit about needs for calcium and vitamin D; little sun exposure because of chronic illness or residing in a nursing home or other institution; vertebral or hip fractures

Laboratory Analysis

↓ Bone density

Impaired Vitamin B$_{12}$ Status

History

Achlorhydria (inadequate hydrochloric acid production); meats and milk avoided because of difficulty chewing and/or swallowing, lactose intolerance, or cost; no supplement usage

Physical Examination

Pallor, weakness, paresthesias (abnormal sensations in feet or legs), difficulty walking, loss of bowel/bladder control

Laboratory Analysis

↓ Hct, ↑ MCV, ↓ plasma vitamin B$_{12}$

Box 5-2   Assessment in Aging—cont'd

Inadequate Zinc Intake

History

Little animal protein or whole-grain intake because of low income or difficulty chewing and/or swallowing; no supplement usage

Physical Examination

Poor sense of taste, distorted taste; dermatitis; poor wound healing; alopecia

Laboratory Analysis

↓ Serum zinc

BMI, Body mass index; *BUN,* blood urea nitrogen; *Hct,* hematocrit; *MCV,* mean corpuscular volume; *TSF,* triceps skinfold.

---

it is in other age-groups. Unlike supplements, food provides a variety of **phytochemicals** and functional components that may have beneficial effects. For example, genistein, a nonnutrient component of soy, apparently reduces the risk of heart disease; soy also provides phytoestrogens (estrogen-like compounds in plants) that are reported to reduce the risk of certain cancers and to provide some relief from menopausal symptoms.

The elderly are, like other age-groups, susceptible to food fads and **nutrition quackery**. They may rely on these beliefs to treat chronic illnesses or other health problems. The elderly need instruction in ways of recognizing quackery. Some characteristics of quackery are heavy reliance on anecdotal and testimonial evidence, rather than clinical trials; insistence that certain foods or supplements can cure disease; and distrust of the food supply as a means of meeting nutritional needs. The National Institute on Aging (NIA) provides information on quackery and a list of reliable health information resources on-line at http://www.niapublications.org/ engagepages/ healthqy.asp. Print copies of the publication are available free from the NIA website or by mail (see Appendix H on Evolve).

A daily multivitamin-multimineral supplement may be beneficial in ensuring adequate intakes. Nutritional supplements for the elderly should not be high in iron because hemochromatosis, an iron storage disorder, is relatively common in North America (Allen KJ et al., 2008). Affected people have progressive increases in their iron stores as they age. In addition, healthy elderly individuals do not have large losses of iron and thus need little from supplements.

Congregate feeding sites for the elderly offer nutritious meals and the social stimulation of gathering to eat with others. The Meals on Wheels program provides balanced meals to the elderly who are home bound.

Hydration. Dehydration or fluid volume deficit is especially likely to occur in the ill elderly person because body water is reduced with aging, from about 55% of body weight in young adults to about 45% in people over 60 years. Therefore any given volume of body fluids represents a greater percentage of body water in the elderly person than it does in the younger adult. Diarrhea, vomiting, or a febrile illness often produces dehydration in the older adult. The sensation of thirst may be diminished in old age, and immobility and confusion may hinder the elderly in getting fluids to drink, further contributing to the risk of dehydration. Some older adults have a narrow margin of safety in their state of hydration because renal or cardiac impairments make them vulnerable to fluid overload. Caregivers should adhere to the following guidelines to prevent dehydration in the elderly patient:

- Assess state of hydration regularly.
- Evaluate fluid intake of the patient receiving tube feedings or total parenteral nutrition. More fluid may be needed than is included in the nutrient solutions. Extra fluid can be administered orally, as an irrigant for the feeding tube, or intravenously.
- Encourage intake of a minimum of 1500 ml fluid, or about 30 ml/kg, per day unless a fluid restriction is needed. If the individual has difficulty remembering how much fluid has been consumed, it may help to fill a pitcher with the needed amount at the beginning of the day, place it in an accessible location, and instruct the person to drink it all by the end of the day.

Coping with altered gastrointestinal function. To reduce the likelihood of constipation, hemorrhoids, and diverticulosis, these guidelines should be followed:

- Encourage intake of at least 25 to 30 g of fiber daily (see Appendix C). Cooked whole grains (oatmeal, brown rice, bulgur, etc.); legumes; and cooked, canned, or very ripe raw fruits and vegetables are good choices if there is difficulty chewing. A fiber supplement (Table 5-3) can be used if dietary intake is inadequate. Fiber should be increased gradually to reduce discomfort, such as excessive flatulence.

■ Increase physical activity as tolerated because this stimulates gastrointestinal motility.

■ Encourage consumption of dried plums (prunes) and prune juice regularly if they are acceptable to the individual, since these products contain a natural laxative. Avoid regular use of laxative medications, on which the individual may become dependent.

■ Encourage an adequate fluid intake.

If achlorhydria, or lack of hydrochloric acid secretion, is present, then the individual may need a vitamin B_{12} supplement because B_{12} absorption is impaired by the lack of gastric acid.

Preserving bone density. For the person at high risk for osteoporosis (e.g., women who undergo early oophorectomy) or already showing signs of osteoporosis, certain medications reduce bone loss. Oral hormone replacement therapy in postmenopausal women is effective in reducing the risk of fractures from osteoporosis, but its long-term side effects include a possible increase in the risk of heart disease and breast and ovarian cancer. Bisphosphonates such as alendronate and risedronate reduce bone resorption and increase bone mass without affecting the rates of heart disease or cancer. Bisphosphonates should not be taken with food or at the same time as a calcium supplement because of potential for impaired absorption of the drug. Selective estrogen receptor modulators (SERMs), such as raloxifene and tamoxifen, appear to reduce the risk of bone loss and vertebral fractures. Calcitonin, which slows bone loss, is approved for treatment of osteoporosis in women who are at least 5 years postmenopausal, but its long-term effects on the risk of fractures are not established. Individuals taking all these antiosteoporosis medications should be instructed to be especially careful to consume adequate vitamin D and calcium.

■ Consume at least 1000 mg of calcium daily (see Figure 3-1).

   ■ Milk and milk products are among the richest sources of calcium, with approximately 300 mg per cup (240 ml). Yogurt and many cheeses (e.g., Swiss, provolone, mozzarella, ricotta)

Table 5-3   Fiber Supplements

Fiber Source	Examples of Products	Adult Recommended Daily Dose	Fiber Content Total	Fiber Content Soluble
Guar gum	Benefiber	2 tsp (3.5 g) up to 3 times daily	3 g/2 tsp	3 g/2 tsp
Psyllium	Metamucil	2-6 capsules up to 3 times daily	0.5 g/capsule	0.3 g/capsule
		2 wafers up to 3 times daily	3 g/wafer	1.5 g/wafer
		1 tbsp up to 3 times daily	3 g/tbsp	2 g/tbsp
	Konsyl Natural Fiber	1 tsp (6 g) up to 3 times daily	5 g/tsp	3 g/tsp
Methylcellulose	Citrucel	1 tbsp (11.5 g) up to 3 times daily	2 g/tbsp	2 g/tbsp
Inulin	Fiber Choice	Up to 12 caplets daily	0.5 g/caplet	0.5 g/caplet
Polycarbophil	FiberCon	2 tablets daily	2 g/tablet	2 g/tablet
	Konsyl Fiber Caplets	2 caplets daily	500 mg/caplet	*
	Equalactin	2 caplets up to 4 times daily	500 mg/caplet	*
		2 caplets up to 4 times daily	500 mg/caplet	*
Mixed fibers†	Ultra-Fiber Plus	1 scoop (10 g) up to 4 times daily	8 g/scoop	3 g/scoop

tbsp, Tablespoon (15 ml); *tsp*, teaspoon (5 ml).

Soluble fiber aids in reduction of cholesterol levels, whereas insoluble fiber is more important in gastrointestinal function.

*Synthetic compound that expands in water to provide bulk but is not fermented by gut bacteria as naturally occurring soluble fibers are.

†Guar gum, oat fiber, polydextrose, purified cellulose, inulin, cellulose gel, fenugreek fiber, rice bran, pectin, fiber, barley beta glucan.

are good calcium sources, but cottage cheese and cream cheese are not calcium rich.

- If lactose intolerance is present, cheese, acidophilus milk, yogurt, or buttermilk can be substituted for milk because these products are lower in lactose than regular milk. Also, lactase enzyme–treated milk is available in most supermarkets, or oral lactase supplements are available to take with milk.
- Use a calcium supplement (e.g., calcium citrate or carbonate) if dietary calcium intake cannot be maintained at the recommended level. Box 5-3 provides guidelines for improving absorption of calcium from the diet or supplements.
- Vitamin D is needed for the absorption of calcium. The recommended intake of vitamin D is higher for the elderly than for any other groups of individuals (10 mcg/day through 70 years, and 15 mcg/day after age 70 years). If vitamin D–fortified milk or another reliable dietary source (see Appendix B) is not consumed daily, the individual may need a supplement.
- Regular weight-bearing physical activity, at least several times weekly, helps to preserve bone.

Box 5-3   Improving Calcium Absorption

- Obtain adequate vitamin D. Vitamin D–fortified milk and breakfast cereals are good sources.
  - Vitamin D is activated in the kidney. Individuals with chronic renal failure may require a supplement of calcitriol, the active form of vitamin D.
- Avoid excessive intake of phosphorus, which competes with calcium for absorption. Limit meat intake to 5 or 6 oz (150 to 180 g) daily and carbonated drinks to no more than 8 to 12 oz daily.
- Increase calcium intake if diet is high in oxalate (e.g., spinach and other deep green vegetables), phytates (e.g., bran and whole grains), or fiber, all of which inhibit calcium absorption.
- Increase calcium intake if using corticosteroid or anticonvulsant medications, which decrease calcium absorption.
- If achlorhydria (lack of hydrochloric acid production) is present and a calcium carbonate supplement is used, take the supplement with meals.

- Vitamin K may be necessary for optimal bone health. Osteoporosis is more common among adults with lower levels of vitamin K, although it is not yet known whether low vitamin K is a cause of osteoporosis (Cashman, 2007). Good sources of vitamin K include deep green leafy vegetables such as spinach and kale, broccoli, leaf lettuce, and oils such as soybean and canola. It may be that higher blood levels of vitamin K are simply a marker of adequate vegetable intake. Supplementation of elderly individuals with vitamin K for 3 years did not reduce bone loss (Booth et al., 2008).

Achieving and Maintaining Desirable Weight

Impaired physical function is more common among overweight and underweight elderly people than among their normal-weight peers. Overweight can impair mobility and contribute to a number of chronic diseases, such as heart disease and diabetes, whereas underweight is associated with debility and can predispose the individual to infectious illnesses.

Overweight

Teaching elderly patients to control their weight can include the following:

- Explain the need for controlling energy intake and/or increasing physical activity level to prevent progressive weight gain as the metabolic rate declines (see Table 5-2). Gradual weight loss or maintenance of body weight is usually possible with intakes of approximately 1200 to 1500 kcal per day for women and 1500 to 1800 kcal per day for men.
- Assist the individual in identifying foods—such as fruits, vegetables, whole grains, and low-fat dairy products—that are relatively low in energy but that make important nutritional contributions; help the individual to create meal plans that use these foods.
- Encourage the elderly person to limit the consumption of foods of low nutrient density (sweets, snack foods) and high-fat items. Fresh, frozen, or juice-pack canned fruits can be used for desserts and snacks. Steaming, microwaving, or baking foods with little or no added fat is preferable to frying.
- Encourage the elderly person to accumulate at least 30 minutes of moderate-intensity exercise at least 5 days per week. The elderly need to be especially careful to warm up before

exercise bouts by stretching and performing light exercise and to decrease the intensity of their exercise gradually at the end of the session, allowing at least a 5- to 10-minute period to cool off. Walking, gardening, and water aerobics are examples of moderate-intensity physical activities that can be useful in weight control. Group activities not only motivate some individuals to maintain an exercise program but also enhance social interactions. Stretching exercises should be performed every day, and strength training should be done at least 2 days per week to increase and maintain muscle mass (CDC, 2008a).

Underweight

Individuals with health or dentition problems or loss of the senses of smell and taste are especially likely to be underweight and malnourished. The health history should include questions about recent unintentional weight loss. Significant weight loss can be defined as loss of 5% of body weight in 1 month, 7.5% in 3 months, or 10% in 6 months. If the cause of poor intake can be determined, it is possible to tailor interventions and teaching to the needs of the individual. Use the following suggestions:

- Try small, frequent feedings rather than three large meals per day if anorexia or severe weakness is present.
- Be aware of potential side effects and interactions of drugs taken regularly (see Appendix G on Evolve). If medication usage appears to be decreasing the appetite, then the health care provider may be able to substitute another drug or reduce the dosage. Toxicity often develops in the older adult at lower dosages than in younger adults, and use of multiple drugs increases the risks of adverse effects. Weight loss may also increase a medication's potency and make a decrease in dosage necessary.
- Assess the individual for the presence of constipation, which may cause anorexia.
- Special diets (low-cholesterol, low-sodium, etc.) may seem tasteless to the individual. Consider liberalizing diet restrictions if intake is poor because the therapeutic diet is unappealing (Niedert, 2005).
- If intake is poor because of declining senses of taste and smell, experiment with low-sodium seasonings, such as herbs, spices,

salt-free seasoning mixes, and lemon juice, to enhance the flavors of foods. Present food in an attractive manner: appealing color combinations, a variety of textures if tolerated by the individual, and not overcooked so that it loses its color or texture.

■ Refer the person to social services for assistance in obtaining food stamps if financial constraints are interfering with obtaining an adequate diet, or encourage participation in the National Nutrition Program for the Elderly, which provides meals at group feeding sites.

■ Encourage the individual to eat with others whenever possible. Group feeding sites (e.g., daily lunches served at senior citizen centers), church functions, or other social activities offer opportunities for socialization. Eating in a social setting can improve appetite.

■ Assess the individual for dental problems, periodontal disease, and/or dysphagia to determine whether this might account for poor intake, and arrange for the individual to obtain proper dental care, including well-fitted dentures, if needed.

■ Involve elderly individuals in the planning of menus for extended care facilities or group feeding sites. Attempt to accommodate the culture(s) and preferences of the participants as much as possible.

■ Light the dining area well so that food can be clearly seen.

■ Provide assistance in eating if necessary. This may range from opening packages of condiments to feeding the person. Plates with high outer rims make it easier for the elderly with physical handicaps to scoop up food. Patience and sensitivity when feeding the individual help preserve dignity and improve intake.

■ Instruct the individual in food purchasing and simple food preparation techniques, if appropriate. Elderly men who have never cooked until late in life are especially vulnerable to nutritional deficits when living alone. The county extension home economist is a good resource for food purchasing and preparation materials, and good educational materials can also be found at the following websites: www.agingwell.state.ny.us/index.htm, http://ohioline.osu.edu/lines/food.html, www.ext.colostate.edu/pubs/columnha/hamenu.html, and http://healthletter.tufts.edu/.

■ If mobility is a problem, then help the person arrange transportation to the market or to feeding sites for the elderly (contact the local agency on aging or a local church or synagogue) or arrange for Meals on Wheels.

Dysphagia

Difficulty swallowing in the older adult may significantly interfere with food and beverage intake. Measures to reduce feeding problems with dysphagia include the following:

- Soft, moist foods, such as mashed potatoes, meat loaf, and omelets, are likely to be easiest to swallow. Foods may need to be chopped, minced, or pureed. Generally, foods are more appealing when they are as close to their normal shape and appearance as possible; therefore, pureed foods should be reserved for those individuals who have difficulty chewing and swallowing chopped or minced foods.
- Thin fluids, such as water and broth, may be difficult to swallow. Commercial thickened fluids (water, juices, milk, tea, etc.) are available, or fluids may be thickened to the desired consistency with the addition of yogurt, mashed potato flakes, or infant cereals.
- A speech pathologist may be able to help the person learn new strategies for swallowing.
- If dysphagia is very severe, enteral tube feeding may be necessary.

Decubitus or Pressure Ulcers

Pressure ulcers are particularly common among relatively immobile individuals and those who are incontinent of urine or stool. Nutrition intervention was effective in reducing the likelihood of pressure ulcers in a large, randomized study in critically ill elderly patients (Reddy et al., 2006). The intervention in that study consisted of a balanced liquid supplement (30% protein, 20% fat, and 50% carbohydrate, in addition to vitamins and minerals) providing 400 kcal daily. Thus it is not possible to determine exactly which nutrients were responsible for the effects.

Conclusion

Nutritional status is an important concern throughout adulthood, since it has important implications for preventing or delaying the onset of chronic illnesses in adults of all ages. Moreover, optimal nutrition has the potential to improve the quality of life and facilitate palliative care in the ill or frail elderly.

REFERENCES

Alberti KG et al: Metabolic syndrome—a new worldwide definition. A consensus statement from the international diabetes federation, *Diabet Med* 23:469, 2006.

Allen KJ et al: Iron-overload-related disease in HFE hereditary hemochromatosis, *N Engl J Med* 358(3):221, 2008.

Bjelakovic G et al: Mortality in randomized trials of antioxidant supplements for primary and secondary prevention: systematic review and meta-analysis, *JAMA* 297(8):842, 2007.

Booth SL et al: Effect of vitamin K supplementation on bone loss in elderly men and women, *J Clin Endocrinol Metab* 93(5):2592, 2008.

Bunout D et al: Height reduction, determined using knee height measurement as a risk factor or predictive sign for osteoporosis in elderly women, *Nutrition* 23(11-12):794, 2007.

Cashman KD: Diet, nutrition, and bone health, *J Nutr* 137(suppl 11): 2507S, 2007.

Centers for Disease Control and Prevention (CDC): Prevalence of Regular Physical Activity Among Adults — United States, 2001 and 2005, *MMWR Morb Mortal Wkly Rep* 56(46):1209, 2007.

Centers for Disease Control and Prevention (CDC): Physical activity for everyone. Available at http://www.cdc.gov/nccdphp/dnpa/physical/everyone.htm. Accessed March 8, 2008a.

Centers for Disease Control and Prevention (CDC): Body mass index. Available at http://www.cdc.gov/nccdphp/dnpa/bmi/index.htm. Accessed March 7, 2008b.

Chumlea WC et al: Stature prediction equations for elderly non-Hispanic white, non-Hispanic black, and Mexican-American persons developed from NHANES III data, *J Am Dietet Assoc* 98(2):137, 1998.

Feldblum I et al: Characteristics of undernourished older medical patients and the identification of predictors for undernutrition status, *Nutr J* 6:37, 2007.

Gray SL et al: Antioxidant vitamin supplement use and risk of dementia or Alzheimer's disease in older adults, *J Am Geriatr Soc* 56(2):291, 2008.

Grundy SM et al: Diagnosis and management of the metabolic syndrome: an American heart association/national heart, lung, and blood institute scientific statement: executive summary, *Circulation* 112(17):e285, 2005.

Kruger J et al: Prevalence of fruit and vegetable consumption and physical activity by race/ethnicity—United States, 2005, *MMWR Morb Mortal Wkly Rep* 56(13):301, 2007.

Labossiere R, Bernard MA: Nutritional considerations in institutionalized elders, *Curr Opin Clin Nutr Metab Care* 11(1):1, 2008.

Lichtenstein AH et al: Diet and lifestyle recommendations revision 2006. A scientific statement from the American Heart Association Nutrition Committee, *Circulation* 114(1):82, 2006.

National Center for Health Statistics: Prevalence of overweight and obesity among adults: United States, 2003-2004. Available at http://www.cdc.gov/nchs/products/pubs/pubd/hestats/overweight/overwght_adult_03.htm. Accessed March 6, 2008.

Niedert KC: Position of the American Dietetic Association: liberalization of the diet prescription improves quality of life for older adults in long-term care, *J Am Diet Assoc* 105(12):1955, 2005.

Otten JJ, Hellwig JP, Meyers LD, editors: *Dietary Reference Intakes: the essential guide to nutrient requirements*, Washington, DC, 2006, National Academies Press.

Pothiwala P et al: Ethnic variation in risk for osteoporosis among women: a review of biological and behavioral factors, *J Womens Health (Larchmt)* 15(6):709, 2006.

Reddy M, Gill SS, Rochon PA: Preventing pressure ulcers: a systematic review, *JAMA* 296(8):974, 2006.

Timlin MT, Pereira MA: Breakfast frequency and quality in the etiology of adult obesity and chronic diseases, *Nutr Rev* 65(6 pt 1):268, 2007.

Tjepkema M: Adult obesity, *Health Rep* 17(3):9, 2006.

U.S. Department of Health and Human Services (USDHHS) and U.S. Department of Agriculture (USDA): *Dietary guidelines for Americans, 2005*, ed 6, Washington, DC, 2005, U.S. Government Printing Office.

Van Lier AM, Roy MA, Payette H: Knee height to predict stature in North American Caucasian frail free-living elderly receiving community services, *J Nutr Health Aging* 11(4):372, 2007.

World Cancer Research Fund, American Institute for Cancer Research (AICR): *Food, nutrition, physical activity, and the prevention of cancer: a global perspective*, Washington, DC, 2007, AICR.

CHAPTER 6

ATHLETIC PERFORMANCE

Most health care generalists encounter few elite athletes, but a number of individuals who are only recreational athletes participate in "extreme" sports and intense physical training. These individuals want and need accurate, reliable nutritional guidance to achieve their best level of performance and maintain optimal health. This chapter summarizes some of the important findings regarding nutrition for the adult athlete participating in regular, vigorous athletic training. A thorough nutrition assessment should be performed as described in Chapter 2. Box 6-1 highlights common or especially serious findings in athletes.

Nutrient Needs and Concerns During Training Energy

Energy needs vary because of the intensity, duration, and frequency of exercise, as well as the effects of age, heredity, lean body mass, body size, and gender. Increased energy needs resulting from exercise can be met through a diet of regular foods. Fat is an important source of energy, and there is no evidence to recommend either an extremely low-fat or a high-fat diet for athletes. Carbohydrates maintain blood glucose concentrations during exercise and replace muscle glycogen; the amount needed depends on factors such as the total energy needs and the type of sport performed. Males usually achieve an adequate intake of carbohydrate to maintain glycogen stores easily, but it may be more difficult for female athletes restricting their energy intakes because of concern about controlling their body fat. Excessive limitation of energy intake contributes to the immunosuppression that is prevalent among elite athletes.

Box 6-1   Assessment in Athletic Performance

Inadequate Energy Intake

History

Frequent or chronic dieting to achieve and maintain low "competitive" weight; extremely strenuous exercise habits (e.g., distance running); exercise-induced anorexia; eating disorder

Physical Examination

↓ Body fat, athletic performance; TSF <5th percentile; BMI <18.5 (for children or adolescents, BMI <5th percentile for age); amenorrhea; delayed growth and development (children and adolescents)

Inadequate Protein Intake

History

Frequent dieting, energy intake so low that protein consumed is utilized for energy; physiologic state requiring ↑ protein: childhood, adolescence, pregnancy, lactation

Physical Examination

Delayed growth and development (children and adolescents); thinning of hair, changes in hair texture

Inadequate Iron Intake

History

Frequent dieting to achieve competitive weight; vegetarian diet that may be marginal in iron; GI blood loss, especially in distance runners

Physical Examination

Pallor; ↓ athletic performance

Laboratory Analysis

↓ Hct, Hgb, MCV, serum Fe, serum ferritin

Continued

Box 6-1   Assessment in Athletic Performance—cont'd

Fluid Volume Deficit

History

Failure to replace fluid losses by drinking during and after athletic endeavors; fluid restriction in an attempt to achieve competitive weight; use of diuretics to achieve competitive weight or produce dilute urine in an effort to confound drug testing

Physical Examination

Weight loss ≥ 2% of baseline body weight; dry, sticky mucous membranes; poor skin turgor; thirst; disorientation; weakness; hypotension

Laboratory Analysis

↑ Serum sodium, Hct, BUN, serum osmolality

BMI, Body mass index; *BUN*, blood urea nitrogen; *GI*, gastrointestinal; *Hct*, hematocrit; *Hgb*, hemoglobin; *MCV*, mean corpuscular volume; *TSF*, triceps skinfold.

Intervention and education. Points to emphasize in teaching have been described in a joint report of the American College of Sports Medicine (ACSM), American Dietetic Association (ADA), and Dietitians of Canada (DC) (2000):

- Energy intake should be adequate to prevent underweight, maximize the training effects, and maintain health. Inadequate energy intakes can reduce muscle mass, result in menstrual dysfunction, contribute to poor bone density, and increase the risk of injury. The athlete's age, gender, heredity, and sport help to determine the optimal amount of body fat, and if fat loss is necessary, it should be carried out before the competitive season. The American Academy of Pediatrics (AAP) Committee on Sports Medicine and Fitness (2005) emphasizes that it is especially important that young athletes not restrict their energy intakes excessively. Male high school athletes should have at least 7% body fat, and adolescent females should have enough body fat to maintain normal menses.
- Carbohydrate intakes of approximately 5 to 7 g/kg body weight per day, with an increase to 7 to 10 g/kg/day for strenuously

exercising endurance athletes, are associated with optimal glycogen stores.

- A moderate- to low-fat diet (20% to 25% of energy from fat) is recommended, but very–low-fat diets (<15% fat) have no advantage.
- If weight loss is needed or desirable to improve athletic performance, plan to accomplish it gradually (no more than 1 to 2 lb/wk [0.5 to 1 kg/wk]), rather than on a crash diet. Reducing intake by 10% to 20% of normal will result in a steady weight loss. Stress healthy eating choices rather than excessive restriction of intake. A registered dietitian with training in sports nutrition can provide valuable guidance.

Protein

It is commonly believed that markedly increased amounts of certain nutrients, particularly protein, are needed to build muscle mass; however, the increase in needs is actually relatively modest. The protein Dietary Reference Intake (DRI) for normal adults is 0.8 g/kg body weight per day, and the needs of most athletes are no more than 50% to 100% greater than this. Amounts close to this can be obtained in the average North American diet, which provides 80 to 110 g protein per day.

Intervention and education. Modest increases in protein intake over the DRI are sufficient for most athletes:

- Endurance athletes (e.g., those involved in activities involving speed and/or distance, such as skaters, runners, and cyclists) need approximately 1.2 to 1.4 g/kg/day, a total of about 98 g for the man who weighs 75 kg (165 lb).
- Athletes performing resistance and strength training (e.g., weight lifters and body builders) need approximately 1.6 to 1.7 g/kg/day.
- Athletes who are vegetarians may need about 10% more protein than nonvegetarians to compensate for less complete digestion of proteins from plant sources (ACSM, ADA, DC, 2000).

Vitamins and Minerals

No evidence exists that markedly increasing vitamin and mineral intake over the DRIs improves athletic performance. B-complex vitamin needs increase during vigorous activity, but they will be met by the increased energy intake needed during heavy exercise. It has been suggested that vigorous exercise increases needs for antioxidant nutrients (e.g., vitamins C and E, carotenes, selenium), but no conclusive evidence supports this.

Vitamin D is important for adequate calcium metabolism and thus for optimal bone mass; and vitamin D levels can be low in athletes from far southern or northern latitudes, where direct sun exposure is reduced, and those who train indoors most of the year. Inadequate intakes of calcium are common, especially among female athletes. Athletic training has the potential to increase bone mineral density (BMD), and this might reduce the risk of osteoporosis in later life. However, the effect on BMD appears to be specific to the type of activity, with sports such as volleyball and squash increasing BMD more than sports such as swimming and weight lifting (Nichols et al., 2007). Amenorrheic female athletes (see "The Female Athlete Triad" on p. 184) are at risk of developing low BMD and need adequate energy and nutrient intake to restore menses.

Vigorous exercise increases iron needs, and iron deficiency is prevalent, especially among female athletes. Possible reasons include increased losses of iron in perspiration during prolonged physical activity, damage to red blood cells in the capillaries of the soles of the feet during running ("foot strike hemolysis") (Schumacher et al., 2002), and increased oxidative damage to the red blood cells. It is also possible that hemolysis is a physiologic process that supplies iron to the muscle to allow increased synthesis of myoglobin (Robinson et al., 2006). Iron deficiency impairs physical performance by interfering with oxygen delivery and allowing lactate accumulation in muscle, which makes the muscle fatigue more quickly (Hinton and Sinclair, 2007).

Intervention and education

- *Vitamin D*: If intake of fortified dairy products is low and the athlete has little regular sun exposure, a supplement providing 5 mcg/day may be needed.
- *Calcium*: If consumption of dairy products and other calcium sources (see Figure 3-1) is poor, a supplement providing 800 to 1200 mg/day will provide the needed calcium.
- *Iron*: Individuals participating regularly in vigorous physical exercise should be instructed in a diet that includes good sources of iron (legumes, meats, whole and enriched grains;

see Appendix B on Evolve), as well as vitamin C, which promotes iron absorption. Female athletes, vegetarians, and distance runners, particularly, may have difficulty maintaining adequate iron nutriture and may need a supplement (Venderley and Campbell, 2006). Absorption of iron from a supplement will be best if it is taken between meals or at bedtime and with fluids other than coffee, tea, or milk.

Performance-Enhancing Supplements

The marketing and use of nutrition-related supplements purported to improve exercise performance are very widespread. Governmental control over the claims made for these supplements is minimal, and thus the athlete, coaches, and trainers must be helped to evaluate these claims. Two commonly used supplements are creatine and chromium.

Creatine phosphate is an important energy source for exercising muscle. Theoretically, increasing the muscle creatine levels should prolong the athlete's ability to perform high-intensity exercise. Some studies suggest that creatine supplements improve performance on short-term, high-intensity tasks such as sprints on stationary bicycles, squash, and elite soccer play. Creatine monophosphate, a form commonly used as a supplement, is associated with a small weight gain (approximately 1 to 2 kg in short-term studies) and fluid retention. Although there are concerns that creatine supplementation might contribute to kidney dysfunction, the risk has not yet been determined (Calfee and Fadale, 2006).

Chromium is an essential trace mineral that is believed by many individuals to increase lean muscle mass and promote fat loss. The research done so far has not supported these beliefs. In one investigation it appeared that chromium picolinate, a common form of chromium supplement, might actually predispose athletes to iron deficits (Lawrence and Kirby, 2002).

Intervention and education. Nutritional aids should be used with caution, and only after careful evaluation. Thorough recommendations for evaluating supplement claims have been published (ACSM, ADA, DC, 2000). In brief, consider the following points:

- *Scientific evidence*: Has the supplement undergone rigorous scientific testing? If so, were the results published in a peer-reviewed journal? Did the research use appropriate control groups, including a double-blind placebo group if possible? Are the studies adequately described? Are the results clear, analyzed with appropriate statistics, and presented in an objective manner? Do they answer the questions of whether the supplement is effective? Do they include the incidence of adverse events among the treatment groups?

- *Claims related to the particular product*: Does the supplement make sense for the sport for which the claim is made; for example, does the advertising imply that the supplement will improve triathlon performance when the product has only shown benefit in short sprints? Is the amount of active ingredient in the supplement comparable with that used in research studies involving this particular ergogenic aid? Do the claims about the product made by the manufacturer or distributor match the scientific evidence?
- *Safety*: Is the product safe over the short and long term? Is it contraindicated for certain groups of people, such as older adults, women who may become pregnant, and those with certain health problems?
- *Legality*: Is the product banned by athletic organizations governing the sport?

The Female Athlete Triad

Physically active females, especially those in sports or dance activities where low body weight is desirable, are at risk for a syndrome known as the *female athlete triad*. The triad describes the relationships among energy availability (intake minus expenditure in exercise), menstrual function, and BMD. The triad exists along a continuum from the desirable state (adequate energy availability, eumenorrhea, and optimal bone health) to seriously pathologic findings (low energy availability with or without an eating disorder, amenorrhea, and osteoporosis [inadequate bone strength with increased risk of fractures]) (ACSM Position Stand, 2007). This problem can occur in both adolescents and adult women. Body building, gymnastics, cycling, triathlon, and running events are some of the sports in which female participants are especially likely to have low body fat.

Intervention and education. Coaches, trainers, and all other individuals working with female athletes need to be aware of the prevalence and signs of the female athlete triad. The triad can impair athletic performance and increase morbidity and mortality among athletes, and these facts can be used to help motivate the athlete and coaching staff to avoid unhealthy weight control practices, such as excessive restriction of intake, as well as purging or use of diuretics or laxatives to maintain a low body weight. The focus should be on healthy food choices rather than body weight. Guidelines for recognizing and treating eating disorders are described in Chapter 19.

Nutrition for Athletic Events
Fluid and Electrolyte Replacement

Adequate replacement of fluid losses during exercise not only improves physical performance but also helps to maintain the health and safety of the exercising individuals. Losses from perspiration are primarily water but also include sodium ($\approx$ 35 mEq/L), potassium, and other minerals. The amount of perspiration loss is affected by intensity of the exercise, temperature and humidity of the environment, and body size, but it can be as great as 1.8 L/hr. Estimated sweat losses for different activities are available in Sawka et al. (2007). Fluids should never be restricted.

Intervention and education. The key nutrition need during exercise is adequate fluid replacement. To maintain hydration, the American College of Sports Medicine (Sawka et al., 2007) states that athletes should do the following:

- *Before exercise*: Drink generous amounts in the 24-hour period before exercise. If the person is normally hydrated and has not exercised vigorously in the previous 8 to 12 hours, prehydration before a bout of exercise is likely to be unnecessary. If fluid deficits are present, the individual should slowly drink beverages (e.g., $\approx$ 5 to 7 ml/kg body weight) at least 4 hours before the exercise task. Hydrating several hours before the event allows urine output to return to normal before exercise. Consuming the fluid with small amounts of sodium-containing foods or salted snacks will help to stimulate thirst and retain the fluid.
- *During exercise*: Follow an individualized plan to limit weight loss during exercise to ≤2% of baseline body weight. This will depend on the activity, the weight and body build of the athlete, and environmental conditions. Weighing before and after exercise is the best way to determine adequacy of fluid replacement

and extent of dehydration. A sports drink may have some advantages over plain water under certain circumstances. Consuming a sports beverage can provide both carbohydrate, which helps to maintain blood glucose and provide energy, as well as adequate electrolytes to replace losses. A general rule of thumb is to consume 0.5 to 1 L of sports beverage per hour, along with sufficient water to prevent excessive dehydration (weight loss). Recommended composition of sports drinks is sodium (≈ 20 to 30 mEq/L), potassium (≈ 2 to 5 mEq/L), and carbohydrate (≈ 50 to 100 g/L). Beverages with greater amounts of carbohydrate can delay gastric emptying.

■ *After exercise*: Normal meals and beverages will usually restore adequate fluid and electrolyte balance. If dehydration during exercise is severe, athletes should consume 1.5 L fluid per kilogram weight loss. Consuming the fluid with salty snacks will help to promote fluid retention and replace sodium losses. Hyponatremia could occur if there were large losses of sodium in perspiration without adequate replacement.

Food Intake Before and During Exercise

No one perfect preexercise meal exists because the optimal meal varies with the event and the athlete. In general, meals before competition or strenuous endeavors should be adequate in fluid to promote hydration, low in fat and fiber to improve gastric emptying and prevent gastrointestinal discomfort, high in carbohydrate to maintain blood glucose and maximize glycogen stores, moderate in protein, and consisting of foods familiar to the athlete (to reduce the risk of intolerance of a new food) (Williams and Serratosa, 2006). Pasta with a low-fat marinara sauce and sandwiches containing sliced chicken or turkey breast and low-fat mayonnaise, served with ample amounts of water, juice, or decaffeinated tea, are examples.

Intervention and education. Performance is improved if the preexercise meal supplies adequate amounts of carbohydrate. Whether carbohydrate intake during short bouts of exercise (1 hour or less) enhances performance is controversial, but carbohydrate is clearly beneficial when exercise lasts 90 minutes or more.

■ Consume 200 to 300 g carbohydrate 3 to 4 hours before exercise to help maintain blood glucose and glycogen stores. One cup of spaghetti with ½ cup low-fat sauce, 3 slices of toasted raisin bread, or one bagel provides this amount of carbohydrate.

- For events lasting 90 minutes or longer, consume carbohydrate, 0.7 g /kg body weight per hour (approximately 30 to 60 g/hr), starting shortly after the beginning of the event. Easy-to-digest carbohydrates that yield glucose or glucose plus fructose are more effective than those providing fructose alone. The carbohydrate can come from a sport drink, a carbohydrate gel, or a solid. Use of carbohydrate-containing beverages allows carbohydrate intake to be combined with fluid replacement. Drinking 600 to 1200 ml/hr of a solution that provides carbohydrate, 4 to 8 g/100 ml (e.g., a commercial sport drink or fruit juice diluted to half strength), will replace fluid losses and provide the needed carbohydrate.
- Following intense exercise, muscle glycogen stores need to be replaced. This process is encouraged by consumption of carbohydrate during the postexercise period: approximately 1 to 1.5 g/kg body weight (e.g., 1 cup cooked pasta and 1 cup fruit juice for an adult) every 2 hours during the waking hours, or a total of approximately 7 to 10 g/kg during the 24-hour period after exercise. Consuming protein along with the carbohydrate will provide amino acids needed for muscle synthesis and repair.

Conclusion

Regular vigorous exercise should be encouraged for its many benefits in weight control and health promotion. Many athletes are interested in nutrition and health, and this interest can be used to encourage them to make wise food choices and maintain a healthy body weight.

REFERENCES

American Academy of Pediatrics (AAP) Committee on Sports Medicine and Fitness: Promotion of healthy weight-control practices in young athletes, *Pediatrics* 116(6):1557, 2005.

American College of Sports Medicine (ACSM), American Dietetic Association (ADA), Dietitians of Canada (DC): Joint position statement: nutrition and athletic performance, *J Am Diet Assoc* 100(12):1543, 2000.

American College of Sports Medicine (ACSM) Position Stand: The female athlete triad, *Med Sci Sports Exerc* 39(10):1867, 2007.

Calfee R, Fadale P: Popular ergogenic drugs and supplements in young athletes, *Pediatrics* 117;e577, 2006.

Hinton PS, Sinclair LM: Iron supplementation maintains ventilatory threshold and improves energetic efficiency in iron-deficient nonanemic athletes, *Eur J Clin Nutr* 61(1):30, 2007.

Lawrence ME, Kirby DF: Nutrition and sports supplements: fact or fiction, *J Clin Gastroenterol* 35(4):299, 2002.

Nichols DL, Sanborn CF, Essery EV: Bone density and young athletic women: an update, *Sports Med* 37(11):1001, 2007.

Robinson Y, Cristancho E, Böning D: Intravascular hemolysis and mean red blood cell age in athletes, *Med Sci Sports Exerc* 38(3):480, 2006.

Sawka MN et al: American College of Sports Medicine Position Stand: exercise and fluid replacement, *Med Sci Sports Exerc* 39(2):377, 2007.

Schumacher YO et al: Hematological indices and iron status in athletes of various sports and performances, *Med Sci Sports Exerc* 34:869, 2002.

Venderley AM, Campbell WW: Vegetarian diets: nutritional considerations for athletes, *Sports Med* 36(4):293, 2006.

Williams C, Serratosa L: Nutrition on match day, *J Sports Sci* 24(7):687, 2006.

OBESITY AND WEIGHT CONTROL

Approximately two thirds of U.S. adults and 60% of Canadian adults are overweight or obese, and one third of U.S. adults and 23% of Canadians can be defined as obese (Tjepkema, 2006; NCHS, 2008). Moreover, approximately 20% to 25% of school-aged children and teens are overweight or obese (Shields, 2006; NCHS, 2008). Because of the prevalence of obesity and the health risks associated with it, it is probably the most serious nutrition problem among developed countries.

Etiology

Most cases of obesity are multifactorial in etiology. Some of the factors are described in the following list.

- *Environment.* The widespread marketing and availability of appealing food combined with a lifestyle with little need for physical activity promote overweight. Familial influences (e.g., using food as a reward, withholding dessert until the plate is clean) help develop eating habits that contribute to overweight. Portion sizes in fast-food and full-service restaurants, as well as the packaging of individual servings (e.g., soft drinks, chips, and other snack foods), have increased in recent years, contributing to excessive intake (Young and Nestle, 2007).
- *Energy expenditure.* Energy expenditure can be divided into three parts: **resting energy expenditure (REE), thermic effect of food (TEF),** and the energy expended in physical activity (see Chapter 2). REE, the energy required for vital body processes such as operation of the heart and lungs, accounts for 60% or more of energy expenditure for most individuals. REE appears to be normal in the obese. TEF, the energy required for digestion, absorption, and disposition of the nutrients in food, is normally about 10% of the total energy expenditure. The obese

have been reported to have low TEF, but this is probably insufficient to be the cause of most cases of obesity. Physical activity, the most variable component of energy expenditure, accounts for about 20% to 30% of the daily energy expenditure for most individuals. The obese tend to be more sedentary than normal-weight people, but this is partially balanced by the fact that the obese require more energy to perform the same tasks as normal-weight individuals. Overall, both adults and children in the United States and Canada are less physically active than is optimal.

- *Genetics*. Children of obese parents are much more likely to be obese than children of normal-weight parents, although it is difficult to separate genetic and environmental influences on body weight in most cases (Durand et al., 2007). Some individuals may have an inherited metabolic makeup that allows them to store fat more efficiently than other individuals do. Recently a genetic variation that can contribute to some cases of obesity and type 2 diabetes was identified (Frayling et al., 2007). It is likely that a number of other genetic mutations play a role in obesity. Plasma concentrations of **leptin**, a hormone released by adipose tissue, normally increase when fat stores are high; this signals to the central nervous system to reduce food intake. In a few dozen people across the world, a defect in leptin secretion has been identified (O'Rahilly, 2007).

- *Neuroendocrine*. Hypothyroidism, Cushing syndrome, and polycystic ovary syndrome are some of the neuroendocrine disorders associated with overweight and obesity. Prader-Willi syndrome, characterized by excessive appetite and inappropriate food-seeking behaviors, can lead to morbid obesity, but it is quite rare. Increased secretion of ghrelin, a hormone released by the stomach, stimulates food intake, but disorders in ghrelin regulation appear to be very rare. Although leptin deficiency (mentioned above) is uncommon, it is possible that some obese individuals are resistant to the effects of leptin. To date, however, no abnormalities in leptin or its metabolism have been found that could explain most cases of human obesity. Other hormones released by the fat cells, including adiponectin and resistin, have a role in body weight regulation, but their importance in contributing to the epidemic of obesity remains unclear (Kong et al., 2006). Consistent lack of sleep is associated with weight gain, although whether this is primarily due to increased food intake or neuroendocrine effects of sleep deprivation is unclear (Patel and Hu, 2008).

■ *Psychology.* Overeating may occur as a response to loneliness, grief, or depression. Overeating may also result from a learned response to external cues, such as food advertising or the fact that it is mealtime, rather than the internal cue of hunger.

■ *Physiology.* Energy expenditure declines with aging, and thus body weight often increases during middle age. Women are especially vulnerable to excess weight gain during pregnancy and the perimenopausal years. Maintaining an active lifestyle can slow the decline in energy expenditure (Simkin-Silverman et al., 2003; Walker, 2007).

Health Risks of Obesity

Obesity is associated with numerous health risks, which are summarized in Table 7-1. Health risks increase progressively with the severity of obesity. In the past, moderate weight gain with aging was believed to be associated with little risk, but recent data indicate that deaths from heart disease and cancer are increased in women who gain only 10 kg (22 lb) or more after the age of 18 years (Hu et al., 2004).

The fat cell, or adipocyte, produces hormonelike substances known as adipokines (Figure 7-1). A number of the adipokines promote an inflammatory response, and thus obesity is a state of

Table 7-1   **Health Problems Caused or Worsened by Obesity**

Type of Problem	Disease, Symptom, or Difficulty
Cardiovascular or respiratory	Hypertension, coronary heart disease, varicose veins, sleep apnea
Endocrine or reproductive	Type 2 diabetes mellitus, insulin resistance, amenorrhea, infertility, preeclampsia
Gastrointestinal	Gallstones, fatty liver
Musculoskeletal and skin	Osteoarthritis, skin irritation and infections, especially in fat folds, striae
Malignancies	Cancer of the colon, rectum, prostate, gallbladder, breast, uterus, and ovaries
Psychosocial	Social discrimination, poor self-image

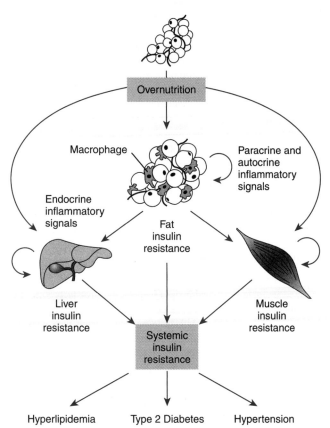

Overnutrition

Macrophage

Paracrine and autocrine inflammatory signals

Endocrine inflammatory signals

Fat insulin resistance

Liver insulin resistance

Muscle insulin resistance

Systemic insulin resistance

Hyperlipidemia   Type 2 Diabetes   Hypertension

Figure 7-1

Overnutrition leads to increased fat cell size and numbers. Although fat is deposited in many parts of the body, three sites that accumulate fat are especially problematic: the liver, skeletal muscle, and visceral (abdominal) adipose tissue. Fatty infiltration of muscle and liver makes these tissues more resistant to insulin action. Macrophages, which are cells of the immune system that are derived from the white blood cells known as monocytes, are attracted to the visceral fat depot. Visceral fat and the macrophages associated with it secrete a number of inflammatory signals or cytokines (also known as adipocytokines or adipokines) that contribute to insulin resistance. The insulin-resistant state is associated with hyperlipidemia, hypertension, and increased likelihood of developing type 2 diabetes.

(Modified with permission from de Luca C, Olefsky JM: Stressed out about obesity and insulin resistance, *Nat Med* 12[1]:41, 2006.)

chronic inflammation. The inflammatory process may contribute to cardiovascular disease and insulin resistance (Kong et al., 2006).

Weight cycling, or "yo-yo" dieting, occurs when individuals repeatedly lose and regain weight. Some studies, but not all, show that weight cycling increases morbidity and mortality among middle and older adults (Luo et al., 2007; Nebeling et al., 2004; Rzehak et al., 2007; Wannamethee et al., 2002), and therefore the benefits of weight loss must be balanced against the possible risks.

Nutrition Care
Assessment

A thorough nutrition assessment should be performed as described in Chapter 2. Box 7-1 highlights common or especially serious findings of obesity and weight control. Obesity refers to an excess of body fat. Visceral, or abdominal, fat (the so-called "apple" shape, or android fat pattern) is a predictor of cardiovascular disease risk. Fat in the hips and thighs (the "pear" shape, or gynecoid fat pattern), on the other hand, is much less likely to be associated with health risk. The waist circumference can be used as an indicator of abdominal fat in individuals with a body mass index (BMI) less than 35. When BMI is greater than 35, abdominal measurement is no longer necessary because health risks are high enough that abdominal obesity is no longer an independent predictor of cardiovascular risk (NIH, NHLBI, NAASO, 2000). Abdominal circumference is measured at the top of the iliac crest, at the end of an exhalation.

Intervention and education. Figure 7-2 provides a treatment algorithm for weight loss. All individuals with a BMI greater than 30 are advised to implement a weight loss strategy. For individuals with a BMI between 25 and 29.9, weight loss is indicated for women with a waist circumference greater than 88 cm (35 inches) and men with a waist circumference greater than 102 cm (40 inches) if they have two or more risk factors (summarized in Box 7-1) for subsequent mortality. Adults with a BMI 25 to 29.9 without concomitant risk factors should also be encouraged to lose weight if they desire to do so (NIH, NHLBI, NAASO, 2000).

When overweight and obesity are identified and the patient and clinician determine that weight loss is needed, the goals of intervention are as follows: (1) decrease body fat, (2) develop healthier

Box 7-1   Assessment in Obesity and Weight Control

Anthropometric and Body Composition Data

- Body mass index (BMI)
- Waist circumference*
- Body fat (bioelectric impedance, dual x-ray electron absorptiometry, air displacement plethysmography) (optional)†

Health History

Risk Factors or Comorbidities Associated with Obesity

- Very high risk: presence of coronary heart disease (CHD), including a history of myocardial infarction, angina pectoris, and coronary artery surgery or other procedures; other atherosclerotic diseases, including peripheral arterial disease, abdominal aneurysm, or symptomatic carotid artery disease; type 2 diabetes; and sleep apnea
- High risk for cardiovascular disease: cigarette smoking; hypertension (systolic blood pressure 140 mm Hg or greater or diastolic blood pressure 90 mm Hg or greater) or current use of antihypertensive medications; serum low-density lipoprotein (LDL)–cholesterol concentration of 160 mg/dl or greater or a borderline LDL concentration (130 to 159 mg/dl) plus two or more other risk factors; serum high-density lipoprotein (HDL)–cholesterol less than 35 mg/dl; impaired fasting glucose (fasting plasma glucose between 110 and 125 mg/dl); family history of premature CHD (myocardial infarction or sudden death experienced by the father or other first-degree male relative at or before 55 years of age or experienced by the mother or other first-degree female relative at or before 65 years of age); or age 45 years or older for men or 55 years or older for women (or postmenopausal)
- Other risk factors: physical inactivity, elevated serum triglycerides (a marker of cardiovascular risk in obese individuals)

Readiness to Lose Weight

- Reasons and motivation for weight loss
- Previous attempts at weight loss—document and evaluate methods and results
- Support expected from family and friends
- Understanding of risks and benefits of weight loss
- Attitudes toward physical activity

Box 7-1   Assessment in Obesity and Weight Control—cont'd

- Time available to devote to physical activity, meal planning, and record keeping
- Potential barriers, including financial limitations, to adoption of change

Diet History

- Usual food intake: meal and snack patterns, portion sizes, food preparation methods
- Activity patterns: type, amount, intensity

From National Institutes of Health, National Heart, Lung, and Blood Institute, and the North American Association for the Study of Obesity: *The practical guide: identification, evaluation, and treatment of overweight and obesity in adults*, Washington, DC, 2000, National Institutes of Health (NIH).

*Men are considered at high risk if the waist circumference is >102 cm (40 in), and women are at high risk if the waist circumference is >99 cm (35 in).

†In clinical management of adult patients, body composition measurements add little information that cannot be obtained from the BMI. See Chapter 2 for a description of methods of assessing body composition.

eating and physical activity habits, (3) prevent loss of lean body mass (LBM) during weight reduction, and (4) maintain weight loss. Weight reduction is achieved by consuming less energy than required to meet energy needs. This can be accomplished with dietary and behavior modification and increased physical activity, as well as medications and surgery. All these methods are discussed in this chapter.

Preventing development of overweight and obesity. It is easier to prevent weight gain than to reduce excess weight. The following points are useful in helping adults avoid weight gain:

- Be aware that health risks are increased even at moderate degrees of overweight.
- Anticipate the likelihood of weight gain with aging, and make lifestyle changes (increase activity level and evaluate and improve eating habits) as needed.
- Be alert to times when weight gain is likely (e.g., when quitting smoking, undergoing unusual stress, or in the perimenopausal period), and plan strategies in advance to prevent weight gain.

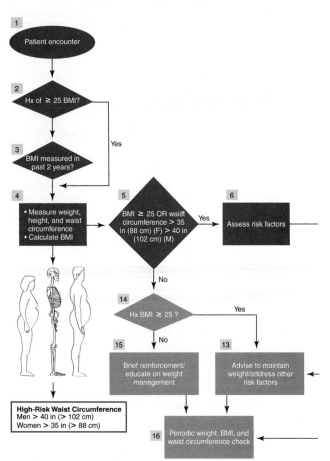

Figure 7-2
Treatment algorithm for overweight and obesity. Body mass index (BMI), waist circumference, presence of health risk factors and comorbidities, and patient willingness to lose weight guide decision making.
(From National Institutes of Health, National Heart, Lung, and Blood Institute, and the North American Association for the Study of Obesity: *The practical guide: identification, evaluation, and treatment of overweight and obesity in adults*, Washington, DC, 2000, National Institutes of Health [NIH].)

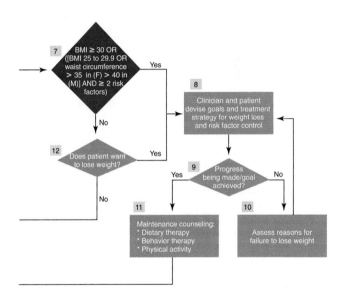

 Examination

Treatment

This algorithm applies only to the assessment for overweight and obesity and subsequent decisions based on that assessment. It does not reflect any initial overall assessment for other cardiovascular risk factors that are indicated.

Some strategies include joining a fitness center, recruiting a group of friends to form a regular walking or biking club, and making more healthful food choices when eating at fast-food restaurants.

Establishing a weight goal. A BMI between 18.5 and 25 for adults (see inside back cover) and no more than the 95th percentile for age and gender in children and adolescents is associated with fewer health risks. Achieving a weight within the desirable range for height may seem overwhelming, especially for severely obese individuals. Even a modest weight loss (5% to 10% of current body weight) can have significant health benefits, however, often reducing blood pressure and fasting blood glucose concentrations (Hainer et al., 2008). Therefore setting a goal of a 5% to 10% weight loss over 6 months may achieve better results than setting a goal of achieving an ideal body weight. Once the 5% to 10% weight loss has been achieved, and the individual is successful in maintaining the weight loss, it may be possible to set another weight loss goal. The obese individual who participates in setting personal weight goals is more likely to be successful in losing weight.

Low-energy weight reduction diets. A weight loss of 0.5 to 1 kg (1 to 2 lb) per week is achievable and safe for most adults. For most adult women an energy intake of 1000 to 1200 kcal/day (4200 to 5040 kJ/day) will promote weight loss at approximately this rate. For men, very active women, and women weighing more than 75 kg, 1200 to 1600 kcal/day (5040 to 6715 kJ/day) will generally promote consistent moderate weight loss. It is difficult to maintain an adequate intake of nutrients on a diet providing less than 1000 to 1200 kcal/day, but short women may have difficulty losing much weight with this energy allowance. They should be encouraged to increase their activity level, rather than reducing their energy intake below 1000 kcal/day (NIH, NHLBI, NAASO, 2000).

The optimal balance of carbohydrate, fat, and protein in a weight reduction diet is a subject of great debate. Low-carbohydrate diets such as the Atkins diet may result in slightly greater weight loss than low-fat diets, at least over the first 6 months of dieting (Nordmann et al., 2006; Gardner et al., 2007). Low-carbohydrate diets appear to have both favorable effects on serum lipids (reducing triglycerides and increasing high-density lipoprotein [HDL]–cholesterol) and unfavorable effects (increasing low-density lipoprotein [LDL]–cholesterol)

(Nordmann et al., 2006). A high-carbohydrate diet with a low glycemic index (one rich in whole grains and high-fiber cereals, which does not markedly elevate blood glucose in the postprandial period) has been reported to have a favorable effect on the serum lipid profile while stimulating weight loss (McMillan-Price et al., 2006). The National Weight Control Registry reports that most of the registrants who have successfully maintained a loss of 30 lb (13.6 kg) or more for at least 1 year follow a low-calorie diet moderate in fat (≈ 29% of energy intake) and carbohydrate (≈ 50%) (Phelan et al., 2006).

Obese individuals often have poor diets, frequently skipping breakfast and consuming foods of low nutrient density (Mendoza et al, 2007; Mota et al., 2008). The eating habits established during weight loss and maintenance efforts should change the quality of the diet in a positive way. There are a variety of ways to plan a healthful low-energy diet based on common foods. Most adults or adolescents can learn to use the *Choose Your Foods: Exchange Lists for Diabetes* available from the American Diabetes Association and the American Dietetic Association, which allow flexibility and are easier than calorie counting. The Dietary Approaches to Stop Hypertension (DASH) diet (see Chapter 1), with an emphasis on making healthful, low-energy choices (e.g., dairy products made with skim milk, whole grains and other good sources of fiber, and ample servings of fruits and vegetables, lean meats, fish, or poultry), can also be used as a tool for wise food selection. Individuals may want to use other diet plans that are found in magazines or books or supported by various commercial or community organizations. Box 7-2 provides guidelines for evaluating weight loss programs.

Practical suggestions for weight loss. Some practical suggestions for the person attempting to follow a low-energy diet include the following:

- Weigh or measure foods initially in order to learn to recognize portion sizes.
- Consume foods rich in fiber. High-fiber foods take longer to consume than low-fiber ones, and satiety (fullness or satisfaction) may be achieved with a reduced energy intake when consuming high-fiber foods. Also, carbohydrates high in fiber tend to have a low glycemic index, meaning they do not increase blood glucose as much as more refined foods. Foods with a low

---

Box 7-2   Characteristics of a Safe and Effective Weight Control Program

---

1. The diet plan includes more than 800 kcal/day.
2. The diet plan includes adequate numbers of servings from all food groups and provides for choices among foods in each group.
3. The plan relies on regular foods, rather than special proprietary products. Foods should be readily available from the supermarket.
4. Claims for weight loss are no more than an average of 1 kg (≈ 2 lb) per week.
5. Exercise or regular physical activity is encouraged.
6. Behavior changes are incorporated.
7. The plan can be adapted to the lifestyle of the individual.
8. The cost of the plan is reasonable.

---

glycemic index do not stimulate as much insulin release as those with a high glycemic index. Some authorities believe that high postprandial insulin levels make it much harder to control body weight, because insulin encourages storage of energy as fat, but the effect of glycemic index on body weight is not fully established.

■ Broil, bake, or steam rather than frying foods. Use herbs, spices, lemon juice, or other low-energy seasonings rather than butter, margarine, olive oil, or salt pork. Choose skim milk and dairy products made with skim milk. Limit foods with "hidden" fat, such as doughnuts, pie crust, croissants, muffins, and other quick breads. If desserts are desired, choose fruit ices, fresh fruit, or low-fat cookies (gingersnaps, newtons) rather than ice cream, cake, pie, or higher-fat cookies.

■ Do not expect rapid, easy weight loss. Weight gain is usually a gradual process, and so is weight reduction. When lapses occur, do not become discouraged; simply resume proper eating habits and physical activity patterns.

■ Include occasional high-energy treats in the eating plan. This approach helps to prevent feelings of deprivation that may lead to binge eating and reduce guilt over indulging in a favorite high-calorie food. It may be necessary to eat high-energy favorite foods under the supervision of a counselor, health care provider, or trusted family member or friend initially, to avoid losing control.

Very–low-calorie diets. Very–low-calorie diets (VLCDs) are those providing 400 to 800 kcal/day. These are intended for obese individuals (BMI >30) under a physician's supervision. Special diet formulas (usually flavored drinks) are available, with the energy being mostly in the form of high-quality protein. This diet is sometimes called a *protein-sparing modified fast*. The usual regimen is to follow the VLCD for 12 to 16 weeks, followed by a gradual reinstitution of regular foods over a period of 3 weeks or longer. Losses of 1.5 to 2.3 kg (3.3 to 5.1 lb) per week occur during the VLCD.

A VLCD should be begun only after a thorough medical examination, and dieters should have regular measurement of serum electrolytes and examinations by a physician. Intake of noncaloric beverages should be at least 2 L/day to prevent dehydration. Gallstones are a possible complication of any rapid weight loss regimen. VLCDs have not been more effective than low-energy weight reduction diets in preventing regain of weight (Tsai and Wadden, 2006).

Fad diets. Diets that promise quick weight loss are popular. Unfortunately, these diets tend to be undesirable for one or more of the following reasons: (1) they are nutritionally inadequate; (2) they require expensive foods or time-consuming food preparation; (3) they are medically unsafe; (4) they do not help the individual change poor eating habits, and thus the weight lost is usually regained; and (5) much of the weight lost is fluid or lean body mass, rather than fat. All weight reduction diets should be evaluated with the criteria in Box 7-2 before beginning the program. In particular, the prospective dieter should remember that weight loss can be achieved without the purchase of expensive diet aids, very rapid weight loss can pose health risks, diet plans that focus heavily on one or a few foods can be nutritionally inadequate, and developing improved eating and lifestyle habits (i.e., recognition of appropriate serving sizes, focusing on healthful food choices, and obtaining regular physical activity) is a key component of a successful weight reduction regimen.

Some popular weight loss plans are summarized in Box 7-3. In a 1-year comparison of the Ornish (very–low-fat), Atkins (low-carbohydrate), Weight Watchers (calorie-restricted), and Zone

Text continued on p. 206.

Box 7-3   Popular Weight Loss Diets

Low-Carbohydrate Diet Plans

Atkins Diet (Dr. Atkins' New Diet Revolution by Robert C. Atkins, MD)

Overview

The diet has four phases: (1) induction, in which daily carbohydrate intake is limited to 20 g "net carbs" (total carbohydrate minus fiber); (2) ongoing weight loss, in which net carb intake is increased weekly (an increment of 5 g/day each week) until weight loss slows to 1 to 2 lb/wk; (3) premaintenance, which occurs when the dieter is within 5 to 10 lb of the weight loss goal, and involves a weekly addition of net carbs of 10 g/day so that weight loss slows to no more than 1 lb (454 g) per week; and (4) lifetime maintenance, which begins when the dieter has maintained his or her weight goal for 1 month and includes an average net carb intake of 40 to 120 g/day.

Comments

The diet encourages aerobic and anaerobic exercise but makes no recommendation about amount. Purchase of Atkins food products, such as snack and breakfast bars, is not required but is encouraged. Very–low-carbohydrate intakes cause ketosis, which can result in fatigue, dehydration, and cognitive impairment. The diet limits nutritious foods, such as whole grains, legumes, fruits, vegetables, and low-fat dairy products. It may be low in fiber and calcium. High protein intake increases uric acid production and can contribute to gout. Increased intake of saturated fats on this diet might contribute to elevated serum low-density lipoprotein (LDL)–cholesterol. Even though the last phase of the diet is termed "lifetime maintenance," the regimen can be difficult to follow because many popular foods, such as pasta, pizza, and desserts, are carbohydrate rich. Some free educational content is available at the website (www.atkins.com).

South Beach Diet (South Beach Diet *by Arthur Agatston, MD*)

Overview

The diet has three phases: (1) 2 weeks with virtually no carbohydrate intake, when only lean meats, poultry and fish, low-fat cheese, eggs, nonstarchy vegetables, nuts, and special South

Box 7-3   Popular Weight Loss Diets—cont'd

Beach desserts are allowed, and a loss of 8 to 13 lb is promised;
(2) the period of ongoing weight loss, when "good carbohydrates," such as fruits, vegetables, and unrefined starches, are
allowed in the context of a low-calorie diet but foods high in
saturated and *trans* fats, refined products such as white flour,
and high sugar foods are banned, and weight loss is approximately 1 to 2 lb/wk; and (3) maintenance, which includes more
of the same foods as during the second phase but still in moderate amounts.

Comments

Aerobic and strengthening exercises are recommended. On-line
help from dietitians and others is available from the website
(www.southbeachdiet.com) for a fee. Special diet products are
not required but are encouraged.

Moderate-Carbohydrate Diet Plans

Zone Diet (The Zone: A Dietary Road Map *by Barry Sears and Bill
Lawren*)

Overview

The diet consists of five meals and snacks daily, with each divided into 40% carbohydrate, 30% protein, and 30% fat. Foods
are categorized into protein, carbohydrate, and fat "blocks."
Eight glasses of water are recommended daily. The foods allowed include lean poultry, seafood, egg whites, low-fat dairy
foods, most fruit and nonstarchy vegetables, oatmeal, barley,
and small amounts of canola and olive oils. A weight loss of 1.5
to 2 lb/wk is suggested.

Comments

Aerobic exercise is recommended daily (30 to 90 minutes, depending on weight goals). Dieters are advised to assess their
state of hunger before each meal or snack and eat whether hungry or not. Although this avoids the hunger that may stimulate
overeating, it does not allow individuals to respond to hunger
cues. The foods allowed are generally nutritious, but the plan
can be cumbersome to manage. Special foods are not required
but are promoted, and diet help is available through a toll-free
number and a website (www.zoneperfect.com).

Continued

Box 7-3   Popular Weight Loss Diets—cont'd

Weight Watchers

Overview

The program has two options: a point system to categorize foods and quantify intake or a core plan with a recommended number of servings daily. In the point system each food is assigned points based on its fat, calories, and fiber per serving, with higher-calorie foods having more points. Based on body size and weight goals, individuals consume a particular number of points daily. Essentially all foods are allowed on the diet, but lean meats and poultry, fruits, vegetables, whole grains, and low-fat dairy products are encouraged. Local group meetings are encouraged; these meetings, directed by a person successful in losing weight, cover recipes and product suggestions, coping strategies, and behavioral techniques. An initial registration fee and monthly fees are required for meeting attendance and use of the tools on the website.

Comments

This diet encourages aerobic exercise. Weight loss is reported to be better among those who attend meetings. Guidance and meal-planning tools are also available on-line at www.weightwatchers.com. Most members are women, and thus men might not feel comfortable at local meetings. However, the website includes specific tools and exercise and diet recommendations for men.

High-Carbohydrate, Moderate- or Low-Fat Diet Plans

Ornish Life Choice Program (Eat More, Weigh Less
by Dean Ornish, MD)

Overview

The program consists of four principles: (1) a very–low-fat, high–complex carbohydrate diet rich in fruits, vegetables, whole grains, beans, and legumes; (2) regular exercise; (3) stress reduction and meditation; and (4) love (learning communication skills and developing commitments and relationships with family and community). Nonfat dairy products and small amounts of plant oils are included. Foods to avoid include meat, poultry, fish, caffeine-containing products, high-fat foods, processed foods, alcohol, sugars, honey, and syrups.

Box 7-3   Popular Weight Loss Diets—cont'd

Comments

Reduction in heart disease risk has been demonstrated in people adhering to the program. Concerns have been expressed that the diet may be so low in fat that essential fatty acid intake is inadequate or absorption of fat-soluble vitamins is impaired. It can be difficult to follow when eating away from home, and not all individuals would want to follow a vegetarian diet. The program is self-directed, with no website or outside support.

Volumetrics (Volumetrics Eating Plan *by Barbara Rolls, PhD*)

Overview

The diet emphasizes foods with greater water content because they have greater volume and increase satiety. Tables of energy densities (EDs) are provided, based on the energy contained in the food divided by its weight in grams. Low-ED foods (Category 1), such as nonstarchy vegetables and fruits, nonfat dairy products, and broth-type soups, can be eaten liberally. Category 2 foods, such as starchy vegetables and fruits (e.g., bananas), grains, fish, skinless poultry, low-fat salad dressings, and pasta, can be eaten daily in controlled portions. Category 3 foods, such as meats, cheese, pizza, regular salad dressings, and ice cream, can be eaten in controlled portions on a weekly basis. Category 4 foods (high ED), such as chips, candy, cookies, and butter, can be eaten in small amounts occasionally. Starting each meal with a low-calorie soup or salad is recommended, to speed up the feeling of satiety. The macronutrient composition is 20% to 30% fat, 15% to 35% protein, and 55% or more carbohydrate. The suggested water intake is 9 cups for women and 13 cups for men.

Comments

Moderate-intensity exercise for 30 to 60 minutes daily is encouraged. The diet is adequate in all respects, based on scientific principles, and rich in fiber. Some recipes in the book require many ingredients and may be daunting to busy cooks, but it is possible to adhere to the program while using simple, readily available foods. The program is self-directed, with no website or outside support.

Continued

Box 7-3   Popular Weight Loss Diets—cont'd

Meal Replacement Plans
Slim-Fast
Overview

The daily food intake consists of Slim-Fast shakes or bars (approximately 180 to 220 kcal each) consumed twice daily, either alone as meal replacements or in combination with regular foods (depending on the caloric allowance) and a third Sensible Meal of approximately 500 kcal, plus snacks providing 3 servings of fruits and vegetables. Dieters are encouraged to strive for a loss of 1 to 2 lb (0.45 to 0.9 kg)/wk.

Comments

Moderate-intensity exercise is encouraged. Free on-line registration (www.slim-fast.com) entitles the dieter to meal and activity planning tools, web-based support from "buddies," and answers from dietitians employed by Slim-Fast. The diet plan could be low in fiber and **nutraceuticals** (nonnutrients in food that may have a variety of health benefits). The intake of regular foods is very low, and thus the diet may not retrain eating habits. Slim-Fast has proven effective in bringing about weight loss in a number of clinical studies (e.g., Truby et al., 2006), but as with many diet plans, maintenance of weight loss has been poor.

(balanced macronutrient) diets, all the diets were associated with modest reductions in weight and serum cholesterol. Dropouts were common with all the diets, especially the Ornish and Atkins diets (Dansinger et al., 2005).

Behavior modification. Behavior modification, in conjunction with a balanced weight reduction diet, helps promote lasting weight loss. It should be a part of all weight loss programs. The following techniques are the primary features of behavior modification programs:

- *Self-monitoring*: recording exercise, food intake, and emotional and environmental circumstances at the time of food consumption to provide a basis for planning changes and for continued monitoring of adherence to lifestyle changes

- *Stimulus control and environmental management*: acquiring techniques to help break learned associations between environmental cues and food intake
- *Positive reinforcement*: a reward system to encourage changes in behavior
- *Contracts*: signed contracts between the therapist and the individual seeking to modify behavior, outlining the consequences if various changes are made or are not made

Box 7-4 provides suggestions for behavioral modification strategies designed to promote weight loss and maintenance. The

---

Box 7-4   Modifying Behavior to Promote Weight Loss or Maintenance

1. Chew food slowly, and put utensils down between bites.
2. Never shop for food on an empty stomach.
3. Make out a grocery shopping list before starting, and do not add to it as you shop.
4. Leave a small amount of food on your plate after each meal.
5. Fill your plate in the kitchen at the start of the meal; do not put open bowls of food on the table.
6. Eat in only one or two places (e.g., the kitchen and dining room table).
7. Never eat while involved in any other activity, such as watching television.
8. Do not eat while standing.
9. Keep a diary of when and where you eat and under what circumstances (e.g., boredom, frustration, anxiety). Be aware of problem circumstances, and substitute another activity for eating.
10. Keep low-calorie snacks available at all times.
11. Reward yourself for weight loss (e.g., buy new clothes, treat yourself to concert tickets or a trip). Establish a stepwise set of goals with a reward for achieving each goal.
12. If you violate your diet on one occasion, do not use that as an excuse to go off the diet altogether. Acknowledge that setbacks happen, and return to your weight control program.
13. When confronted with an appealing food, remember that this will not be your last chance to have the food. Content yourself with a small portion.

individuals who are most successful in losing weight and maintaining weight loss tend to be those who develop personalized methods of controlling food intake and increasing energy expenditure (Phelan et al., 2006). As an example, overly rapid food consumption is one cause of overeating. The feeling of satiety takes 20 minutes or more to develop in a hungry person, and the person who eats a meal in less time may overeat simply because he or she does not yet feel full. To slow the eating rate, the individual can eat with friends or family and talk with them during meals, lay utensils down after each bite, chew each bite thoroughly, and eat many leafy salads and other foods of low energy density.

Physical activity. Activities involving gross movements of large muscles promote fat loss while conserving LBM. Aerobic exercise is especially effective in reducing visceral fat. Many individuals on weight reduction diets find that, after an initial period of weight loss, their weight plateaus. The primary reason is that energy expenditure decreases as weight decreases. An increase in physical activity can reduce the likelihood of the plateau effect. Moderate physical activity for 30 minutes most days of the week is sufficient to achieve cardiovascular benefits, but more exercise is required to promote weight loss. For best results the dieter must obtain about 60 min/day of moderate-intensity exercise, and 60 to 90 min/day may be required to maintain weight loss (USDHHS and USDA, 2005). Table 5-1 provides a guide to energy expenditure during exercise.

Although a regular exercise regimen is invaluable, increasing energy expenditure in the activities of daily living can also facilitate weight loss and maintenance. For example, park farther from the door, use stairs rather than the elevator, and bicycle or walk rather than driving on errands when possible.

Medications. Most medications used for weight loss fall into two general categories: those with anorexic properties, generally stimulators of the sympathetic nervous system, and those that reduce nutrient absorption. The prescription drug sibutramine (Meridia) suppresses appetite and also increases energy expenditure, as does phenylpropanolamine (in over-the-counter products such as Acutrim and Dexatrim). Rimonabant (Acomplia or Zimulti; not available in the United States) reduces appetite by blocking the brain's cannabinoid receptors. Orlistat (Xenical) acts by inhibiting the release of gastric and pancreatic lipases and thereby blocking the digestion and absorption of approximately one third of the fat consumed. Alli, a version of orlistat that is available without a prescription, provides one half of the dose of the prescription capsule. Several drugs approved for use in control of hyperglycemia in diabetes are associated with moderate weight loss. These include metformin, an insulin-sensitizing agent that also reduces intestinal carbohydrate absorption; acarbose, an inhibitor of carbohydrate digestion; and exenatide and pramlintide, both of which delay gastric emptying.

Weight loss medications are usually used in conjunction with other methods (low-energy diets, exercise programs, behavior modification) to promote weight loss. Medications increase the likelihood that the obese will lose at least 10% of their initial body weight, and therefore they reinforce the effects of lifestyle changes designed to promote weight loss; however, the total amount of weight loss caused by medications by themselves is only moderate—2 to 10 kg (4 to 22 lb) in most reports—and the weight plateaus after about 6 months (Franz et al., 2007). Weight regain is common after medications are stopped. Because obesity is a long-term problem, short-term use of medications has little benefit. Long-term use of medications is currently recommended only for carefully selected patients, particularly those who have obesity-related health problems, and not for the general obese population.

Orlistat can reduce absorption of fat-soluble vitamins (A, D, E, and K) and carotenoids. People using this medication should take a multivitamin containing the fat-soluble vitamins daily, at least 2 hours before or after taking orlistat. Other side effects of orlistat include oily spotting, increased flatus, oily or fatty stools, fecal urgency, increased number of bowel movements, and fecal incontinence. These are usually temporary, but they may be worsened by a high-fat diet (greater than 30% of energy intake) or a very–high-fat intake at a single meal or snack.

Bariatric surgery. An individual with a BMI above 40, or a BMI above 35 plus a serious obesity-related complication, who has failed to lose weight with more conventional methods may be considered for obesity surgery. Two strategies are used: restrictive procedures, which limit the capacity of the stomach to store food and cause the individual to feel full quickly, and malabsorptive procedures, which bypass a portion of the intestine. In the increasingly popular gastric banding procedure, an inflatable band is placed around the stomach to create a 15- to 30-ml pouch; the size of the pouch outlet can be adjusted by altering the amount of fluid in a reservoir attached to the band (Figure 7-3, *A*). In gastroplasty (or gastric stapling; Figure 7-3, *B*), the stomach is partitioned to create a small pouch (30 to 60 ml). The use of a vertical band around the pouch outlet (vertical banded gastroplasty) reinforces it and reduces the risk of stretching the outlet. Gastric bypass (Figure 7-3, *C*) combines the restrictive approach with some degree of malabsorption. A gastric pouch is created and connected to the jejunum, bypassing the distal stomach and the duodenum. The biliopancreatic diversion technique (Figure 7-3, *D*) uses a larger gastric pouch (200 to 250 ml), with bypass of much of the small bowel, maintaining a food channel of 50 to 100 cm of ileum. The standard biliopancreatic diversion creates an anastomosis of the ileum to the stomach, whereas the biliopancreatic diversion with duodenal switch creates an anastomosis of the ileum to the duodenum.

Overall, bariatric surgeries are successful in reducing weight by approximately 21% to 38%, sufficient to reduce the symptoms of diabetes, cardiovascular disease, hypercholesterolemia, obstructive sleep apnea, and hypertension, as well as many other complications of obesity, in most individuals (Mango and Frishman, 2006). Gastric bypass and biliopancreatic diversion procedures produce the greatest weight loss, and adjustable gastric banding produces the least. Weight loss usually ceases within 12 to 24 months after surgery, but it may continue for longer if patients participate in a follow-up program that emphasizes lifestyle practices for weight control. The surgical procedures in themselves can produce disappointing results unless combined with lifestyle changes to promote weight loss. Especially with the restrictive procedures, it is possible to gain weight by continually sipping high-energy liquids. Three small solid meals daily appear to yield the best results.

Complications after bariatric surgery. The malabsorptive procedures are especially likely to be associated with nutritional problems. Some of the most common concerns are as follows:

▪ *Dumping syndrome.* Consumption of simple carbohydrates is likely to cause dumping syndrome after gastric bypass or biliopancreatic diversion because of the rapid movement of osmotically

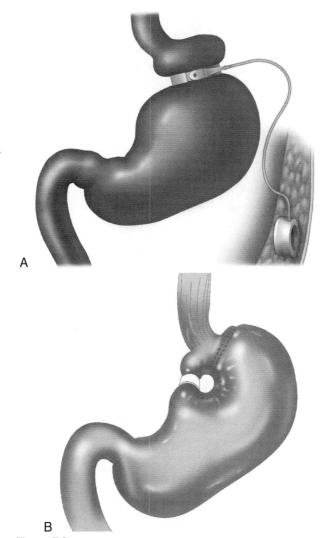

A

B
Figure 7-3
Surgical approaches to weight control. **A**, Gastric banding.
B, Vertical banded gastroplasty.

Continued

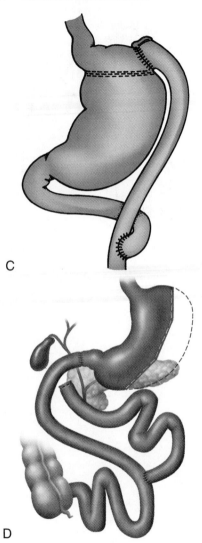

Figure 7-3, cont'd
C, Roux-en-Y gastric bypass. The stomach is stapled completely horizontally; the jejunum is resected from the duodenum and connected to the upper gastric pouch; the distal duodenal stump is connected to the jejunum to permit drainage of intestinal secretions. **D,** Biliopancreatic diversion.

active particles into the small bowel. The symptoms of dumping syndrome include dizziness, sweating, nausea, abdominal cramping, weakness, tachycardia, and diarrhea. Limiting intake of simple sugars, such as candy and sugar-sweetened beverages, reduces the likelihood of dumping syndrome.

- *Iron.* Gastric acid promotes iron absorption, and the small gastric pouch produces less acid; in addition, iron is normally absorbed in the duodenum and upper jejunum, which are partially or totally bypassed. Patients often need a supplement (iron sulfate 325 mg/day) to avoid iron deficiency.
- *Calcium.* Calcium malabsorption is especially likely with the biliopancreatic diversion because it is associated with steatorrhea. A supplement providing the Dietary Reference Intake (DRI) for calcium will help to avert deficiency and osteoporosis.
- *Vitamin B_{12}.* Vitamin B_{12} deficiency may occur because the stomach produces less acid and intrinsic factor—both of which are required for vitamin B_{12} absorption—than normal. Oral supplements of pharmacologic amounts of vitamin B_{12} may be absorbed well enough to prevent deficiency.
- *Protein-energy malnutrition.* This is particularly likely following the biliopancreatic diversion, with steatorrhea (3 to 5 loose stools daily) being a common finding.

A variety of problems not related to nutrition are encountered with these surgeries. Wound infections, wound dehiscence, and venous and pulmonary thrombosis are relatively common in the early postoperative period. With gastric banding, gastric prolapse is possible but infrequent. With the other surgeries, leaks along the staple lines or at the sites of anastomosis can occur. Hernia and ulcers are two of the most common complications with the biliopancreatic diversion. Patients need to be observed for the rest of their lives to detect complications and monitor weight control.

Weight maintenance. After weight is lost, by whatever means, the goal becomes maintenance of the loss. Instead of thinking of weight control in terms of dieting, which is a temporary practice, the individual must think of it as a permanent lifestyle change. He or she can never return to old eating habits, or the weight will be regained. A study of individuals successful in maintaining a loss of at least 13.6 kg (30 lb) revealed that successful maintainers had certain common characteristics: frequent self-monitoring of their weight and dietary intake, i.e., keeping food records; adherence to a low-energy diet; regular physical activity, usually at least 60 to 90 min/day, of moderate-intensity exercise; consumption of breakfast; and minimal television watching (Hill and Wyatt, 2005; Phelan et al., 2006; Raynor et al., 2006). Weight maintenance does become easier over time; 3 to 5 years after weight loss, fewer weight control strategies were required than during or immediately after weight loss.

Overweight in childhood. In dealing with obese children, frequently the goal is to achieve weight maintenance; as the child grows in stature, weight for height then becomes more appropriate. One teaching technique for preschool and young school-age children is the "traffic light" plan (Goldfield and Epstein, 2002; Johnston and Steele, 2007). Foods less than 20 kcal/serving are green, or GO, foods and can be used freely. Green foods include seasonings and a few vegetables, such as asparagus and lettuce. Yellow foods are the primary foods in the diet; they can be eaten with CAUTION. Examples are corn, oranges, grilled chicken, skim milk, and English muffins. Red, or STOP, foods are high in energy. No more than four servings of red foods are to be eaten per week. Some examples of red foods are scalloped potatoes, fruit in heavy syrup, fried chicken, whole milk, and doughnuts. A modification of the traffic light plan categorizes foods based on their fat content, since the foods highest in fat tend to be the ones highest in total energy. Foods with 0 to 3 g fat/serving are considered green foods, those with 4 to 5 g fat/serving are yellow, and those with more than 5 g fat/serving are red foods according to this categorization. Parents need to be made aware how important it is for them to make available nutritious food choices and model healthy eating and activity habits. Schools are another important influence on children's eating and exercise, and cafeteria meals and vending machines should provide nutritious, low-energy food choices. The increasing use of fast food and sweetened soft drinks is a special concern (St-Onge et al., 2003; Warner et al., 2006). The American Academy of Pediatrics (2004) has recommended that the sale of soft drinks be restricted in schools.

Conclusion

Overweight and obesity are among the most serious health problems in the world today. Various tools are available for treatment, including low-calorie diets, medications that decrease appetite or interfere with nutrient digestion or absorption, and bariatric surgery. Unfortunately, even if weight loss is successful, maintenance of the loss is difficult. Use of behavioral modification techniques and support from family, friends, and professionals improve attempts at weight maintenance, but improved strategies are needed. A useful guide for professionals working with overweight and obese individuals is available from the National Institutes of Health (NIH, NHLBI, NAASO, 2000).

REFERENCES

American Academy of Pediatrics Committee on School Health: Soft drinks in schools, *Pediatrics* 113:152, 2004.

Dansinger ML et al: Comparison of the Atkins, Ornish, Weight Watchers, and Zone diets for weight loss and heart disease risk reduction: a randomized trial, *JAMA* 293(1):43, 2005.

Durand EF, Logan C, Carruth A: Association of maternal obesity and childhood obesity: implications for healthcare providers, *J Community Health Nurs* 24(3):167, 2007.

Franz MJ et al: Weight-loss outcomes: a systematic review and meta-analysis of weight-loss clinical trials with a minimum 1-year follow-up, *J Am Dietet Assoc* 107(10):1755, 2007.

Frayling TM et al: A common variant in the FTO gene is associated with body mass index and predisposes to childhood and adult obesity, *Science* 316(5826):889, 2007.

Gardner CD et al: Comparison of the Atkins, Zone, Ornish, and LEARN diets for change in weight and related risk factors among overweight premenopausal women: the A TO Z Weight Loss Study: a randomized trial, *JAMA* 297(9):969, 2007.

Goldfield GS, Epstein LH: Management of obesity in children. In Fairborn CG, Brownell KD, editors: *Eating disorders and obesity: a comprehensive handbook*, ed 2, New York, 2002, Guilford Press.

Hainer V, Toplak H, Mitrakou A: Treatment modalities of obesity: what fits whom? *Diabetes Care* 31 Suppl 2:S269, 2008.

Hill JO, Wyatt HR: Role of physical activity in preventing and treating obesity, *J Appl Physiol* 99(2):765, 2005.

Hu FB et al: Adiposity as compared with physical activity in predicting mortality among women, *N Engl J Med* 351(26):2694, 2004.

Johnston CA, Steele RG: Treatment of pediatric overweight: an examination of feasibility and effectiveness in an applied clinical setting, *J Pediatr Psychol* 32(1):106, 2007.

Kong AP, Chan NN, Chan JC: The role of adipocytokines and neurohormonal dysregulation in metabolic syndrome, *Curr Diabetes Rev* 2(4):397, 2006.

Luo J et al: Body size, weight cycling, and risk of renal cell carcinoma among postmenopausal women: the Women's Health Initiative (United States), *Am J Epidemiol* 166(7):752, 2007.

Mango VL, Frishman WH: Physiologic, psychologic, and metabolic consequences of bariatric surgery, *Cardiol Rev* 14(5):232, 2006.

McMillan-Price J et al: Comparison of 4 diets of varying glycemic load on weight loss and cardiovascular risk reduction in overweight and obese young adults: a randomized controlled trial, *Arch Intern Med* 166(14):1466, 2006.

Mendoza JA, Drewnowski A, Christakis DA: Dietary energy density is associated with obesity and the metabolic syndrome in U.S. adults, *Diabetes Care* 30(4):974, 2007.

Mota J et al: Relationships between physical activity, obesity and meal frequency in adolescents, *Ann Hum Biol* 35(1):1, 2008.

National Center for Health Statistics (NCHS): Prevalence of overweight and obesity among adults: United States. 2003-2004. Available at http://www.cdc.gov/nchs/products/pubs/pubd/hestats/overweight/overwght_adult_03.htm. Accessed March 9, 2008.

National Institutes of Health (NIH), National Heart, Lung, and Blood Institute (NHLBI), North American Association for the Study of Obesity (NAASO): *The practical guide: identification, evaluation, and treatment of overweight and obesity in adults,* Washington, DC, 2000, National Institutes of Health (NIH).

Nebeling L et al: Weight cycling and immunocompetence, *J Am Dietet Assoc* 104:892, 2004.

Nordmann et al: Effects of low-carbohydrate vs low-fat diets on weight loss and cardiovascular risk factors: a meta-analysis of randomized controlled trials, *Arch Intern Med* 166(3):285, 2006.

O'Rahilly S: Human obesity and insulin resistance: lessons from experiments of nature, *Biochem Soc Trans* 35(pt 1):33, 2007.

Patel SR, Hu FB: Short sleep duration and weight gain: a systematic review, *Obesity (Silver Spring)* 16(3):643, 2008.

Phelan S et al: Are the eating and exercise habits of successful weight losers changing? *Obesity (Silver Spring)* 14(4):710, 2006.

Raynor DA et al: Television viewing and long-term weight maintenance: results from the National Weight Control Registry, *Obesity (Silver Spring)* 14(10):1816, 2006.

Rhezak P et al: Weight change, weight cycling and mortality in the ERFORT Male Cohort Study, *Eur J Epidemiol* 22(10):665, 2007.

Shields M: Overweight and obesity among children and youth, *Health Rep* 17(3):27, 2006.

Simkin-Silverman LR et al: Lifestyle intervention can prevent weight gain during menopause: results from a 5-year randomized clinical trial, *Ann Behav Med* 26(3):212, 2003.

St-Onge MP, Keller KL, Heymsfield SB: Changes in childhood food consumption patterns: a cause for concern in light of increasing body weights, *Am J Clin Nutr* 78:1068, 2003.

Tjepkema M: Adult obesity, *Health Rep* 17(3):9, 2006.

Truby H et al: Randomised controlled trial of four commercial weight loss programmes in the UK: initial findings from the BBC "diet trials," *BMJ* 332(7553):1309, 2006.

Tsai AG, Wadden TA: The evolution of very-low-calorie diets: an update and meta-analysis, *Obesity (Silver Spring)* 14(8):1283, 2006.

U.S. Department of Health and Human Services (USDHHS) and U.S. Department of Agriculture (USDA): *Dietary guidelines for Americans, 2005*, ed 6, Washington, DC, 2005, U.S. Government Printing Office.

Walker LO: Managing excessive weight gain during pregnancy and the postpartum period, *J Obstet Gynecol Neonatal Nurs* 36(5):490, 2007.

Wannamethee SG, Shaper AG, Walker M. Weight change, weight fluctuation, and mortality, *Arch Intern Med* 162:2575, 2002..

Warner ML et al: Soda consumption and overweight status of 2-year-old Mexican-American children in California, *Obesity (Silver Spring)* 14(11):1966, 2006.

Young LR, Nestle M: Portion sizes and obesity: responses of fast-food companies, *J Public Health Policy* 28(2):238, 2007.

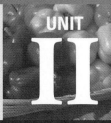

NUTRITION SUPPORT

Nutrition support is the use of oral, enteral, or parenteral feedings as a part of the therapeutic regimen. **Enteral feedings** are those given into the gastrointestinal (GI) tract, either by mouth or by tube. **Parenteral**, or intravenous, **feedings** may be given through a central venous catheter or peripheral vein. Parenteral feedings seem to be most beneficial in patients who are malnourished (Jeejeebhoy, 2007). In critically ill patients with intact GI tracts, enteral feedings reduce the risk of infection compared with parenteral feedings (Dhaliwal and Heyland, 2005). Enteral feedings also have at least a theoretic advantage in stimulating GI immune tissue and hormone release and in allowing nutrients to reach the liver by means of the portal vein, the physiologic route of delivery (Genton and Kudsk, 2003; Deacon, 2005). Patients who cannot tolerate sufficient nutrients through the enteral route often receive a combination of the two types of feedings. The choice of route and type of nutrition support should be based on the individual patient's needs. Figure II-1 shows an example of a decision tree that might be used for determining the appropriate form of nutrition support. Whichever route of nutrient delivery is used, overfeeding and hyperglycemia are associated with an increased risk of complications and should be avoided (Jeejeebhoy, 2007).

Nutrition support is a specialized treatment modality, and multidisciplinary nutrition support services or teams operating in an evidenced-based manner deliver this treatment in the safest, most efficacious, and most cost-effective manner (Schneider, 2006). The teams often include one or more physicians, nurses, dietitians, and pharmacists (and sometimes other professionals, such as physical therapists and social workers) with advanced skills in nutrition assessment and delivery of nutrition support.

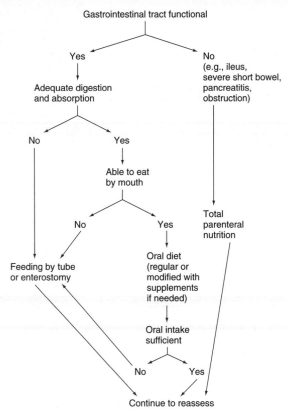

Figure II-1

Determining the optimal form of nutrition support. Caregivers continually reassess the individual and change the type of nutrition support as needed.

REFERENCES

Deacon CF: What do we know about the secretion and degradation of incretin hormones? *Regul Pept* 128(2):117, 2005.

Dhaliwal R, Heyland DK: Nutrition and infection in the intensive care unit: what does the evidence show? *Curr Opin Crit Care* 11(5):461, 2005.

Genton L, Kudsk KA: Interactions between the enteric nervous system and the immune system: role of neuropeptides and nutrition, *Am J Surg* 186(3):253, 2003.

Jeejeebhoy KN: Enteral nutrition versus parenteral nutrition—the risks and benefits, *Nat Clin Pract Gastroenterol Hepatol* 4(5):260, 2007.

Schneider PJ: Nutrition support teams: an evidence-based practice, *Nutr Clin Pract* 21(1):62, 2006.

ENTERAL NUTRITION

Enteral nutrition refers to the use of the gastrointestinal (GI) tract to provide nutrients. Enteral feedings can be supplied in one of three ways: (1) diets of regular or modified foods delivered orally; (2) nutritional supplements given by mouth; and (3) tube feedings.

Modified Diets

Modified diets are used by individuals with specific difficulties in consuming, digesting, absorbing, or metabolizing foods usually included in regular, unmodified diets. Some typical modified diets are summarized in Appendix J on Evolve. Additional information is given in the chapters in Unit III.

Oral Supplements

Oral supplements are useful for individuals who can digest and absorb nutrients. They are most effective for people who are consuming some foods but cannot take in enough because of anorexia or increased metabolic demands resulting from trauma, burns, infection, or other causes.

Types of Supplements

Some individuals prefer home-prepared foods, such as shakes and eggnogs. Commercial formulas, or medical nutrition products, that contain protein, carbohydrates, fat, vitamins, and minerals may also be used and may be more appropriate for individuals requiring dietary modification (Table 8-1). Some medical nutrition products are available in the form of fortified bars, soups, frozen desserts, cookies, cereals, or puddings.

Modular products (Table 8-2) providing specific nutrients (usually carbohydrates, lipids, or protein) can be added to foods such as cooked or dry cereals, mashed potatoes, applesauce,

Text continued on p. 229

Table 8-1 Enteral Feeding Products*

Product and Manufacturer	kcal/ml	Osmolality (mOsm/kg H₂0)	Pro/CHO/Fat (g/L)	Free Water (ml/L)	Approximate ml Needed to Meet Vitamin/Mineral DV†
Polymeric Products					
Oral Supplements for Clear Liquid Diets					
Boost Breeze[4]	1.06	750	46/216/0	784	‡
Enlive![1]	1.25	825	42/272/0	800	‡
Hormel Solutions Nutritional Juice Drink[3]	1.1	NA	34/254/0	NA	‡
Carnation Instant Breakfast Juice Drink[4]	1.0	990	39/236/0	812	‡
Standard Oral Supplements					
Boost Drink[4§]	1.01	610-670	42/171/17	833	1180
Boost Plus[4]	1.52	630-670	58/187/58	771	946
Carnation Instant Breakfast Lactose Free[4]	1.0	480-490	35/131/36	840	2100
Ensure[1¶]	1.06	590-600	36/160/24	800	948
Ensure Plus[1]	1.5	680	54/208/46	750	1185
Great Shake[3]	1.7	NA	51/186/85	720	‡
NuBasics Plus Drink[4]	1.5	620	52/176/65	720	1400
Resource Support[4]	1.5	800	87/175/50	762	‡

Calorie-Dense Formulas (2 kcal/ml or More) for Oral Feeding Unless Otherwise Stated

Carnation Instant Breakfast Lactose Free VHC[4]	2.25	950	90/197/122	672	‡
MedPass 2.0[3]	2.0	NA	83/237/20	675	‡
Nutren 2.0[4] (tube feeding)	2.0	745	80/196/104	700	750
Plus-2 3 (contains lactose)	2.0	NA	75/183/100	NA	‡
Resource 2.0[4] (oral or tube feeding)	2.0	790	84/219/88	700	948
Resource Shake Plus[4] (contains lactose)	2.0	1430	62/287/67	654	‡
TwoCal HN[1] (oral or tube feeding)	2.0	725	84/218/91	700	948

Standard Formulas, Primarily for Tube Feeding

Fibersource[1§]	1.2	490	43/170/39	814	1165
Fibersource HN[1§]	1.2	490	53/160/39	814	1165
Isocal[4]	1.06	270	34/135/44	840	1890
Isocal HN[4]	1.06	270	44/124/45	850	1180
Isosource[4]	1.2	490	43/170/39	819	1165
Isosource HN[4]	1.2	490	53/160/39	818	1165
Jevity[1§]	1.06	300	44/155/35	835	1321
Jevity 1.5[1§]	1.5	525	64/216/50	760	1000
Nutren 1.0[4]	1.0	315-370	40/127/38	850	1500
Nutren 1.5 Fiber[4§]	1.5	475-600	60/169/68	760	1000
Nutren ProBalance[4§]	1.2	350-450	54/156/41	810	1000
Osmolite[1]	1.0	300	44/144/35	842	1321

Continued

Table 8-1 Enteral Feeding Products*—cont'd

Product and Manufacturer	kcal/ml	Osmolality (mOsm/kg H₂O)	Pro/CHO/Fat (g/L)	Free Water (ml/L)	Approximate ml Needed to Meet Vitamin/Mineral DV†
Osmolite 1.5[1]	1.5	525	63/204/49	762	1000
Ultracal[1§]	1.06	300	45/142/39	830	1120
Elemental and Semielemental Formulas for Tube Feeding					
Crucial[4]	1.5	490	94/134/68	770	1000
Impact[4]	1.0	375	56/130/28	853	1500
Optimental[1]	1.0	540	51/139/28	832	1432
Peptamen[4]	1.0	270	40/127/39	850	1500
Peptamen AF[4§]	1.2	390	76/107/55	810	1500
Peptinex 1.0[4]	1.0	320	50/160/17	828	1500
Peptinex DT[4§]	1.0	460-550	50/164/17	830	1500
Perative[1§]	1.3	460	67/180/37	790	1155
Vital HN[1]	1.0	500	42/185/11	867	1500
Vivonex T.E.N.[4]	1.0	630	38/210/3	853	2000

Disease- or Condition-Specific Formulas

Diabetes Formulas

Boost Diabetic[4]§	1.06	400	58/84/49	847	1180
Diabetisource AC[4]§	1.2	450	60/100/59	818	1250
Glucerna[1]§	1.0	355	42/96/54	853	1420
Glucerna Select[1]§	1.0	470	50/96/54	839	1420
Mighty Shakes No Sugar Added[3]	1.7	NA	58/167/83	NA	‡
Nutren Glytrol[4]§	1.0	280	45/100/48	840	1400
Resource Diabetishield (clear liquid)[4]	0.63	380	29/125/0	890	‡

Renal Formulas

Nepro[1]§	1.8	585	81/167/96	725	948
Novasource Renal[4]	2.0	700	74/200/100	709	1000
Nutren Renal[4]	2.0	650	70/205/104	700	750
RenalCal[4]	2.0	600	34/290/82	700	1000
Suplena[1]§	1.8	600	45/205/96	735	948

Pulmonary Formulas

Novosource Pulmonary[4]	2.0	700	74/200/100	709	1000
Oxepa[1]	1.5	535	63/105/94	785	946
Pulmocare[1]	1.5	475	63/106/93	785	947

Continued

Table 8-1   Enteral Feeding Products[*]—cont'd

Product and Manufacturer	kcal/ml	Osmolality (mOsm/kg H_2O)	Pro/CHO/Fat (g/L)	Free Water (ml/L)	Approximate ml Needed to Meet Vitamin/ Mineral DV[†] Comments
Critical Care/Surgery/Wound Healing Formulas					
Impact Advanced recovery[4][§]	1.4	930-1000	76/190/39	772	[‡]
Impact Glutamine[4][§]	1.3	630	78/150/43	808	1000
IsoSource VHN[4][§]	1.0	300	62/130/29	847	1250
Nutren Replete[4][¶]	1.0	300-350	62/113/34	845	1000
Pivot 1.5 Cal[1][§]	1.5	595	94/172/51	759	1000
Promote[1][¶]	1.0	340	62/130/26	839	1000
Pediatric Formulations	kcal/ml	Osmolality (mOsm/ kg H_2O)	Pro/CHO/Fat (g/100 kcal)	Free Water (ml/L)	Comments
Elemental Infant Formulas (<12 mo)					
EleCare[5] (unflavored)	0.67	350	3.1/10.7/4.8	895	Oral or tube
Enfamil Pregestimil with MCT[6]	0.67	280	2.8/10.2/5.6	895	

Children 1-10 yr

Oral Formulas

Enfamil Kindercal[6]¶	1.06	440-520	30/135/44	850	
NutriPals Balanced Nutrition Drink[1]	0.62	NA	29/79/21	NA	
Pediasure[1]	1.0	480-560	30/131/38	845	Oral or tube
Resource Just for Kids[4]¶	1.0	390-440	30/110/50	853	Oral or tube
Resource Just for Kids 1.5 Cal[4]¶	1.5	390	42/165/75	720	Oral or tube

Standard Formulas for Tube Feeding

Nutren Junior[4]¶	1.0	350	30/110/50	850	Tube or oral
Pediasure Enteral[1]¶	1.0	335	30/133/40	854	Tube or oral

Elemental Formulas Primarily for Tube Feeding

Neocate One +[7]	1.0	610	2.5/14.6/3.5	800
Pediatric Peptinex DT[4]¶	1.0	290	30/138/39	852
Peptamen Junior[4]¶	1.0	260	30/138/38	850
Vivonex Pediatric[4]	0.8	360	24/130/24	893

DV, Daily Value; *NA*, not available.

Manufacturers: [1] Abbott Laboratories, [2] Axcan Pharma, [3] Hormel Health Labs, [4] Nestle Nutrition, [5] Ross Products, [6] Mead Johnson Nutritionals, [7] SHS North America. This is only a representative listing of the many products available and is not meant to imply endorsement of any product. Products are lactose free unless indicated otherwise.

† Daily values are for adults, unless the product is specified for children.

‡ Not intended as a total feeding.

§ Fiber containing.

¶ Available in an essentially identical form with fiber.

Table 8-2   Modular Components for Enteral Feeding
(Oral or Tube)

Type of Module	Nutrient Content	
	Protein (g) per g Powder (except as noted)	Kcal/g Powder (except as noted)
Protein		
Beneprotein[1]	0.9	3.6
ProPass[2]	0.8	3.8
Pro-Stat 64[3]	0.5/ml*	2.0/ml*
Unjury (unflavored)[4]	0.9	3.5
Protein and Carbohydrate		
HiProCal[2]	0.4	3.7
Protein, Carbohydrate, and Fat		
Multimix[2]	0.4	3.8
ProNutra[5]	0.5	3.7
Carbohydrate		
Polycose powder[6]	—	3.8
Polycose liquid[6]	—	2/ml*
	Fat (g/ml)	Kcal/ml
Fat		
Benecalorie[1]†	0.7*	7.0*
Epulor[7]	0.8*	7.0*
MCT oil[1]‡	0.9*	7.7* (or 8.3/g)
Microlipid[1]	0.5l*	4.5*
	Total Fiber per g or ml Product	Kcal/g or ml
Fiber		
Benefiber[1]	0.8 g/g powder	3.2/g powder
FiberBasics Instant Soluble Fiber[2]	0.9 g/g powder	3.8/g powder
Fiber-Stat[3]	0.4 g/ml*	1.1 g/ml*

Manufacturers: [1]Nestle, [2]Hormel Health Labs, [3]Medical Nutrition USA, [4]Prosynthesis, [5]NuMedTec, [6]Abbott, [7]VistaPharm.
*Liquid product; values are expressed per milliliter.
†Not intended for tube feeding.
‡Does not contain essential fatty acids, which are required nutrients.

juices, tea, coffee, shakes, soups, salad dressings, and sandwich fillings. Modular carbohydrates are especially versatile because they can be added to many soft foods or liquids without altering their flavor or texture. Modular products are especially useful for enhancing the protein and/or energy provided by infant formulas.

Delivery of Oral Supplements

Liquid supplements are best tolerated if consumed slowly, taking 180 to 360 ml over 15 to 45 minutes. Liquid supplements contain readily digested carbohydrate. As a result, they can cause **dumping syndrome**, with abdominal cramping, weakness, tachycardia, and diarrhea, if they are consumed rapidly. Most liquid supplements taste best if they are chilled or served over ice. Fat is an important energy source; supplements containing at least a moderate amount of fat ($\approx$ 30% of energy) are desirable unless contraindicated or poorly tolerated, as with acute pancreatitis or massive small bowel resection.

Enteral Tube Feedings

Enteral tube feedings may be needed for the following reasons (Smith and Elia, 2006):

■ Inability to consume adequate food because of mechanical problems with eating, psychologic disorders, or unconsciousness. Tube feedings may be used to supplement or replace oral feedings; examples include head and neck tumors, esophageal stricture or obstruction, coma, anorexia of chronic illness, anorexia nervosa, hyperemesis gravidarum, neurologic disorders interfering with swallowing, and premature birth with inefficient suckling or uncoordinated suck and swallow.

■ Increased nutritional requirements that are not met by oral feedings alone; examples include severe trauma and burns. Infants with congenital heart disease might also need supplemental tube feedings.

■ Maldigestion or malabsorption requiring unpalatable modified formulas or making continuous feedings necessary to maintain adequate nutritional status; examples include pancreatic or biliary insufficiency, short bowel syndrome, inflammatory bowel disease, and protracted diarrhea with malnutrition.

Types of Tube Feeding Formulas

Polymeric or intact protein formulas

When the GI tract is functional, nutritionally complete **polymeric formulas** can be used (see Table 8-1). These contain proteins such as casein or lactalbumin; carbohydrates in the form of sugars, hydrolyzed starches, or dextrins; and varying amounts of fat. Most commercially prepared formulas are lactose free because lactose intolerance is common among adults, especially individuals of African, Native American/First Nation, or Asian descent, as well as individuals with malabsorption.

The ratio of energy to protein (nitrogen) content is one consideration in choosing a formula. The optimal ratio in healthy adults is approximately 150 nonprotein kcal to 1 g of nitrogen, and most standard commercial formulas provide approximately this ratio. In critically ill and metabolically stressed individuals, nitrogen needs are increased, and the ratio is reduced (Shils et al., 2006). In children the ratio is higher than in adults to provide the energy needed for growth. Adults with renal and hepatic failure may also need a higher ratio to ensure that adequate fat and carbohydrate are available to meet energy needs, so that the nitrogen in the feeding is available for tissue synthesis.

Fiber is included in some polymeric formulas. Insoluble forms of fiber, such as wheat bran and psyllium, increase the fecal mass and reduce the likelihood of constipation. Soluble fibers such as gums and pectin decrease serum cholesterol and postprandial blood glucose concentrations. Also, some of the soluble fiber is fermented to short-chain fatty acids by colonic bacteria. The short-chain fatty acids are absorbed along with sodium and water in the colon, possibly reducing the likelihood of diarrhea (Wiesen et al., 2006).

The form of fat in the formula can be an important factor determining tolerance of the feeding. The fat in polymeric formulas is usually in the form of vegetable oils or a combination of vegetable oils and **medium-chain triglycerides (MCTs)**. MCTs contain fatty acids 8 to 12 carbons in length. They are used as a calorie source because they are easily digested and absorbed compared with the long-chain triglycerides (LCTs) found in vegetable oils. MCTs do not include the essential fatty acids, so formulas provide at least a small amount of fat (approximately 3% of total energy intake) in the form of long-chain essential fatty acids.

Fat digestion and absorption

Fat is a key nutrient to consider when planning enteral feedings for the patient with impaired digestion or absorption. Absorption of fat (see Figure 1-3), particularly fat in the form of LCTs, requires the following factors:

■ *Lipase*: LCTs are too large and too insoluble in the watery intestinal secretions to be absorbed intact. Usually the two outer fatty acids are removed, leaving the inner fatty acid attached to glycerol and creating a monoglyceride (one fatty acid attached to glycerol). Lipases released in the mouth and the stomach may be important in infancy. Much of the fat digestion in adults and older children is performed by lipase released by the pancreas, however. Release of pancreatic lipase is likely to be low in individuals with cystic fibrosis, **pancreatitis,** and other diseases affecting exocrine pancreatic function. Because MCTs are smaller and more water miscible than LCTs, lipase activity is less important with MCTs.

■ *Bile salts*: Bile salts (produced in the liver and stored in the gallbladder) combine with fatty acids and monoglycerides to form **micelles**, forming an emulsion of the fats with the digestive secretions in the bowel. Bile salts can cause micelle formation because they have both water-soluble and fat-soluble components. The fatty acids and the fat-soluble part of the bile salt are in the center of the micelle, and the water-soluble portion of the bile salt and the glycerol portion of the monoglycerides are on the outer part of the micelle. Long-chain fatty acids are relatively insoluble in water, but by forming an emulsion with the bile salts, their solubility is improved enough to allow them to pass through the unstirred water layer that lies just over the intestinal mucosal cells. Because medium-chain fatty acids are smaller and more soluble in water than long-chain fats, they do not require thorough micelle formation to pass through the unstirred water layer.

■ *Bowel surface area for absorption*: The jejunum is responsible for much of the fat absorption, and the ileum is needed for bile salt reabsorption. Reabsorbed bile salts are returned to the liver for reuse. Conditions such as surgical removal of the jejunum, inflammatory bowel disease, or radiation damage to the bowel can interfere with fat absorption. Ileal resection or damage impairs bile salt reabsorption and can deplete the body's pool of bile salts. Because absorption of MCTs is less dependent on bile salts than absorption of LCTs, MCTs can be useful in treating fat malabsorption that occurs when bowel surface area is diminished.

In addition, LCTs must be formed into chylomicrons (including a protein coating and a lipid core) inside the intestinal cell and extruded into the lymphatic circulation. The absorption of MCTs is more similar to the absorption of protein and carbohydrate than it is to the absorption of LCTs. Not only is micelle formation less important for MCTs than for LCTs, but also MCTs do not have to be packaged as chylomicrons in order to be soluble enough to enter the circulation. The majority of fatty acids from MCTs are released directly from the intestinal cells into the portal vein blood, just as the amino acids and monosaccharides are, instead of entering the lymph system with the LCTs.

Elemental (predigested) formulas

Many individuals with maldigestion and malabsorption tolerate polymeric formulas, particularly those containing MCTs; however, those with severe impairment of digestion and absorption may require **elemental** or **predigested formulas** (see Table 8-1). Elemental formulas are either very low in fat or provide much of their fat in the form of MCTs to improve fat absorption, and elemental formulas contain protein hydrolysates (partially hydrolyzed or digested proteins), peptides (short chains of amino acids), and/or free (crystalline) amino acids. Free amino acids and small peptides are absorbed by different mechanisms, and thus having both components in a formula might improve absorption. Elemental formulas are more expensive than the polymeric ones. They are appropriate for selected patients with short bowel syndrome or other malabsorptive disorders, such as pancreatitis, severe enteropathy associated with acquired immunodeficiency syndrome (AIDS), and inflammatory bowel disease.

Disease- or condition-specific formulas

Specialized formulas have been developed for many different disease or metabolic conditions, including AIDS, glucose intolerance or diabetes, hepatic encephalopathy, pulmonary disease, renal failure, trauma and critical illness, and wound healing. It is important to evaluate patients carefully to determine whether there is a real need for a specialized product. These condition-specific products can be characterized in the following manner:

- *AIDS and severe malabsorption*: Concentrated in energy, low in fat or high in MCT to reduce fat malabsorption. These formulas are typically taken by mouth and thus are flavored.
- *Glucose intolerance*: Fiber containing (10 to 15 g/L) to help reduce the blood glucose response to feeding; high in monounsaturated fatty acids and low in saturated fat. These formulas are high in fat (40% to 49% of total energy) and moderate to low in carbohydrate (30% to 45% of energy). In comparison, the American Diabetes Association (ADA) (2004) recommends that most diabetic individuals consume a diet supplying less than 30% fat, with 55% to 60% of energy as carbohydrate. However, these recommendations are primarily intended for individuals eating a diet of regular foods, where high-fat diets are likely to be associated with excessive energy, cholesterol, and saturated fat intake. In the formulas for glucose intolerance, monounsaturated fat and carbohydrate together provide approximately 60% to 70% of total energy, the saturated fat content is low, and protein provides 15% to 20%, consistent with the recommendations (ADA, 2004) for diabetic individuals without renal failure. Individualized assessment is required to determine whether these formulas meet the needs of a patient with renal impairment. Also, it might be necessary to choose a formula with a lower fat content for patients with gastroparesis, because high-fat diets can worsen the delay in gastric emptying in individuals with this disorder (Hasler, 2007).
- *Hepatic encephalopathy*: Concentrated in energy to allow fluid restriction, low protein (11% to 15% of total energy), high in branched-chain amino acids (approximately 50% of the protein equivalent vs. the 20% in standard formulas) and low in aromatic amino acids and methionine, low in sodium, low to moderate in fat (13% to 27%) to compensate for impaired fat absorption. These formulas are not indicated for patients without encephalopathy.
- *Pulmonary disease*: Concentrated in energy to allow fluid restriction; moderate to low in carbohydrate to reduce carbon dioxide production; contain MCT to enhance fat absorption; fortified with antioxidants (vitamins A, C, beta-carotene, and possibly selenium) to reduce oxidative damage during oxygen therapy.

Although carbohydrate does result in greater carbon dioxide production than fat, excessive energy intake is a greater risk for carbon dioxide production than a high-carbohydrate diet. Oxepa, a specialized product for patients with acute respiratory distress syndrome (ARDS), contains increased levels of omega-3 fatty acids and antioxidants. In clinical trials this product appeared to have benefit for ARDS patients (Bongers and Griffiths, 2006).

- *Renal disease*: Concentrated in energy to allow fluid restriction; products for use predialysis are low in protein (6% to 7% of total energy) with emphasis on essential amino acids, and products for use during dialysis are moderate in protein (approximately 14% to 15% of total energy); moderate to low in vitamins A and D and high in folic acid and vitamin B_6; restricted in sodium, potassium, phosphorus, and magnesium; contain carnitine to improve fat metabolism. Protein status of patients should be carefully evaluated because the renal formulas may be inadequate in protein for some dialysis patients.

- *Surgery, trauma, stress, and critical illness*: High protein (>20% of total energy intake), low nonprotein kilocalorie/nitrogen ratio. These formulas are generally enriched in antioxidants and nutrients especially important in healing (including some or all of the following: vitamins A, C, and E; beta-carotene; selenium; zinc) and may contain increased levels of branched-chain amino acids, glutamine, and omega-3 fatty acids, as well as nucleotides. Immune-enhancing formulas are usually enriched in arginine, as well as constituents previously listed. They contain low levels of omega-6 fatty acids, which have proinflammatory properties. It has been difficult to identify benefits of "stress formulas" for surgical and critical care patients in general, perhaps because the patients are very heterogeneous and generally a specific formulation, rather than a single nutrient, has been tested (Heyland and Dhaliwal, 2005; Bongers and Griffiths, 2006). It appears that glutamine may have benefit for elective surgery patients and those who have experienced burns or trauma. However, arginine supplementation actually seems to increase mortality among septic patients.

- *Wound healing*: High protein, low nonprotein kilocalorie/ nitrogen ratio, enriched in arginine. Many contain fiber or other complex carbohydrates.

- *Presurgery and postsurgery*: Clear liquid nutritional supplements containing protein, vitamins, electrolytes, and minerals.

Other formula characteristics
Energy density and fluid content

Many formulas provide 1 kcal/ml because adults need approximately 1 ml of water per kilocalorie consumed, or about 30 ml/kg/day. However, energy-dense formulas containing 1.5 to 2 kcal/ml are available for individuals needing fluid restrictions. The hydration status of patients receiving these concentrated formulas must be closely monitored, with more free water given as required.

Table 8-3 provides a guideline for calculating fluid requirements for maintenance needs; these must be adjusted based on estimated losses from sources such as wounds, ostomies, vomiting, diarrhea, and GI drainage. Careful intake and output records are essential in estimation of these losses. Intermittent fever does not alter fluid requirements very much, but prolonged fever increases fluid needs about 12% for every degree above 37° C (or 7% for every degree above 98.6° F). If a deficit in fluid intake occurs in adults and adolescents, the volume of replacement fluid needed (in addition to that needed for maintenance) can be calculated from the ratio of the normal serum sodium concentration (approximately 140 mEq/L [140 mmol/L]) to the patient's actual serum sodium, as follows:

Fluid deficit in liters = 0.6 × Body weight (kg) − [(Normal serum sodium/Patient sodium) × 0.6 × Body weight (kg)]

Table 8-3   Maintenance Fluid and Electrolyte Requirements*

Infants, Children, and Adults	Water (ml)	Na+ (mEq/kg)†	K+ (mEq/kg)†
Infants/ Children		2-4	1-3
≤10 kg	100/kg		
11-20 kg	1000 + 50/kg over 10 kg		
>20 kg	1500 + 20/kg over 20 kg		
Adults	1500 + 20/kg over 20 kg	2-3	2-3

*Must be increased when losses are greater than normal.
†1 mEq Na (sodium) = 23 mg; 1 mEq K (potassium) = 39 mg.

In infants and young children, the most accurate method of estimating fluid deficit is by weight loss:

Fluid deficit in liters = Usual weight (kg) − Present weight (kg)

Where the usual weight is unavailable or unclear, clinical signs (see Table 2-7) can be used for estimation of the amount of fluid deficit.

Osmolality

Osmolality refers to the number of osmotically active particles per kilogram of water in a solution. A formula is considered to be isotonic or isosmolar if its osmolality is similar to that of plasma (approximately 300 mOsm/kg). It is hypertonic or hyperosmolar if its osmolality is greater than that of plasma. It was once thought that hyperosmolar solutions were a common cause of diarrhea. For this reason, formulas were diluted to quarter or half strength when tube feedings were initiated, and the strength was gradually increased. Evidence now indicates that hyperosmolality by itself is unlikely to cause diarrhea and use of diluted formula only delays the delivery of adequate nutrients to the patient (Edes et al., 1990; Heimburger et al., 1994; Wiesen et al., 2006). In some patients with other causes for diarrhea, use of a hyperosmolar formula might worsen diarrhea, however.

Nonnutritive components of formulas

The normal gut flora is altered during serious illness and during the use of antibiotics, and this makes the patient more vulnerable to diarrhea and possibly to systemic infections. A number of nonnutritive components are added to formulas in an effort to support the growth of beneficial bacteria, which help to control the growth of pathogenic bacteria in the gut. Probiotics are preparations supplying beneficial bacteria, such as bifidobacteria or lactobacilli. Prebiotics are substances such as soluble fibers and similar carbohydrates (e.g., oligofructose) that are fermented by gut bacteria and stimulate the growth of beneficial bacterial species. Synbiotics are a combination of probiotics and prebiotics (Wiesen et al., 2006).

Feeding Tubes

Routes for tube feedings

Tube feedings may be given into the esophagus, stomach, or small intestine. Figure 8-1 illustrates the gastric and intestinal locations. Nasogastric (NG) and nasoduodenal (ND)/nasojejunal (NJ) tubes are

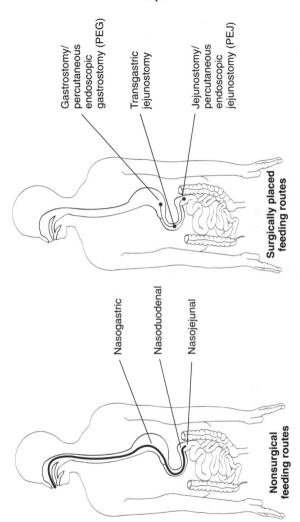

Figure 8-1
Types of enteral feeding routes.
(From Rolin Graphics. In Grodner M, Long S, Walkingshaw BC: *Foundations and clinical applications of nutrition: a nursing approach*, ed 4, St Louis, 2007, Mosby.)

often used for short-term feedings; and esophagostomy, gastrostomy, and jejunostomy are frequently chosen for long-term feedings. Percutaneous endoscopic gastrostomies (PEGs) are especially popular.

Nasogastric tubes (or orogastric in infants)

Advantages: tube easily inserted; allows use of almost all the GI tract; suited to intermittent feedings

Disadvantages: tube easily dislodged, especially with altered sensorium; potential for pulmonary aspiration and for development of sinusitis and otitis media

Nasoduodenal or nasojejunal tubes

Advantages: theoretically decrease the likelihood of pulmonary aspiration, although clinical investigations to date have not found conclusive evidence of a significant benefit of small bowel feedings in prevention of aspiration (Ho et al., 2006; Kattelmann et al., 2006); useful in individuals with delayed gastric emptying; allow for simultaneous gastric decompression and small bowel feeding

Disadvantages: more difficult to insert tube than NG; bypasses the stomach, a barrier to infection; usually necessitates continuous feedings given with a pump; can cause dumping syndrome; tube easily dislodged; potential for development of sinusitis and otitis media

Gastrostomy

Advantages: more difficult to dislodge tube than NG; usually has a larger diameter than NG, allowing use of more viscous formulas (e.g., home blended); easily hidden by clothing (and gastric button device fits flush against the skin, with no tube protruding except during feedings); conventional surgical gastrostomies can bypass esophageal obstruction, but placement of PEG tubes requires a patent esophagus; a jejunostomy tube can be inserted through a gastrostomy

Disadvantages: potential for irritation and erosion of skin around insertion site; bleeding and infection of the insertion site (usually in the immediate postinsertion period)

Jejunostomy

Advantages: same as for ND/NJ; can bypass upper GI obstruction; more difficult to dislodge tube than with ND/NJ; can be inserted percutaneously

Disadvantages: potential for erosion of skin around insertion site from leakage of intestinal contents, which contain digestive enzymes; bypasses the stomach, a barrier to infection; usually requires continuous feedings given through a pump; feedings can cause dumping syndrome; bleeding and infection of the insertion site (usually in the immediate postinsertion period)

Selection of feeding tubes

Nonreactive tubes are soft, nonirritating tubes made of polyurethane, silicone rubber, or similar materials. Tubes for NG and ND/NJ feedings range in size from 5 to 12 French (F) (1F ≈ 0.34 mm). Stylets are available to facilitate insertion of many of these pliable tubes. Nonreactive tubes can be left in place for several weeks without stiffening.

Insertion of nasogastric and nasoduodenal/nasojejunal tubes (Figure 8-2)

1. Select an appropriately sized tube. Generally, 8F tubes, sometimes called "small-bore" or "fine-bore," are suitable for adults and children. If thick fluids are to be used, then a 10F to 12F tube may be needed. Most infants can use 6F or 8F tubes, but premature infants may need 5F tubes.
2. Explain the procedure to the individual. Patients may be reassured by the information that tube insertion is not painful, although it may cause gagging. Have the person sit up, if possible, and lean the head forward. If not contraindicated, lidocaine spray for the throat makes tube insertion more comfortable.
3. Mark the length of tube to be inserted. For adults the following equation is a guide to the appropriate length of tube:

   Length for NG insertion = ([Nose to ear to xiphoid process
   measurement (cm) − 50 cm] ÷ 2) + 50 cm

   For children, one suggested method is as follows:

   Length for NG insertion = 6.7 + 0.226 (Height in cm)
   + 3 cm + Distance from distal tip to feeding pores on tube (cm)

4. Lubricate the tip of the tube with water-soluble lubricant. Gently advance the tube through the nostril parallel to the roof of the mouth and then down the esophagus. Inhalable nasal decongestants used before tube insertion can make the process more comfortable. The patient can help by sipping fluids, unless

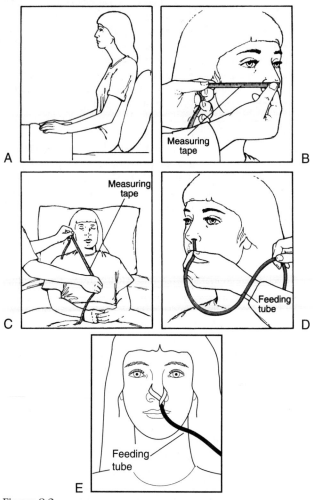

Figure 8-2
Insertion of a feeding tube. **A,** Place the patient in Fowler position before tube insertion, if possible, so that gravity can facilitate passage of the tube. **B** and **C,** Measure the distance nose to ear and then to xiphoid process, and calculate length of tube needed. **D,** Encourage patient to sip fluids or chew ice chips while the tube is gently advanced. **E,** Tape tube securely in place.
(**A** to **D** from Beare PG, Myers JL, editors: *Principles and practice of adult health nursing*, St Louis, 1990, Mosby. **E** redrawn from Beare PG, Myers JL, editors: *Principles and practice of adult health nursing*, St Louis, 1990, Mosby.)

they are contraindicated, or swallowing while the tube is being advanced.

5. If the individual begins to cough or choke during the insertion, the tube may be in the trachea. Remove it, and try again.

6. When the proper length of tube has been inserted, secure the tube to the nose with tape.

7. If ND/NJ placement is desired, insert a sufficient length of tubing (85 cm appears adequate for most adults). Prokinetic agents such as metoclopramide or erythromycin administered before beginning the insertion of the tube increase the likelihood that the tube will pass spontaneously through the pylorus. A variety of techniques have also been recommended by experienced practitioners, including rotating the tube slightly while advancing it gradually through the stomach, placing the individual in the right lateral decubitus position, insufflation of air into the stomach while advancing the tube, electromyogram, electrocardiogram, and use of an external magnet (Haslam and Fang, 2006). Fluoroscopic or endoscopic techniques may be used to place the tube.

8. Confirm tube placement before administering feedings.

Confirming tube placement

An abdominal radiograph is the recommended method for confirming initial tube placement before feedings are started, if the tube was not inserted using fluoroscopy or endoscopic guidance. Auscultation over the left upper quadrant of the abdomen while insufflating air through an NG tube is sometimes used, but this method cannot be recommended because of the potential for hearing air when the tube tip is positioned in the respiratory system (de Aguilar-Nascimento and Kudsk, 2007).

After the initial radiographic confirmation, methods to confirm that a tube remains in the correct position during the course of enteral feeding include the following:

■ *External length of feeding tube*. At the time the initial radiograph confirms that the tube is properly positioned, a marking should be placed on the tube where it exits the nose or mouth. If this marking subsequently is found to have moved a substantial amount external to its original location, this suggests tube displacement. In a small group of patients, an increase in external tube length more than 13 cm occurred when the tube moved and shifted from the small bowel to the stomach or from the stomach to the esophagus (Metheny et al., 2005). The distal end of the tube can move from the small bowel to the stomach and coil in the stomach without a change in external tube length, however.

- *pH of the tube aspirate.* A fall in pH from 7 or above to 5 or below, using pH paper, often indicates that the tube has moved from the small bowel to the stomach. A rise from pH 5 or below to 7 can indicate that the tube has moved from the stomach to the esophagus. The pH measurement can be combined with measurement of the aspirate bilirubin concentrations, using bilirubin-detecting test strips (Metheny et al., 2000). If pH is above 5 and bilirubin is less than 5 mg/dl, this indicates probable respiratory tract placement. A pH below 5 and bilirubin below 5 mg/dl indicate that the tube tip is in the stomach. A pH above 5 and bilirubin above 5 mg/dl indicate intestinal placement of the tube tip.

Delivery of tube feedings

Continuous feedings

Continuous feedings, feedings delivered over the entire day or some portion of the day (usually 10 to 12 hours), are used in certain circumstances:

- Duodenal or jejunal feedings because continuous feedings reduce the risk of dumping syndrome
- Decreased absorptive area (e.g., chronic diarrhea, short bowel syndrome, acute radiation enteritis, and severe malnutrition with atrophy of the villi) because continuous feedings may increase the total amount tolerated
- Some cases of severe stress with normal GI function. (Burn patients, for instance, have been found to have less diarrhea and more adequate intake if given continuous, rather than intermittent, feedings.)

Although continuous NG or gastrostomy feedings may be beneficial in certain situations, they keep the gastric pH continuously high and appear to increase the risk of pneumonia in very ill patients. The less acid gastric pH might allow increased growth of bacteria and yeast in the stomach, and these organisms can colonize the trachea and cause pneumonia. In addition, aspiration pneumonia related to reflux of feedings or gastric fluid is relatively common in seriously ill and elderly patients. Transpyloric feedings (delivered into the small bowel) have a theoretic advantage over intragastric feedings in reducing the risk of pulmonary aspiration, although clinical studies have not always found a decrease in aspiration with transpyloric vs. gastric feedings (Ho et al., 2006; Kattelmann et al., 2006; Metheny, 2006). To reduce the risk of pneumonia during tube feedings, use aseptic or scrupulously clean technique in administering tube feedings and administer feedings in closed feeding sets. Keep the patient in a semirecumbent position (head elevated 30 to 45 degrees) as much as possible. Patients who must remain flat in bed, such as those with head or neck injuries, are at risk of aspiration, as are those with neurologic deficits or those requiring sedation. During mechanical ventilation, the mouth and upper airway can become colonized with pathogenic organisms. Scrupulous mouth cleansing, as well as frequent or continual suctioning of subglottic secretions, reduces the risk of pneumonia.

It has long been thought that gastric residual volumes should be measured on a regular schedule; however, the nonreactive tubes tend to collapse when suction is applied to them and often do not yield accurate volumes. Moreover, regular measurement of residuals increases the likelihood of clogging the tube because gastric acid can coagulate the protein in the formula. Therefore measuring gastric residuals is currently undergoing critical examination by many clinicians. If residual volumes are measured, the tube should be thoroughly flushed with water afterward. The practice of stopping feedings for large residuals (defined in different ways in different institutions and by individual practitioners but generally at least 200 ml) interferes with adequate nutrient delivery. An occasional, isolated finding of large residuals is common even among patients who tolerate feedings well, although a trend toward consistently large residuals may indicate delayed gastric emptying caused by sepsis, poorly controlled hyperglycemia, or other clinical problems. Once the correctable causes of delayed gastric emptying have been addressed, use of prokinetic medications such as metoclopramide or erythromycin can be effective in improving feeding tolerance in patients who still exhibit problems. Transpyloric feedings stimulate gastric secretion and can result in large gastric volumes. Gastric decompression with a sump tube may be necessary during transpyloric feeding to reduce accumulation of gastric secretions and risk of pulmonary aspiration. Monitoring the patient frequently for gastric distention, bloating, and increase in abdominal girth is an important part of care. Accepting an isolated residual of 250 ml or more and carefully evaluating the clinical situation before stopping or holding feedings when there are repeated gastric residuals of 250 ml or more improve the adequacy of nutritional intake (Kattelmann et al., 2006).

Intermittent feedings

Feedings given every 2 to 4 hours are preferred for certain patients:

- Confused individuals who, if left unattended, are in danger of dislodging the tube
- Stable long-term patients, especially home patients, in whom continuous feedings interfere with normalization of lifestyle

Intermittent feedings are better tolerated if given by slow drip rather than by rapid bolus infusion. Usually 300 to 400 ml can be tolerated several times daily if each feeding is infused over at least 20 to 30 minutes. Abdominal discomfort, diarrhea, tachycardia, and nausea during or shortly after feedings signal that the flow is too rapid or the volume too large.

Promoting comfort

Comfort can be increased by the following methods:

- Encourage intake of food and fluids if not contraindicated. (Many people are initially afraid that they cannot eat while the tube is in place.)
- Provide adequate fluid. Most formulas for adults provide 1 kcal/ml. This may not provide adequate fluid for some patients. If the individual cannot drink fluid and is not fluid restricted, then provide extra water by tube. For example, irrigate the tube after each feeding or every 4 to 6 hours with 30 to 60 ml or more of water.
- Provide regular mouth care and stimulation of saliva flow. Important comfort measures include rinsing the mouth with water or mouthwash; brushing the teeth; sucking hard candy or chewing gum in moderation, if not contraindicated (particularly candy or gum containing xylitol or other sugar substitutes, to reduce the risk of dental caries); and gargling with warm saltwater to relieve sore throat.
- Use a nonreactive tube with the smallest possible diameter if the tube is placed through the nose, and secure the tube so that it does not move back and forth.

Assessing Response to Nutrition Support

Anthropometric measurements, physical assessment, and hematologic and biochemical measurements are used in assessing response to nutrition support. A thorough nutrition assessment should be performed as described in Chapter 2. Table 8-4 highlights common or especially serious responses to nutrition support.

Preventing and Correcting Complications of Enteral Nutrition

Enteral nutrition support is sometimes perceived as less risky than total parenteral nutrition, but tube feedings are associated with several serious and challenging complications. Measures for the prevention or correction of tube feeding complications are described in Table 8-5.

Malnourished individuals receiving either enteral or parenteral feedings are at risk of developing the **refeeding syndrome** (Kraft et al., 2005). One major contributor to the refeeding syndrome is hypophosphatemia. As muscle and fat are lost in starvation, fluid and minerals, including phosphorus, are also lost. During refeeding, especially with high-carbohydrate feedings, insulin levels rise and cellular uptake of glucose, water, phosphorus, potassium, and other nutrients is stimulated. Serum levels of phosphorus subsequently fall, which can lead to cardiac dysrhythmias; congestive heart failure; hemolysis; muscular weakness; seizures; acute respiratory failure; and a variety of other complications, including sudden death. Hypokalemia, hypomagnesemia, and vitamin (thiamin) deficiency may occur for similar reasons. Glucose intolerance and fluid overload often accompany the refeeding syndrome. Caregivers should be aware of patients who are at risk for refeeding syndrome, especially those with kwashiorkor or marasmus (see Chapter 2), anorexia nervosa, morbid obesity with recent massive weight loss, and prolonged fasting. In these individuals it is especially important to monitor blood levels of electrolytes, phosphorus, glucose, and magnesium carefully, particularly during the first week of refeeding; keep careful records of fluid intake and output; record weight daily; and monitor heart rate frequently. Severely malnourished patients are often bradycardic. With overfeeding and an increase in the intravascular volume, heart rate increases; a rate of 80 to 100 beats/min in a previously bradycardic patient may be a sign of significant cardiac stress.

Text continued on p. 251

Table 8-4   Assessing Response to Nutrition Support

Parameter	Frequency of Measurement*	Purpose/Comments
Anthropometric Measurements		
Weight	Daily	Indicator of efficacy and fluid status; patients should have steady gain or weight maintenance, as appropriate; use usual or IBW for guide to desirable weight; a gain of >0.1-0.2 kg (>0.25-0.5 lb)/day usually indicates fluid retention
Length or Height (pediatrics only)	Monthly	Indicator of efficacy; see growth charts (Appendix D on Evolve) for expected growth pattern
Physical Assessment		
Fluid Balance	Daily	Overhydration: check for edema of dependent body parts, shortness of breath, rales in lungs, fluid intake consistently > output; dehydration: look for poor skin turgor, dry mucous membranes, complaints of thirst, output > intake (measure stool volumes if liquid), >10% difference between blood pressure when lying and standing
GI Motility (tube-fed individuals) (i.e., presence of bowel sounds,	Every 2-4 hr during initiation of feedings; every 8 hr	Indicators of GI motility and feeding tolerance

	signs of abdominal distention, passage of flatus or stool, nausea or vomiting)	when stable	

Hematologic and Biochemical Measurements

Serum Glucose	3 times daily until stable, then 2-3/wk	Assess glucose tolerance; determine need to adjust infusion rate of enteral or parenteral feeding or administer insulin
Serum Electrolytes	Daily until stable, then 2-3/wk	Indicates need for modification of fluid/electrolyte intake
BUN	1-2/wk	Increased: inadequate fluid intake, renal impairment, or excessive protein intake; decreased: inadequate protein intake possible
Serum Ca, P, Mg	1-2/wk	Ensure stability; avoid refeeding syndrome
Complete Blood Count	1/wk	Indicator of adequacy of Fe, protein, folate, and vitamin B_{12}; see Chapter 2 for more information
Serum Triglycerides (during TPN)	After each ↑ in lipid dosage; 2-3/wk when stable	Elevated levels indicate inadequate lipid clearance and possibly a need for reduction in lipid dosage
Serum Transferrin or Prealbumin†	1/wk	Indicator of efficacy in maintaining or improving protein nutriture

BUN, Blood urea nitrogen; *Ca*, calcium; *Fe*, iron; *GI*, gastrointestinal; *IBW*, ideal body weight; *Mg*, magnesium; *P*, phosphorus; *TPN*, total parenteral nutrition.

*These are suggested frequencies only. Individual patients may need more or less frequent assessment. Stable home patients need laboratory analyses on a much less frequent schedule.

†Altered by the acute-phase reaction, overhydration or underhydration, renal or liver disease. Therefore they have limited value in critically ill patients or those with organ failure. However, they can be useful markers during nutritional rehabilitation.

Table 8-5   Management of Tube Feeding Complications

Complication	Possible Cause	Suggested Interventions
Pulmonary aspiration*	Feeding tube in esophagus or respiratory tract	Confirm proper placement of tube before administering any feeding; check tube placement at least every 4-8 hr during continuous feedings; consider intermittent feedings (Chen et al., 2006).
	Regurgitation of formula	Consider giving feeding into small bowel rather than stomach in high-risk patients; keep head elevated 30-45 degrees during feedings; stop feedings temporarily during treatments such as chest physiotherapy.
Diarrhea	Antibiotic therapy	Antidiarrheal medications may be ordered if the possibility of infection with *Clostridium difficile* has been ruled out; *Lactobacillus* or *Saccharomyces boulardii* is sometimes given enterally in an effort to establish benign gut flora.
	Hypertonic medications (e.g., KCl) or medications containing sorbitol	Dilute enteral medications well; evaluate sorbitol content of medications, particularly elixirs and syrups.
	Malnutrition/hypoalbuminemia	Use continuous rather than bolus feedings; consider a formula high in MCT.
	Bacterial contamination	Use scrupulously clean formula preparation and administration techniques; refrigerate home-prepared, reconstituted, or opened cans of formula until ready to use, and use all such products within 24 hr; consider use of closed systems, which reduce risk of contamination.

Predisposing illness (e.g., short bowel syndrome, inflammatory bowel disease, AIDS)	Use continuous feedings; consider a formula with MCT and/or soluble fiber.
Lactose intolerance	Use a lactose-free formula.
Fecal impaction	Perform digital examination to rule out fecal impaction with seepage of liquid stool around the obstruction.
Intestinal mucosal atrophy	Consider use of formula rich in MCT or containing prebiotics, probiotics, or synbiotics (Wiesen et al., 2006).
Constipation	
Lack of fiber	Consider fiber-containing formula; ensure that fluid intake is adequate; stool softeners may be beneficial.
Tube occlusion	
Administration of medications through tube	Avoid crushing tablets and administer medications in elixir or suspension form whenever possible; irrigate feeding tube with water before and after giving medications; never mix medication with enteral formulas because this may cause clumping of formula.
Sedimentation of formula	Irrigate tube with water every 4-8 hr during continuous feedings and after every intermittent feeding; irrigate tubes well after measuring gastric residuals (if applicable), since gastric juices left in the tube may cause precipitation of formula. Instilling pancreatic enzymes into the tube can remove or prevent some occlusions. A mechanical device (a flexible plastic probe with screw threads [DeClogger, Bionix Medical Technologies]) is available for removal of clogs in larger tubes, such as PEGs.

Continued

Table 8-5   Management of Tube Feeding Complications—cont'd

Complication	Possible Cause	Suggested Interventions
Delayed gastric emptying	Serious illness, diabetic gastroparesis, prematurity, surgery, high-fat content of formula, hyperglycemia	Consult with physician regarding whether feedings can be administered into the small bowel, a lower-fat formula can be used, or erythromycin, metoclopramide, or other prokinetic agents can be administered to stimulate gastric emptying; improve glycemic control if hyperglycemia exists (Horowitz et al., 2002).
Hyperglycemia	Excessive glucose in feedings/fluids, glucose intolerance caused by stress/sepsis, diabetes or prediabetes, drug therapy (e.g., corticosteroids)	Monitor serum glucose several times daily until stable and regularly thereafter; correct underlying illness if possible, reduce enteral or parenteral feedings if excessive, consider use of insulin, consider lower carbohydrate formula or formula containing soluble fiber.

AIDS, Acquired immunodeficiency syndrome; *KCl,* potassium chloride; *MCT,* medium-chain triglycerides; *PEGs,* percutaneous endoscopic gastrostomies.

A variety of metabolic complications (hypernatremia and hyponatremia, hyperkalemia and hypokalemia, hypercalcemia and hypocalcemia, hyperphosphatemia and hypophosphatemia, etc.), as well as deficiencies or excesses of vitamins and minerals, occur in patients receiving enteral and parenteral nutrition. For this reason, adequacy of electrolytes, calcium, phosphate, magnesium, zinc, and other nutrients must be assessed regularly (frequently during the early stages, less frequently in stable long-term patients) for the duration of nutrition support.

*Signs and symptoms of pulmonary aspiration include tachypnea, shortness of breath, hypoxia, and infiltrate on chest radiographs.

Home Care

A discharge planner or social worker should be involved in preparation for home care, assisting in arranging for supply sources and third-party coverage of costs. Education of the individual and family who are going to deliver tube feedings at home includes the following:

- Clean technique
- Caring for the access device (if applicable: insertion of feeding tube and care of the tube, care of the feeding stoma site; irrigation of tube after feeding)
- Preparation of the enteral formula if necessary
- Safe administration of the formula, including operation of the enteral feeding pump if one is used
- Appropriate feeding schedule and volume
- Obtaining the necessary formula and supplies
- Signs and symptoms of complications; measures to take if these occur
- Self-monitoring; including measuring weight regularly and evaluating state of hydration

Conclusion

Tube feedings provide a method for enteral feeding even in selected patients with severe disorders of digestion and absorption. However, the fact that the feedings are delivered into the GI tract does not mean that they are completely safe or without side effects. Careful patient selection, assessment of nutrition needs, attention to standards of care in delivery of feedings, and monitoring of the response are essential steps in safe and effective enteral feedings.

REFERENCES

American Diabetes Association (ADA): Evidence-based nutrition principles and recommendations for the treatment and prevention of diabetes and related complications, *Diabetes Care* 27 (suppl 1):36, 2004.

Bongers T, Griffiths RD: Are there any real differences between enteral feed formulations used in the critically ill? *Curr Opin Crit Care* 12(2):131, 2006.

Chen YC et al: The effect of intermittent nasogastric feeding on preventing aspiration pneumonia in ventilated critically ill patients, *J Nurs Res* 14(3): 167, 2006.

de Aguilar-Nascimento JE, Kudsk KA: Use of small-bore feeding tubes: successes and failures, *Curr Opin Clin Nutr Metab Care* 10(3):291, 2007.

Edes TE, Walk BE, Austin JL: Diarrhea in tube-fed patients: feeding formula not necessarily the cause, *Am J Med* 88(2):91, 1990.

Haslam D, Fang J: Enteral access for nutrition in the intensive care unit, *Curr Opin Clin Nutr Metab Care* 9(2):155, 2006.

Hasler WL: Gastroparesis: symptoms, evaluation, and treatment, *Gastroenterol Clin North Am* 36(3):619, 2007.

Heimburger DC, Sockwell DG, Geels WJ: Diarrhea with enteral feeding: prospective reappraisal of putative causes, *Nutrition* 10(5):392, 1994.

Heyland D, Dhaliwal R: Immunonutrition in the critically ill: from old approaches to new paradigms, *Intensive Care Med* 31(4):501, 2005.

Ho KM, Dobb GJ, Webb SA: A comparison of early gastric and post-pyloric feeding in critically ill patients: a meta-analysis, *Intensive Care Med* 32(5):639, 2006.

Horowitz M et al: Gastric emptying in diabetes: clinical significance and treatment, *Diabet Med* 19(3):177, 2002.

Kattelmann KK et al: Preliminary evidence for a medical nutrition therapy protocol: enteral feedings for critically ill patients, *J Am Diet Assoc* 106(8):1226, 2006.

Kraft MD, Btaiche IF, Sacks GS: Review of the refeeding syndrome, *Nutr Clin Pract* 20(6):625, 2005.

Metheny NA: Preventing respiratory complications of tube feedings: evidence-based practice, *Am J Crit Care* 15(4):360, 2006.

Metheny NA et al: Indicators of tube site during feedings, *J Neurosci Nurs* 37(6):320, 2005.

Metheny NA, Smith L, Stewart BJ: Development of a reliable and valid bedside test for bilirubin and its utility for improving prediction of feeding tube location, *Nurs Res* 49:302, 2000.

Shils M et al, editors: *Modern nutrition in health and disease*, ed 10, Philadelphia, 2006, Lippincott Williams & Wilkins.

Smith T, Elia M: Artificial nutrition support in hospital: indications and complications, *Clin Med* 6(5):457, 2006.

Wiesen P, Van Gossum A, Preiser JC: Diarrhoea in the critically ill, *Curr Opin Crit Care* 12(2):149, 2006.

CHAPTER 9

PARENTERAL NUTRITION

The term *parenteral nutrition* describes a continuum of intravenous (IV) nutrient delivery. At its simplest, parenteral feeding may involve only IV provision of fluid and electrolytes. At the other end of the continuum lies total parenteral nutrition (TPN), or delivery of all nutrients by IV infusion.

Intravenous Fluid and Electrolytes

Water makes up approximately 60% of body weight in healthy adults. The intracellular compartment contains about two thirds of body water, and the extracellular compartment contains the remaining one third. Interstitial fluid and lymph make up the majority of extracellular fluid, with the blood, or intravascular space, accounting for approximately one third. Other extracellular body fluids, such as peritoneal, synovial, cerebrospinal, and pleural fluids, as well as gastrointestinal secretions, total only about 1 L of fluid at any one time. However, the daily flux (secretion and reabsorption) of gastrointestinal secretions amounts to as much as 6 L. Elderly adults and obese people contain less water per kg body weight than younger, nonobese individuals and therefore can become dehydrated more quickly. Infants contain a greater proportion of water than adults (70% to 80% of body weight).

The body fluids contain solutes, which can be divided into electrolytes (ions that will conduct an electric current) and nonelectrolytes, such as glucose and urea. The predominant extracellular electrolytes are sodium and chloride, and these are contained in many IV solutions. The predominant intracellular electrolytes are potassium and phosphate. Other important electrolytes include calcium, magnesium, and bicarbonate (or total CO_2). Deficits or excesses of electrolytes can result from inadequate or excessive levels in IV and TPN solutions, as well as clinical disorders (Box 9-1). Caretakers should be alert to signs of these disorders in patients receiving IV therapy.

Box 9-1   Summary of Electrolyte Disorders

Hyponatremia

- Possible causes: increased renal sodium excretion (diuretic use, chronic renal failure, adrenal insufficiency); syndrome of inappropriate antidiuretic hormone secretion (SIADH), excess free water intake
- Signs/symptoms: weakness, fatigue, muscle cramps, confusion, anorexia, nausea, vomiting, headaches, seizure, coma

Hypernatremia

- Possible causes: gastrointestinal fluid losses (copious diarrhea, vomiting, nasogastric suction), fluid loss in excess of sodium loss (osmotic diuresis, e.g., in hyperglycemia; diuretics; excessive sweating), hyperaldosteronism, Cushing syndrome
- Signs/symptoms: thirst, agitation, lethargy, tachycardia, decreased blood pressure, fever, oliguria, dry sticky mucous membranes, flushed skin

Hypokalemia

- Possible causes: intracellular shift (acute alkalosis, administration of glucose and insulin, **anabolism**), increased losses (vomiting, diarrhea, small bowel or biliary fistula), excessive renal excretion (diuretic or glucocorticoid treatment, hyperaldosteronism, magnesium deficiency)
- Signs/symptoms: weakness, paralytic ileus, cardiac conduction defects (flattened T wave, depressed ST segment, prominent U wave)

Hyperkalemia

- Possible causes: tissue destruction (hemolysis, massive tissue injury, tumor lysis, catabolism), acidosis, renal failure, adrenal insufficiency, heparin therapy (especially combined with potassium-sparing diuretics, angiotensin-converting enzyme inhibitors, or nonsteroidal antiinflammatory drugs)
- Signs/symptoms: weakness, cardiac toxicity (peaked T waves, prolonged P–R interval and widened QRS, loss of P wave, progressing to ventricular fibrillation)

Hypocalcemia

- Possible causes: thyroidectomy or parathyroidectomy, acute pancreatitis, hyperphosphatemia, magnesium depletion,

Box 9-1 Summary of Electrolyte Disorders—cont'd

chronic renal failure, chronic vitamin D deficiency; transient hypocalcemia can occur in sepsis, burns, acute renal failure, massive transfusions
- Signs/symptoms: muscle spasms, carpopedal spasm, facial grimacing, laryngeal spasm, convulsions, prolonged Q–T interval, dysrhythmias, poor responsiveness to digitalis

Hypercalcemia
- Possible causes: malignancy, hyperparathyroidism, excess of vitamins A or D
- Signs/symptoms: bone pain, weakness, lethargy, confusion, paresthesias, renal stones, cardiovascular alterations (Q–T interval shortened in moderate hypercalcemia; Q–T interval lengthened in severe hypercalcemia)

Hypophosphatemia
- Possible causes: intracellular anabolic shifts (recovery from malnutrition and burns), diabetic ketoacidosis (during treatment), alcoholism, renal loss (hypomagnesemia, hypokalemia, recovery from acute renal failure), prolonged vomiting, diarrhea, vitamin D deficiency, respiratory alkalosis
- Signs/symptoms: acute muscular weakness, occasionally with respiratory muscle paralysis; ataxia; confusion; seizures; coma; hemolysis; platelet dysfunction with bruising

Hyperphosphatemia
- Possible causes: renal failure, hyperthyroidism, intracellular to extracellular shifts (rhabdomyolysis, sepsis, malignant hyperthermia, chemotherapy)
- Signs/symptoms: soft tissue calcifications, e.g., in kidney

Hypomagnesemia
- Possible causes: gastrointestinal losses (malabsorption from pancreatic insufficiency, short bowel syndrome, inflammatory bowel disease, etc.; prolonged nasogastric suction or vomiting; fistulas), poor intake (alcoholism, protein-energy malnutrition), increased urinary losses (diabetic ketoacidosis or poorly controlled hyperglycemia, drugs that increase urinary excretion such as loop diuretics, cisplatin, amphotericin, aminoglycosides, cyclosporine)

Continued

Box 9-1   Summary of Electrolyte Disorders—cont'd

Hypomagnesemia

■ Signs/symptoms: muscle spasms, tetany, weakness, hypocalcemia, hypokalemia resistant to correction, tachycardia, atrial fibrillation

Hypermagnesemia

■ Possible causes: renal failure, adrenocortical insufficiency (Addison disease), hypothermia, excessive intake of magnesium-containing antacids, enemas, and laxatives or magnesium sulfate
■ Signs/symptoms: nausea, vomiting, flushing, diaphoresis, muscular weakness or paralysis, hypotension, soft tissue calcification, loss of patellar reflex

---

The two primary types of IV solutions are colloids and crystalloids. The colloids contain cells, proteins, or synthetic macromolecules that do not cross the capillary membrane readily, and therefore they primarily expand the intravascular volume. Blood products are the most commonly used colloids. The crystalloids contain dextrose (glucose) and/or electrolytes (Table 9-1); these can cross the capillary membrane and therefore can increase the volume of other fluid compartments, in addition to the blood volume. Isotonic electrolyte solutions (e.g., normal saline) can enter all the extracellular fluid. Patients receiving colloids and isotonic electrolyte solutions should be monitored for fluid overload. In addition to expanding the extracellular fluid, hypotonic saline solutions (0.45% saline) and solutions of dextrose in water contribute fluid to the intracellular space. This is known as providing "free water," and fluids that have this ability can replace deficits of total body water. Hypotonic fluids should not be administered in the presence of increased intracranial pressure or third-space fluid shift (loss of fluid into a body compartment where it is unavailable to either the intracellular or extracellular fluid, e.g., ascites, abnormal sequestration of fluid in the interstitial space in burns or trauma, trapping of fluid because of lymphatic or venous obstruction).

Fluids and electrolytes are needed for maintenance (to replace ongoing excretion in urine, normal feces, and sweat, as well as

Table 9-1 Common Crystalloid Solutions

Solution	Glucose (g/L)	Electrolyte Composition (mEq/L)		Uses/Comments
		Na$^+$	Cl$^-$	
Dextrose in water				Used to replace total body water losses (ECF and ICF) and treat hypernatremia; do not provide any electrolytes; D$_{10}$W is hypertonic when infused, but the glucose is rapidly metabolized, and the solution is then hypotonic to cells; D$_5$W provides 170 kcal/L; D$_{10}$W provides 340 kcal/L
5% (D$_5$W)*	50	—	—	
10% (D$_{10}$W)*	100			
Saline				Used to replace hypotonic fluid losses, e.g., increased sweating or insensible losses, osmotic diuresis in diabetic ketoacidosis (used after initial restoration of ECF volume in ketoacidosis); used as a maintenance solution although it does not replace all electrolytes
0.45%*	—	77	77	
0.9% (normal saline)	—	154	154	Used to expand intravascular volume and replace ECF losses, e.g., initial correction of hypovolemia in diabetic ketoacidosis; contains Na$^+$ and Cl$-$ in excess of plasma concentrations; the only IV fluid that can be infused with blood products

Continued

Table 9-1 Common Crystalloid Solutions—cont'd

Solution	Glucose (g/L)	Electrolyte Composition (mEq/L)		Uses/Comments
		Na⁺	Cl⁻	
Dextrose in saline				Similar in usage to the saline-only products; provide 170 kcal/L
5% in 0.2% (D₅¼NS)*	50	38.5	38.5	
5% in 0.45% (D₅½NS)*	50	77	77	
5% in 0.9% (D₅NS)	50	154	154	
Multiple electrolyte solutions				Similar in electrolyte composition to normal plasma except they contain no magnesium
Ringer's	—	147	156	Contains (in mEq/L) 4 K⁺ and 5 Ca⁺⁺; contains more Cl⁻ than plasma; used to expand intravascular volume and replace ECF losses
Lactated Ringer	—	130	109	Closely resembles composition of plasma; contains (in mEq/L) 4 K⁺, 3 Ca⁺⁺, 28 base (as lactate); used to treat losses from burns and lower gastrointestinal tract; should not be used in lactic acidosis

Ca ++, Calcium; *Cl*−, chloride; *ECF*, extracellular fluid, e.g., plasma, lymph, peritoneal fluid; *ICF*, intracellular fluid; *IV*, intravenous; *K* +, potassium; *Na* +, sodium. Normal plasma concentrations are as follows: sodium, 135-145 mEq/L; chloride, 95-105 mEq/L; 1 mEq = 1 mmol for sodium and chloride.
*Provide free water.

insensible losses through skin and lungs) and to replace any abnormal losses. Maintenance losses are normally replaced with crystalloid solutions, such as 0.45% saline, even though this solution does not contain electrolytes other than sodium and chloride. Thus other electrolytes must be monitored and replaced as needed. In normal adults, daily urine output is approximately 1.5 L, and skin (sweat and insensible), gastrointestinal, and lung losses total approximately 1.2 L. Maintenance needs (per unit of body weight) are higher in infants and small children than in adults (see Table 8-3). In particular, caring for low–birth-weight infants under radiant warmers can greatly increase insensible losses; insensible losses are essentially electrolyte free, requiring hypotonic replacement fluids (see Table 9-1). Where there are abnormal fluid losses (polyuric renal failure, osmotic diuresis with diabetic ketoacidosis, burns, severe diarrhea, fistula drainage, etc.), the composition of the fluid lost determines the appropriate composition of replacement fluids. The composition of some common body fluids is given in Table 9-2.

IV glucose and electrolyte solutions are nutritionally inadequate. If an adult's oral nutrient intake is inadequate or is expected to be inadequate for more than 5 to 7 days, enteral or parenteral feedings providing nitrogen as protein or amino acids, vitamins, minerals, and adequate amounts of energy and electrolytes are needed.

Total Parenteral Nutrition

TPN is usually recommended when oral or tube feedings are expected to be contraindicated or inadequate for more than 5 to 7 days in adults and children. A neonate with an illness that delays oral or enteral feedings should receive parenteral nutrition as soon after birth as possible. TPN is most commonly used for one of two reasons:

1. The gastrointestinal tract is unable to digest or absorb adequate nutrients. Examples include intractable vomiting, severe diarrhea, prematurity, some cases of abdominal trauma, prolonged ileus, and massive small bowel resection.
2. There is a need for bowel rest. Examples include enteral fistulas and acute inflammatory bowel disease that does not respond to other therapies.

Table 9-2   Electrolyte Composition of Various Body Fluids (mEq/L or mmol/L)

Fluid	Sodium	Potassium	Chloride	Bicarbonate
Gastric	65 (20-80)	10 (5-20)	100 (90-150)	0
Bile	150 (120-160)	4 (3-8)	100 (80-120)	35 (30-40)
Pancreatic	140 (120-150)	7 (5-15)	80 (75-120)	75 (60-110)
Small bowel				
Midbowel	140 (80-150)	6 (5-15)	100 (90-130)	30 (20-40)
Terminal ileum	140 (80-150)	8 (5-30)	60 (20-115)	70
Diarrhea	50 (10-90)	35 (10-80)	40 (10-110)	50 (30-55)
Sweat	45	5	580	

Data from Feldman M, Friedman LS, Brandt LJ: *Sleisenger and Fordtran's gastrointestinal and liver disease*, ed 8, Philadelphia, 2006, Saunders; Behrman RE, Kliegman RM, Jensen HB: *Nelson textbook of pediatrics*, ed 17, Philadelphia, 2004, Saunders; Doherty GM, Way LW, editors: *Current surgical diagnosis and treatment*, ed 12, New York, 2006, McGraw-Hill.

Values are mean, with approximate range, where available, in parentheses.

In most instances, initiation of TPN is contraindicated when the gastrointestinal tract is functional, enteral feedings are expected to be adequate within 5 days, or death from the underlying disease is imminent.

Routes and Devices for Delivery of Parenteral Nutrition

Parenteral nutrition may be delivered through peripheral or central veins. Use of peripheral parenteral nutrition (PPN) depends on the adequacy of peripheral venous access. Blood flow through the peripheral veins is not as great as that through the large central veins, and thus PPN is not as rapidly diluted into the bloodstream as centrally delivered TPN. This limits the concentrations of the glucose and amino acid solutions used in PPN. TPN delivered into the central veins can contain higher concentrations of glucose and amino acids, but it requires the placement of an indwelling central venous catheter (CVC), which can be associated with serious infectious and mechanical complications.

Peripheral venous catheters

Peripheral venous catheters are usually inserted in the upper extremities, although lower extremity veins are used in infants. Hypertonic (hyperosmolar) fluids are irritating when delivered through small peripheral veins (discussed in the following text). A rough estimate of the osmotic concentration (in mOsm/kg) of a parenteral nutrition solution can be obtained from the following formula (Davis, 1997):

$$(100 \times \text{Amino acid percentage}) + (50 \times \text{Carbohydrate percentage}) + (2 \times \text{Total electrolyte additives in mEq})$$

Short catheters (7.6 cm [3 in] or less)

Advantages: few mechanical or infectious complications, other than the risk of superficial phlebitis; inexpensive and easy to place at the bedside

Disadvantages: Require good peripheral venous access; not useful for prolonged therapy; may be difficult to deliver adequate energy to stressed individuals or those with high energy needs because peripheral veins do not generally tolerate solution concentrations above 900 mOsm/kg (although with simultaneous infusion of lipid emulsions as much as 1000 to 1200 mOsm/kg may be tolerated), which limits dextrose concentrations to about

10% and amino acid concentrations to 5%; cannot be used for solutions with pH less than 5 or more than 9; not suitable for TPN in patients needing fluid restriction; in adult patients the catheters should be removed and replaced routinely (no more frequently than every 72 to 96 hours) to reduce the risk of infection and phlebitis, but no recommendation is made for routine replacement in children (CDC, 2002).

Midline catheters (15 to 25 cm [6 to 10 in])

Midline catheters are inserted in the antecubital fossa into the basilic or cephalic veins; they do not enter a central vein and thus are peripheral catheters.

Advantages: Similar to short cannulas; longer life than the short catheters (no recommendation is made for routine replacement of midline catheters, and they have lasted as long as 2 to 4 weeks); preferred over short catheters when IV therapy will likely last 6 days or longer (CDC, 2002).

Disadvantages: Fluid, dextrose, amino acid, osmolality, and pH limitations are similar to those of short catheters; site infections and phlebitis possible; some anaphylactoid reactions have occurred with catheters made of elastomeric hydrogel.

Central venous catheters

CVCs are usually inserted into the superior or inferior vena cava by means of the subclavian, internal or external jugular, or femoral veins. These catheters provide a reliable IV route for long-term access (weeks to years), and they allow use of extremely hypertonic solutions (≥1800 mOsm/kg) with high dextrose and amino acid concentrations and solutions with low or high pH. Most of the catheters are made of Teflon, silicone rubber, or polyurethane. A variety of types are available; the Groshong-type catheter provides a 3-way valve that prevents reflux of blood into the catheter and reduces clotting.

Peripherally inserted central catheters

Peripherally inserted central catheters (PICCs) are long (51 cm [20 in] or longer in many adults) catheters threaded through peripheral veins, usually the basilic, cephalic, or brachial, into the superior vena cava.

Advantages: Can be inserted at the bedside or in the clinic in many cases; allow delivery of very hypertonic solutions without the risk of pneumothorax; can be used for patients receiving long-term treatment and at home; less risk of infection than the nontunneled CVCs; multilumen PICCs are available to facilitate delivery of different solutions and/or blood drawing.

Disadvantages: Complications include phlebitis and potential central vein thrombosis, catheter-related sepsis, and catheter fracture (with potential for embolization).

Nontunneled central venous catheters

These catheters are primarily for temporary use (up to a few weeks). They are available in either single-lumen or multilumen styles. Most catheter-related bloodstream infections occur with these catheters, but it must be noted that they are used frequently in critically ill patients with a variety of risk factors for infection.

Advantages: Can be inserted at the bedside in many cases; easily removed. Multilumen catheters reduce the risk of drug incompatibilities when more than one medication must be given at once and allow for blood sampling through the CVC. Multilumen catheters are best suited to adults and older children because they are generally too large in diameter for infants and small children.

Disadvantages: Complications include pneumothorax, air embolism, central vein thrombosis, superior vena cava syndrome, catheter-related sepsis, and catheter embolization (rare); not as appropriate as other CVCs for home patients.

Tunneled central venous catheters

Tunneled catheters are usually inserted into the subclavian, internal jugular, or femoral veins, and the proximal end is tunneled under the skin away from the insertion site (Figure 9-1). A cuff on the catheter encourages the subcutaneous tissues to adhere to the catheter.

Advantages: Infection rate is lower than with nontunneled CVCs (Maki et al., 2006); not easily dislodged after the subcutaneous tissues have had time to adhere to the cuff; easier for the patient to care for than nontunneled CVCs and well suited to home use; may not require a dressing once the insertion site has healed.

Disadvantages: Complications are the same as for nontunneled CVCs, except for the lower risk of infection. More difficult to remove than nontunneled CVCs.

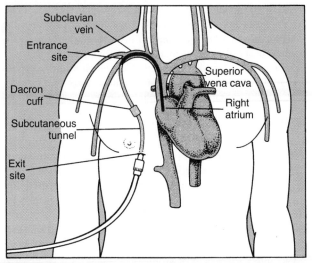

Figure 9-1
Hickman central venous catheter. The proximal end is tunneled under the subcutaneous tissue to increase stability. A Dacron cuff on the catheter provides a roughened surface, which encourages subcutaneous tissue to adhere to the catheter and further secure it.
(From Beare PG, Myers JL, editors: *Principles and practice of adult health nursing*, St Louis, 1990, Mosby.)

Totally implantable catheter

The totally implantable catheter is a tunneled catheter with a subcutaneous infusion port attached. Before each infusion, a noncoring needle is inserted through the skin and into the septum on the port.

Advantages: Useful for intermittent therapy (e.g., chemotherapy, selected patients needing intermittent fluid therapy or TPN); require flushing only every 28 days if not in use; no routine site care and no dressing is needed; lower infection rates than nontunneled catheters (Maki et al., 2006); more cosmetically appealing than other CVCs; long lasting (predicted life span of the port is approximately 2000 punctures); well suited to home patients.

Disadvantages: All the disadvantages of CVC, except need for site care; requires a needle to access the port; thus some mild discomfort is likely with access; risk of extravasation of infusate if the needle slips out of the port; a tunneled CVC or PICC line is preferable when therapy is continuous rather than intermittent.

Umbilical catheters

Umbilical catheters, used in newborns, are inserted into either an umbilical artery or an umbilical vein.

Advantages: Access easy to establish. Use of an arterial catheter allows access for monitoring blood gases as well as parenteral feeding/fluid administration.

Disadvantages: Risk of infection/sepsis, bleeding, obstruction of circulation to the lower extremities (removal of the catheter is recommended with any sign of vascular insufficiency). The recommended life span of these catheters is short, with arterial catheters being removed in 5 days or less and venous catheters in 14 days or less (CDC, 2002).

Catheter Care

Insertion

Insertion of peripheral catheters can be done with clean technique (i.e., clean but not sterile gloves) and no mask. Central catheters, including PICC lines, require sterile technique with full barrier precautions (gown, mask, gloves, and drapes).

The skin should be thoroughly disinfected before catheter insertion. Chlorhexidine 2% is preferred for adults and older children, but povidone-iodine, tincture of iodine, or 70% alcohol can also be used (CDC, 2002). The patient should be questioned about allergies before using these preparations, particularly iodine-containing solutions

Catheter dressings

Peripheral and central catheters can be covered by a gauze and tape or transparent semipermeable polyurethane dressing. Either type of dressing should be replaced if it becomes damp, soiled, or loosened. One dressing has no apparent advantage over the other in terms of infection control, but gauze and tape dressings require more frequent routine changes (every 2 days vs. weekly for semipermeable) and thus more time for care (Byrnes and Coopersmith, 2007). The transparent dressings have the additional advantage of allowing visual inspection of the insertion site. However, because of their absorbent nature, gauze and tape dressings may be preferable for patients with diaphoresis or oozing of blood at the insertion site. The catheter should not be submerged in water, but showering can be permitted if the catheter is protected with a waterproof covering. Dressings on tunneled and totally implanted catheters should be changed weekly until the insertion site heals, after which no dressing may be needed.

Good hand cleansing before any contact with the dressing or infusion sets is essential. Clean gloves can be worn during changes of peripheral catheter dressings, whereas sterile gloves are needed for central catheter (including PICC) dressing changes. During dressing changes the skin should be cleaned with a disinfectant, as for catheter insertion. No topical antibiotic ointment or cream should be used at the catheter insertion site, because this raises the risk for growth of fungi and antibiotic-resistant bacteria (CDC, 2002).

Monitoring and maintaining the catheter

Consistent, well-trained nursing staff reduces the risk of infection. The catheter site should be monitored routinely through the dressing, with the frequency depending on the patient's status (e.g., critical care vs. stable home patient). Pain on palpation, purulent drainage, and fever of unexplained origin in a patient with a CVC suggest catheter-related infection and deserve further evaluation. Peripheral catheters should be removed at any sign of phlebitis (erythema, warmth, tenderness, or palpable hardness of the vein) or infection at the site.

CVCs are normally flushed with a heparin-containing solution when not in use. Routine flushing of the catheter while in use may reduce the risk of thrombosis (CDC, 2002). CVC catheters with a heparin-bonded coating are also available. Some CVCs are permeated with antimicrobial or antiseptic substances (e.g., chlorhexidine/silver sulfadiazine, silver/platinum, minocycline/rifampin). Chlorhexidine catheters are not approved for infants weighing 3 kg or less because of uncertainty about safety in that population. Although the antibiotic-containing catheters raise concerns about antibiotic-resistant microorganisms, they do appear to reduce the risk of catheter-related bloodstream infections in critical care patients (Ryder, 2006; Ramritu et al., 2008). The chlorhexidine/silver sulfadiazine catheters are also more effective than uncoated catheters in reducing bloodstream infections (Maki et al., 2006; Ramritu et al., 2008).

Parenteral Nutrition Solutions

The estimated nutrient needs of stable patients needing TPN are shown in Table 9-3. Crystalline amino acids provide the nitrogen (protein) needed. Specialized amino acid solutions are available for

Table 9-3   Estimated Daily Nutrient Needs of TPN Patients[a]

Component	Adults	Term Infants	Children over 1 yr
	(per kg per day)	(per kg per day)	(per kg per day)
Amino acids (g)	0.8-1 (maintenance)	2-2.5	1.5-2 (children)
	1.2-2 (catabolic)		0.8-2 (adolescents)
Energy (kcal)[b]	25-30[c]	90-120 (<6 mo)	75-90 (1-7 yr)
		80-100 (6-12 mo)	60-75 (7-12 yr)
			30-60 (>12-18 yr)
Fluid (ml)	25-40	100	See note on p. 269
	(total)	(per kg per day)	(per kg per day)
Electrolytes and Minerals			
Na (mEq)	≥60	2-3	3-4
K (mEq)	≥60	1-2	2-4
Mg (mEq)	8-20	0.3-0.7	0.2-0.3
Ca (mg)	200-300	60-70[d]	20-60
Phosphate (mg)	600-1200	50-55[d]	40-45
Zinc (mg)	2.5-5[e]	0.25 <3 mo	0.05 (max 5/day)
		0.10 >3 mo	
Copper (mg)	0.3-0.5	0.02	0.02 (max 0.3/day)
Chromium (mcg)[f]	10-15	0.2	0.2 (max 5/day)

Continued

Table 9-3 Estimated Daily Nutrient Needs of TPN Patients[a]—cont'd

Component	Adults (per kg per day)	Term Infants (per kg per day)	Children over 1 yr (per kg per day)
Manganese (mcg)[g]	60-100	1	1 (max 50/day)
Selenium (mcg)	40-80	2	2 (max 30/day)
Molybdenum (mcg)	— (total)	0.25 (total)	0.25 (max 5/day) (total)
Vitamins (per day)[h]			
A (retinol) (mg)[i]	1	0.7	0.7
D (ergocalciferol or cholecalciferol) (mcg)	5	10	10
E (alpha-tocopherol) (mg)	10	7	7
K (phylloquinone) (mcg)	150	200	200
C (ascorbic acid) (mg)	200	80	80
Folic acid (mcg)	600	140	140
Niacin (mg)	40	17	17
Thiamin (B_1) (mg)	6	1.2	1.2
Riboflavin (B_2) (mg)	3.6	1.4	1.4

Pyridoxine (B$_6$) (mg)	6	1
Cyanocobalamin (B$_{12}$) (mcg)	5	1
Pantothenic acid (mg)	15	5
Biotin (mcg)	60	20

From *Federal Register* 65(77):21200, 2000; National Advisory Group on Standards and Practice Guidelines for Parenteral Nutrition: Safe practices for parenteral nutrition formulation, *JPEN J Parenter Enteral Nutr* 22:49, 1998; Shils ME et al: *Modern nutrition in health and disease*, ed 9, Philadelphia, 1999, Lippincott Williams & Wilkins.

TPN, Total parenteral nutrition.

[a]Amounts of constituents must be individualized; the levels listed are "usual" ranges.

[b]Glucose monohydrate, used in IV solutions, contains 3.4 kcal/g.

[c]Estimated range only. See Table 2-6 for the Harris-Benedict equations for calculation of energy expenditure. Indirect calorimetry provides the most accurate estimate.

[d]Calcium and phosphate not to exceed 500 to 600 mg/L and 400 to 450 mg/L, respectively, to prevent precipitation.

[e]For maintenance needs; add 2 mg daily during acute periods of hypermetabolism; add 12 mg for each liter of small bowel losses and 17 mg/kg of stool or ileostomy losses.

[f]Decrease or omit with increasing severity of renal dysfunction.

[g]Excreted in bile; omit in patients with obstructive jaundice and cholestasis.

[h]Adult vitamin dosages are for individuals 11 years of age and older.

[i]1 mg of vitamin A = 3300 USP units; 0.7 mg = 2300 USP units.

NOTE: Children's approximate fluid needs are based on body weight as follows: ≤10 kg, 100 ml/kg/day; 11-20 kg, 1000 ml + 50 ml/kg over 10 kg; >20 kg, 1500 ml + 20 ml/kg over 20 kg.

use in renal and hepatic failure and for infants. Renal solutions contain the essential amino acids only. Patients with renal failure need both essential and nonessential amino acids, and therefore use of these special formulations should be limited to short periods. Amino acid formulations for hepatic failure are low in aromatic amino acids and methionine and higher in branched-chain amino acids than the standard formulations. They are designed for patients with hepatic encephalopathy. Standard adult amino acid solutions are not ideal for infants. In particular, they contain too little tyrosine, glutamine, and cysteine for optimal growth. The amino acid solutions for infants are designed to resemble the amino acid composition of human milk. The proper age to switch from an infant to an adult amino acid solution is not established, but most institutions use the infant formulation until the child is at least 1 year of age.

Glucose (dextrose) is an important energy source, but adults cannot oxidize glucose more rapidly than approximately 5 mg/kg/min. If glucose is infused at a faster rate, then the excess may be used to form lipids. Thus a 70-kg adult should receive no more than about 500 g of glucose daily. Lipid is given as a source of essential fatty acids and energy, as well as to provide balance to the nutritional intake. PPN solutions are similar to those delivered centrally in their electrolyte, mineral, and vitamin composition but, as described earlier, are restricted in the amount of glucose and amino acids they may contain.

Lipid emulsions, containing triglycerides, phospholipids, and glycerol, are available as 10%, 20%, and 30% preparations. These contain 10, 20, or 30 g fat/100 ml and provide 1.1, 2, or 2.9 kcal/ml, respectively. IV lipid should be limited to 2.5 to 3 g/kg/day for adults and no more than 3 to 4 g/kg/day for children, and lipid emulsions should supply a maximum of 60% of the energy intake (Intralipid and Liposyn III package inserts). Lipid emulsions may be administered separate from ("piggy-backed" with) or mixed with the glucose–amino acid solutions. Lipid emulsions support the growth of *Candida* species and many bacteria better than glucose–amino acid solutions do and thus should be administered with scrupulous aseptic technique (Didier et al., 1998).

TPN solutions also include multivitamin mixtures, minerals, and trace elements. Iron is not typically included. Most patients receive TPN for 3 months or less, and deficiency is unlikely if iron stores were adequate before beginning TPN. Long-term TPN patients and those with poor stores who cannot absorb oral iron must receive parenteral iron. Three forms are available: iron dextran, sodium ferric gluconate, and iron sucrose. The latter two are approved by the U.S. Food and Drug Administration only for patients with chronic kidney disease receiving erythropoietin therapy (package inserts). All three preparations can be delivered intravenously, and iron dextran can also be administered by deep (Z-track) intramuscular injection. Iron dextran requires a test dose before administering a full dose because of the risk of anaphylactoid reaction. When iron dextran is added to glucose–amino acid mixtures, there is a risk of precipitate formation. If it is included in a TPN solution, iron should be added immediately before the solution is administered, the solution should be visually inspected for precipitate before administration and periodically during infusion, and a 0.2- or 1.2-μm filter should be used. Molybdenum is not usually administered to adults receiving TPN, and other elements believed to have a role in human nutrition (boron, tin, etc.) are also omitted, largely because of lack of knowledge of absolute requirements and concern for possible toxicity. Careful ongoing monitoring of physical signs and symptoms is essential in identifying micronutrient deficiencies that may occur, particularly in long-term TPN patients and those who receive or absorb little or no oral intake. Electrolytes are included in TPN and may be modified as needed to replace losses or compensate for electrolyte retention.

Carnitine, a derivative of the amino acid lysine, stimulates entry of long-chain fatty acids into the mitochondria so that they can be oxidized as an energy source. Carnitine is found in foods of animal origin and is synthesized by healthy adults and children, but TPN solutions do not contain carnitine unless supplemented with it. Infants, especially preterm infants, and older children and adults who receive long-term TPN might not synthesize adequate amounts of carnitine (Crill and Helms, 2007). Signs of deficiency include cardiomyopathy, muscle weakness, lethargy, hypoglycemia, encephalopathy, delayed growth, and seizures. Carnitine supplements are available to be given orally or added to TPN solutions when deficiency is suspected or anticipated.

TPN solutions may include numerous nonnutritive additives, particularly drugs used to prevent or control the potential complications of TPN. Common additives are insulin, heparin (used both to reduce the likelihood of thrombosis and to stimulate lipoprotein lipase [the enzyme responsible for removing fatty acids from triglycerides, allowing them to be used by cells and thus improving utilization of lipid emulsions]), and histamine-H_2 blockers (used because gastric acid secretion is frequently increased in TPN patients, especially those with short bowel syndrome).

Administration of Total Parenteral Nutrition

TPN may be infused continuously or cyclically. Continuous infusions are used for the critically ill and most other hospitalized patients. Cyclic TPN is usually infused for several hours and then discontinued until the next day (e.g., 12 hours on TPN, then 12 hours off). Cyclic TPN allows the patient receiving long-term TPN more flexibility and freedom and may improve liver function (Kumpf, 2006); it is especially well suited to home patients. In administering either continuous or cyclic TPN, follow these guidelines:

■ Examine TPN solutions and lipid emulsions for precipitation, separation, or signs of contamination (e.g., fungal growth) before hanging them.
■ Handle TPN solutions, administration sets, and the peripheral or central catheter with aseptic technique.
■ A filter with 0.22-μm pores can be used for amino acid–glucose mixtures, and a filter with 1.2-μm pores can be used for lipid-containing solutions. Filters have not been proven to be necessary for infection control, because solutions can be filtered to remove contaminants and particulates in the pharmacy in a more cost-efficient manner (CDC, 2002). However, an air-eliminating filter may reduce the risk of air embolus.

Assessing Response to Total Parenteral Nutrition

Anthropometric measurements, physical assessment, and hematologic and biochemical measurements are used in assessing response to nutrition support (see Table 8-4). Hyperglycemia, imbalances of electrolytes, and acid-base disturbances are common complications of TPN delivery. Fluid and electrolyte status must be carefully monitored. In the patient receiving long-term TPN, adequacy of vitamin and trace mineral status must be assessed regularly by thorough physical examination as well as use of appropriate biochemical testing (see Table 2-2). A positive nitrogen balance occurs when there is nitrogen retention within the body, presumably for protein synthesis, and is an indicator of adequate protein delivery. Nitrogen balance determination requires a 24-hour record of protein intake (the amino acids delivered in TPN plus the protein consumed in enteral and/or oral feedings) in addition to 24-hour collection of urine and feces. If fecal losses are low, skin and fecal losses together are often estimated as 4 g/day. Nitrogen losses from unusual sources (e.g., large exudative skin lesions, ungrafted burns, fistula drainage) must be measured or estimated.

Nitrogen balance = [24-Hour protein intake (g) × 0.16] − [24-Hour urine urea nitrogen (g) + Fecal nitrogen (g)]

Preventing and Correcting Complications of Parenteral Nutrition

Table 9-4 summarizes complications of parenteral nutrition and lists measures for their prevention or correction. In addition to the complications listed, excess or deficits of electrolytes (see Box 9-1) and acid-base disorders are relatively common and require close monitoring. Hyperglycemia in patients receiving TPN is associated with an increase in adverse outcomes, including infections, cardiac complications, organ failure, and death (Cheung et al., 2005; Lin et al., 2007). It may be necessary to reduce the rate of TPN infusion, decrease the proportion of total kcal provided by glucose (i.e., reduce the amount of glucose in the solution while increasing the amount of lipid emulsion delivered), or treat the patient with insulin to control blood glucose concentrations. The refeeding syndrome, which can occur in malnourished patients given either enteral or parenteral nutrition, is described in Chapter 8.

Patients receiving long-term TPN are susceptible to the development of a number of serious complications, including biliary dysfunction (acalculous cholecystitis, bile sludging, and cholelithiasis), hepatic steatosis, and metabolic bone disease. Cholecystitis may occur because of inadequate stimulation of gallbladder contraction in individuals with little or no food intake. The most important measure to prevent the problem is to encourage oral intake if indicated. Steatosis, or fatty liver, may occur because of overfeeding but also appears to be associated with elevation of the inflammatory cytokines. Avoiding overfeeding; providing an appropriate balance of protein, carbohydrate, and fat; and correcting underlying inflammatory processes, if possible, are proposed remedies (Guglielmi et al., 2006). Oral or enteral intake, if tolerated, is beneficial in preventing steatosis; cycling of TPN (e.g., 12 hours on and 12 hours off) has also been used in an effort to decrease the risk of steatosis. Metabolic bone disease, including osteomalacia and

Table 9-4 TPN Complications

Complication	Signs/Symptoms	Prevention/Interventions
Catheter site infection	Erythema, warmth, inflammation, and pus at the catheter insertion site	Insert catheter with maximal barrier precautions (gown, mask, gloves, drapes) and strict aseptic technique; use aseptic technique in maintaining the insertion site; monitor insertion site regularly; culture site and administer antibiotics as appropriate if infection is apparent.
Catheter-related sepsis	Fever, chills, glucose intolerance, positive blood culture; bacterial colony counts in blood from the catheter 5-10 times higher than in blood obtained from a peripheral site	Insert catheter with maximal barrier precautions (gown, mask, gloves, extensive drapes) and strict aseptic technique; maintain an intact dressing; change if contaminated by vomitus, sputum, etc.; use aseptic technique whenever handling catheter, IV tubing, and TPN solutions; hang a single bottle of TPN no longer than 4 hr and lipid emulsion no longer than 12 hr; use a a 0.22-μm filter with solutions that do not contain lipids or a 1.2 -μm filter with solutions that contain lipids; avoid using single-lumen, nontunneled catheter for blood sampling and infusion of non-TPN solutions if possible. If sepsis is apparent, notify physician and obtain cultures as ordered; the catheter will likely be removed.
Air embolism	Dyspnea, cyanosis, tachycardia hypotension, possibly death	Use Luer lock system; Groshong catheter, which has valve at tip, can reduce risk of air embolism; use an inline,

		air-eliminating filter; have patient perform Valsalva maneuver during tubing changes; if air embolism is suggested, place patient in left lateral decubitus position and administer oxygen; immediately notify physician, who may attempt to aspirate air from the heart.
Central venous thrombosis	Unilateral edema of neck, shoulder, and arm; development of collateral circulation on chest; pain in insertion site	Follow measures to prevent sepsis; *Staphylococcus aureus* bacteremia is especially likely to be associated with thrombosis (Crowley et al., 2008); repeated or traumatic catheterizations are most likely to result in thrombosis; treatment usually includes anticoagulation; if symptoms are not too severe, thrombolytic therapy may be attempted, but catheter removal is usually necessary.
Catheter occlusion or semiocclusion	No flow or sluggish flow through the catheter; or infusion through the catheter possible, but blood cannot be aspirated from the catheter	Flush catheter with heparinized saline if infusion is stopped temporarily; if catheter appears to be occluded, attempt to aspirate the clot; thrombolytic agent may restore patency if clotted or occluded by fibrin sheath.
Hypoglycemia	Diaphoresis, shakiness, confusion, loss of consciousness	Do not discontinue TPN abruptly; taper rate over several hours; use pump to regulate infusion so that it remains ±10% of ordered rate; if hypoglycemia is suggested, then administer oral carbohydrate; if oral intake is contraindicated or patient is unconscious, a bolus of IV dextrose may be used.

Continued

Table 9-4 TPN Complications—cont'd

Complication	Signs/Symptoms	Prevention/Interventions
Hyperglycemia	Thirst, headache, lethargy, increased urination	Monitor blood glucose frequently until stable; the patient may require reduction in the glucose content of TPN and/or in-sulin treatment if the problem is severe.
Hypertriglyceridemia	Serum triglyceride concentrations elevated (especially serious if >400 mg/dl); serum may appear turbid	Monitor serum triglycerides after each increase in rate and at least 3 times weekly until stable in patients receiving lipid emulsions; reduce lipid infusion rate or administer low-dose heparin with lipid emulsions if elevated levels are observed.

IV, Intravenous; *TPN,* total parenteral nutrition.

osteopenia, occurs primarily in patients receiving long-term TPN. The etiology is not definitely known, but possible contributors include vitamin D toxicity, inadequate provision of calcium in TPN because of the difficulty in including enough of both calcium and phosphorus without causing precipitation of calcium phosphate, chronic metabolic acidosis, aluminum contamination of parenteral nutrition components, and the patient's underlying disease or treatment (e.g., corticosteroids). Correction of metabolic acidosis if present and use of acidic amino acid mixtures (which increase the solubility of calcium and phosphorus in the TPN solution) reduce the risk of bone disease (Acca et al., 2007). The U.S. Food and Drug Administration has placed limits on the amount of aluminum that can be contained in products for use in TPN.

Preparing the Patient and Family for Home Parenteral Nutrition

Preparation for home TPN is a multidisciplinary process, usually involving the physician, nurse, dietitian, pharmacist, and social worker. Topics that must be covered in patient teaching include the following:

- Aseptic technique
- Caring for the access device, including irrigation and heparinization of the catheter, site care, and dressing changes, if applicable
- Making additions to the TPN solution (if necessary)
- Initiating, administering, and discontinuing the TPN infusion, including operation of the infusion pump
- Signs and symptoms of complications and management of those complications; self-monitoring (e.g., monitoring of blood glucose, regular weighing, checking body temperature as needed, evaluating state of hydration)
- Financial, third-party payer, and supply issues related to delivery of home TPN

Conclusion

TPN is life saving in many instances, but it poses infectious, mechanical, and metabolic hazards. A team approach with appropriate patient selection, careful assessment of nutrition needs, attention to standards of care, and frequent monitoring of safety and response improves outcome.

References

Acca M et al: Metabolic bone diseases during long-term total parenteral nutrition, *J Endocrinol Invest* 30 (Suppl 6):54, 2007.

Byrnes MC, Coopersmith CM: Prevention of catheter-related blood stream infection, *Curr Opin Crit Care* 13(4):411, 2007.

Centers for Disease Control and Prevention: Guidelines for the prevention of intravascular catheter-related infections, *MMWR Recomm Rep* 51(RR-10):1, 2002.

Cheung NW et al: Hyperglycemia is associated with adverse outcomes in patients receiving total parenteral nutrition, *Diabetes Care* 28(10):2367, 2005.

Crill CM, Helms RA: The use of carnitine in pediatric nutrition, *Nutr Clin Pract* 22(2):204, 2007.

Crowley AL et al: Venous thrombosis in patients with short- and long-term central venous catheter-associated Staphylococcus aureus bacteremia, *Crit Care Med* 36(2):385, 2008.

Davis A: Initiation, monitoring, and complications of pediatric parenteral nutrition. In Baker BB, Baker RD, Davis A, editors: Pediatric parenteral nutrition, New York, 1997, Chapman & Hall.

Didier ME, Fischer S, Maki DG: Total nutrient admixtures appear safer than lipid emulsion alone as regards microbial contamination: growth properties of microbial pathogens at room temperature, JPEN *J Parent Ent Nutr* 22(5):291, 1998.

Guglielmi FW et al: Total parenteral nutrition-related gastroenterological complications, *Dig Liver Dis* 38(9):623, 2006.

Kumpf VJ: Parenteral nutrition-associated liver disease in adult and pediatric patients, *Nutr Clin* Pract 21(3):279, 2006.

Lin et al: Hyperglycemia correlates with outcomes in patients receiving total parenteral nutrition, *Am J Med Sci* 333(5):261, 2007.

Maki DG, Kluger DM, Crnich CJ: The risk of bloodstream infection in adults with different intravascular devices: a systematic review of 200 published prospective studies, *Mayo Clin Proc* 81(9):1159, 2006.

Ramritu P et al: A systematic review comparing the relative effectiveness of antimicrobial-coated catheters in intensive care units, *Am J Infect Control* 36(2):104, 2008.

Ryder M: Evidence-based practice in the management of vascular access devices for home parenteral nutrition therapy, *JPEN J Parenter Enteral Nutr* 30(suppl 1):82-93, 98-89, 2006.

SELECTED BIBLIOGRAPHY

A.S.P.E.N. Board of Directors and Clinical Guidelines Task Force: Guidelines for the use of parenteral and enteral nutrition in adults and pediatric patients, *J Parenter Enteral Nutr* 26 (suppl 1):33SA, 2002.

Steiger E: Consensus statements regarding optimal management of home parenteral nutrition (HPN) access, *JPEN J Parenter Enteral Nutr* 30 (suppl 1):94, 2006.

Ukleja A, Romano MM: Complications of parenteral nutrition, *Gastroenterol Clin North Am* 36(1):23, 2007.

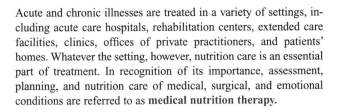

MEDICAL NUTRITION THERAPY

Acute and chronic illnesses are treated in a variety of settings, including acute care hospitals, rehabilitation centers, extended care facilities, clinics, offices of private practitioners, and patients' homes. Whatever the setting, however, nutrition care is an essential part of treatment. In recognition of its importance, assessment, planning, and nutrition care of medical, surgical, and emotional conditions are referred to as **medical nutrition therapy.**

METABOLIC STRESS: CRITICAL ILLNESS, TRAUMA, AND SURGERY

Critical illness and wound healing are stressors that result in **hypermetabolism,** or markedly increased energy expenditure. Nutrition care is a priority to minimize nutritional deficits during the period of hypermetabolism and to promote repair during convalescence.

The Stress Response

Injury and critical illness are accompanied by a stress response. The stress response is directed at two important tasks:

- *It produces energy to meet the increased metabolic needs from surgery and injury.* Increased secretion of glucagon, epinephrine, norepinephrine, and corticosteroids results in breakdown of glycogen, fat stores, and body proteins, especially in skeletal muscles. The net effect in severe injury is increased urinary nitrogen loss, muscle wasting, and weight loss.
- *It maintains the blood volume.* Antidiuretic hormone (ADH) secretion increases during the stress response, decreasing urine output and increasing fluid retention. In hypovolemia, increased aldosterone secretion occurs, and this also stimulates retention of sodium and fluid.

Impaired host defenses make the critically ill and injured person vulnerable to infection. Sepsis, the systemic response to infection, is believed to occur because of the release of inflammatory mediators such as cytokines, eicosanoids, and the hormones mentioned previously. The **systemic inflammatory response syndrome (SIRS),** which includes sepsis, can occur in the absence of infection, when the presence of ischemic and necrotic tissue (e.g., trauma, burn, pancreatitis) stimulates a severe inflammatory response (Lenz et al., 2007). Sepsis and SIRS result in hypermetabolism, insulin resistance and hyperglycemia, and increased protein catabolism and lipid release from the adipose tissue. Lean body mass can be rapidly lost during severe inflammation.

Nutrition Care

The goal of nutrition care is to prevent or correct nutritional deficits that could impair healing.

Assessment

A thorough nutrition assessment should be performed as described in Chapter 2. Box 10-1 highlights common or especially serious findings of metabolic stress. A careful physical examination and nutritional history may be the most useful tools for determining nutritional risk in the ill or injured patient, because other parameters are unreliable in unstable patients. Changes in fluid balance in the acutely ill patient can alter anthropometric measurements. Moreover, serum protein concentrations are affected by many factors, including fluid balance, inflammation, the acute-phase response, and organ failure. In response to injury or infection, inflammatory mediators, such as cytokines, redirect liver protein metabolism from the synthesis of proteins such as albumin, transferrin, and prealbumin (transthyretin) and toward the formation of the acute-phase reactants, such as fibrinogen, C-reactive protein, complement 3 (C3), and haptoglobulin. Concentrations of serum albumin, transferrin, prealbumin, and retinol binding protein usually fall in the early period after injury or surgery (reverse acute-phase reaction), although decreased synthesis may not be the primary reason (especially for albumin, which has a long half-life). Hemodilution from fluid resuscitation and fluid retention causes "capillary leak" of the proteins into the interstitial space, and having the patient in the recumbent position before blood sampling is carried out can falsely lower serum proteins because of redistribution of body fluid (Johnson et al., 2007). (Fluid in the interstitial compartment, particularly in the lower extremities, returns to the bloodstream during bedrest.) Thus the early changes in serum proteins are unrelated to nutritional status.

Once the patient's clinical status has stabilized and adequate nutritional intake has been achieved, rising levels of prealbumin and retinol binding protein may be early indicators of the resolution of the acute phase and the beginning of a response to nutrition therapy (Raguso et al., 2003; Devoto et al., 2006). A fall in the concentrations of C-reactive protein, a marker of inflammation and stress, also signals the end of the acute-phase response (Johnson et al., 2007).

Box 10-1   Assessment in Metabolic Stress

Protein-Energy Malnutrition (PEM) or Protein-Calorie Malnutrition (PCM)

History

Increased needs caused by hypermetabolism from trauma, burns, surgery, fever, sepsis, pneumonia, or other infection; catabolic effects of corticosteroid therapy (head injury); weight loss before surgery, especially if >2% in 1 wk, >5% in 1 mo, >7.5% in 3 mo, or >10% in 6 mo; poor intake caused by anorexia, intestinal obstruction or ileus, nausea or vomiting, and alcoholism; increased losses caused by small intestinal resection, gastrectomy, fistula, burns (loss of serum proteins through damaged capillaries)

Physical examination

Muscle wasting; weight <10th percentile or BMI <18.5; edema

Laboratory analysis

Not usually helpful in the early phase of care; after the acute phase, prealbumin and nitrogen balance can be used to evaluate efficacy of nutrition support

Altered Carbohydrate Metabolism

History

Catabolism caused by trauma or burns; corticosteroid therapy

Physical examination

Muscle wasting

Laboratory analysis

↑ Serum glucose; glucosuria

Vitamin Deficiencies

C

History

Increased needs caused by trauma, burns, or major surgery; poor intake caused by anorexia

Continued

Box 10-1   Assessment in Metabolic Stress—cont'd

Physical examination

Gingivitis; petechiae, ecchymoses; delayed wound healing

Laboratory analysis

↓ Serum or leukocyte vitamin C

B Complex

History

Increased needs caused by fever or hypermetabolism; poor intake (same causes as PEM)

Physical examination

Glossitis; cheilosis (cracking at the corners of the mouth); peripheral neuropathy; dermatitis

Mineral Deficiencies

Iron

History

Blood loss, acute or chronic; poor intake (same causes as PEM); impaired absorption, especially after gastrectomy

Physical examination

Pallor; spoon-shaped nails; tachycardia

Laboratory analysis

↓ Hct, Hgb, MCV; ↓ serum iron and ferritin

Zinc

History

Increased losses from burns (loss of albumin to which zinc is bound), fistula or surgical drainage, open abdomen, or diarrhea; increased needs for healing of wounds; poor intake (same causes as PEM)

Physical examination

Poor sense of taste, distorted taste; poor wound healing; alopecia; dermatitis

Box 10-1   Assessment in Metabolic Stress—cont'd

Laboratory analysis

↓ Serum zinc

Fluid and Electrolyte Imbalances

Fluid Deficit

History

Increased losses from burns, persistent vomiting or diarrhea, gastric suction without adequate replacement, fever, tachypnea, fistula drainage, transient diabetes insipidus following head injury, use of radiant warmers or phototherapy (infants); poor intake caused by intestinal obstruction, coma, or confusion, causing failure to recognize or communicate thirst, use of tube feedings (especially in obtunded individuals) without adequate fluid

Physical examination

Poor skin turgor; acute weight loss; oliguria (adult: <20 ml/hr; infant or child: <2-4 ml/kg/hr; infant <6 days: <1-3 ml/kg/hr); hypotension; dry skin and mucous membranes; sunken fontanel (infants)

Laboratory analysis

Serum sodium >150 mEq/L; ↑ serum osmolality, urine specific gravity, Hct, BUN

Potassium Excess

History

Loss of potassium from damaged cells into extracellular fluid caused by burns or crushing injuries (early, usually within first 3 days)

Physical examination

Irritability; nausea, diarrhea; weakness

Laboratory analysis

↑ Serum potassium

Continued

Box 10-1   Assessment in Metabolic Stress—cont'd

Potassium Deficit

History

Increased losses caused by burns or crushing injury (after the early response), diarrhea, or vomiting; refeeding syndrome

Physical examination

Weakness; ↓ serum potassium, inverted T wave on ECG

Phosphorus

History

Aggressive refeeding (especially high-carbohydrate feedings, as in TPN) in malnourished individuals; alcoholism; increased losses from severe diarrhea or vomiting; hyperventilation related to causes such as sepsis, pain, anxiety, diabetic ketoacidosis

Physical examination

Tremor, ataxia; irritability progressing to stupor, coma, and death

Laboratory analysis

↓ Serum phosphate

BMI, Body mass index; *BUN,* blood urea nitrogen; *ECG,* electrocardiogram; *Hct,* hematocrit; *Hgb,* hemoglobin; *MCV,* mean corpuscular volume; *TPN,* total parenteral nutrition.

Intervention and education

Nutrient needs

Fluids and electrolytes. Daily maintenance requirements for fluid and electrolytes are summarized in Table 8-3. Increased losses, such as those from nasogastric suction, diaphoresis, and profuse diarrhea (short bowel syndrome), may substantially increase needs. Careful records of fluid output provide a guide to fluid and electrolyte replacement. Fluid deficits in infants and small children can be estimated from changes in body weight: fluid deficit (L) = usual weight (kg) − current weight (kg). For adults, fluid deficit can be estimated from serum sodium: fluid deficit (L) = 0.6 × body weight (kg) − [(140/patient's serum sodium concentration) $\times$ 0.6 $\times$ body weight (kg)], where sodium is in mEq/L or mmol/L, and 140 represents a normal serum sodium. Fluid resuscitation is a critical part of early burn care. Although standardized formulas are frequently used for estimating fluid resuscitation volumes, hemodynamic monitoring provides a more accurate assessment of the needs of the burn patient.

The syndrome of inappropriate antidiuretic hormone secretion (SIADH) is especially likely to occur in individuals with closed head injury. In this condition, serum sodium is unusually low, usually less than 126 mEq/L. SIADH does not result from sodium deficit but instead from fluid retention. It can usually be corrected by fluid restriction.

Energy. Energy needs of injured or postoperative individuals vary widely because of a number of injury- and treatment-related effects (Table 10-1), and indirect calorimetry is the most accurate method for measuring energy needs. It should be repeated regularly (as often as twice weekly) as the patient's condition changes. Where indirect calorimetry is not available, estimates of energy expenditure in the initial period following injury are made with a variety of formulas. The following is a summary of some of these formulas:

- The Harris-Benedict equations (see Table 2-6) to estimate basal energy expenditure (BEE). If the Harris-Benedict equations are used, the results are often multiplied by "injury factors" that attempt to estimate total daily energy expenditure. Injury factors commonly range from 1.1 times the BEE, for each degree of fever consistently over 98.6° F (37° C), to 1.2 to 1.4 times the BEE, for moderate to severe trauma or head injury (injury severity score of 25 to 30; see http://www.trauma.org/archive/scores/iss.html).
- The Mifflin–St. Jeor equations (see Table 2-6).
- Estimates of initial energy needs of patients with trauma to the central nervous system (CNS) are as follows:
  - Severe head injury causes increased energy expenditure or hypermetabolism, at least partly because it stimulates a marked increase in the release of catecholamines, with a resulting increase in oxygen consumption. Posturing, seizures, hyperventilation, and fever further increase the metabolic

Table 10-1   Factors That Impact Energy Expenditure in Patients with Trauma, Burns, or Major Surgery

	Increase	Decrease
Physiologic Factors		
Age		✓
Burn or wound size	✓	
Fever*	✓	
Malnutrition		✓
Pain	✓	
Pancreatitis	✓	
Spinal cord injury		✓
Traumatic brain injury, severe, unsedated	✓	
Traumatic brain injury, severe, sedated		✓
Effects of therapy		
Mechanical ventilation	✓	
Physical therapy	✓	
Pharmacologic Effects		
Barbiturates		✓
Corticosteroids	✓	
Neuromuscular blockade		✓
Propofol (continuous infusion)		✓
Vasoactive agents	✓	

*Sepsis or wound infection has little additional effect outside of fever.

rate. Pharmacologic paralysis, frequently used in treatment of severe head injury, reduces oxygen demand and energy expenditure. For patients with severe closed head injury (Glasgow Coma Scale <8), the following apply:

- Adult needs are approximately 140% of measured resting energy expenditure (≈30 kcal/kg/day) if there is no pharmacologic paralysis.
- Energy needs with pharmacologic paralysis can be estimated as 100% of measured resting energy expenditure (≈25 kcal/kg/day) (Jacobs et al., 2004).
- Energy needs of spinal cord injury patients decline because of the decrease in muscle energy use (Jacobs et al., 2004).
    - Quadriplegia: 20 to 22 total kcal/kg/day (or 55% to 90% of predicted BEE by Harris-Benedict equation).

- Paraplegia: 22 to 24 total kcal/kg/day (80% to 90% of predicted BEE by Harris-Benedict equation).

■ For burn patients, weekly indirect calorimetry is strongly encouraged, because needs change over the course of treatment and in response to complications and resolution of those complications. However, in the absence of indirect calorimetry, daily energy needs can be estimated as 1440 kcal/m^2 total body surface area or by a formula that takes into account the size of the burn: 1000 kcal/m^2 total body surface area + (25 × % body surface area burned) (Dickerson et al., 2002; Frankenfield, 2006).

Ongoing assessment is necessary to allow for adjustment of nutrition support as needed. Overfeeding sick and injured patients contributes to increased morbidity—for example, hyperglycemia, infection, and prolonged need for ventilatory assistance and intensive care. In no case should carbohydrate be delivered at a higher rate than 5 mg/kg/min, and stressed patients may not tolerate delivery rates this high. Hyperglycemia in perioperative and intensive care patients predisposes patients to infection and prolonged hospital stays. The most effective measures to control hyperglycemia are avoiding overfeeding and using insulin if needed (Debaveye and Van den Berghe, 2006; Powell-Tuck, 2007). Energy needs decline as healing takes place, and needs should be reassessed repeatedly, preferably with the use of indirect calorimetry, in order to adjust intake appropriately.

Protein. In adults, protein needs are estimated to be 1.25 g/kg daily for most trauma, and up to 2 g/kg/day in severe burns (Jacobs et al., 2004). For children, protein needs are approximately 2 to 3 g/kg/day.

Vitamins and minerals. Needs for most vitamins and minerals increase in metabolic stress; however, energy needs are also high, and if energy needs are met, adequate amounts of most vitamins and minerals are usually provided. Vitamin C, vitamin A or β-carotene, zinc, and iron intakes may need special attention, however.

Vitamin C, zinc, iron, and copper are all needed for collagen synthesis, an important part of wound healing. Zinc is required for DNA and protein synthesis, and zinc deficiency results in diminished wound strength and delayed epithelial coverage of the wound. Iron deficiency is relatively common because of blood loss and inadequate intake, and very severe deficiency can impair both collagen synthesis and oxygen transport to wounds and damaged tissues. In addition to their roles in healing, vitamins C and E, selenium, and zinc play a role as antioxidants. Metabolic stress is associated with increased production of "free radicals," which are especially reactive atoms with one or more unpaired electrons that can damage cells, proteins, and DNA by altering their chemical structures. Free radicals and other oxidants are believed to contribute to the development of adult respiratory distress syndrome. An adequate intake of antioxidant nutrients may help to limit oxidant damage. Micronutrient supplementation may also enhance immunity in injured patients. For example, supplementation with zinc, selenium, and copper reduced the risk of nosocomial pneumonia in a small but well-controlled study in patients with major burns (Berger et al., 2006).

Micronutrient needs in stressed patients are not well established, but the following is a guide to doses that have been used in critically ill and injured patients (Heyland et al., 2005; Berger and Shenkin, 2006).

- *Vitamin C*: 500 to 1000 mg daily.
- *Zinc*: 10 to 35 mg daily. Unusually high small or large bowel output requires zinc replacement; estimated zinc needs are 12 mg/L of small bowel drainage and 17 mg/kg of diarrheal stool or ileostomy drainage. Exudate from burns is also rich in zinc. Large doses of zinc provide no benefit unless deficiency or unusual losses are present, and, in fact, high intakes of zinc can have oxidant effects and suppress immune function.
- *Selenium*: 200 to 1000 mcg/day.
- *Iron*: 25 to 50 mg elemental iron daily if ferritin levels are low.

Nutrition support. Nutrition support is recommended for patients who will be unable to eat for at least 7 days before and after surgery and for those that are unable to consume at least 60% of their nutrient needs by mouth for more than 10 days. If surgery is not an emergency, preoperative nutrition support should be provided to patients at high nutritional risk for at least 10 to 14 days before surgery; ideally preoperative nutrition support should be given at home. Patients at high risk include those that have lost 10% to 15% of their body weight in the last 6 months, BMI <18.5 kg/m^2, serum albumin concentration <3.0 g/dl but no evidence of liver or renal disease, signs of muscle wasting and/or loss of subcutaneous fat, poor nutrient intake for 2 weeks or more, and/or GI symptoms daily or frequently for at least 2 weeks (Weimann et al., 2006).

Early enteral feeding (in comparison with either no artificial nutrition support or total parenteral nutrition [TPN]) has been shown in some studies to improve outcome in critically ill and injured patients, including those with abdominal trauma and colorectal surgery. However, meta-analysis evaluations of the randomized studies of enteral nutrition compared with no nutrition support or with TPN have not found differences in mortality among the treatments, even though infectious complications were less frequent in enterally fed patients (Gramlich et al., 2004; Koretz et al., 2007; Peter et al., 2005). The beneficial effects of enteral feeding may result from better maintenance of the gastrointestinal (GI) tract as a barrier to infection. In animal studies, lack of enteral nutrients causes GI mucosal atrophy and promotes translocation of microorganisms from the GI tract across the damaged gut and into the circulation. The importance of translocation in humans remains unclear (Gramlich et al., 2004). However, the GI tract is an important component of the immune system and contains significant amounts of gut-associated lymphoid tissue (GALT). Thus enteral feeding may result in fewer infections because it is more effective in maintaining or improving the GI tract's immune function. Also, TPN is likely to be associated with more infections because it provides a direct route for microorganisms to enter the bloodstream.

Delay in gastric emptying is common in acutely ill and injured patients, and this limits the amount of enteral formula that can be delivered into the stomach. Patients with traumatic brain injury and spinal cord injury are especially likely to have difficulty with gastric emptying, and their feeding tolerance may be improved if they are given duodenal or jejunal, rather than gastric, feedings. However, patients with unstable hemodynamic status and those who require pressor therapy to maintain adequate blood pressure are vulnerable to ischemic bowel damage. If patients at high risk for bowel ischemia are to be fed enterally, they need to be carefully monitored. The following guidelines have been suggested (McClave and Chang, 2003; Kutayli et al., 2005):

■ *Enteral formula selection*: Isotonic, as opposed to hypertonic, formulas are likely to be best tolerated. Fiber-containing formulas should be avoided because they serve as a substrate for bacterial growth. Glutamine-enriched formulas may be beneficial, whereas arginine enrichment is likely to provide no benefit or even be harmful (Heyland and Dhaliwal, 2005).

■ *Monitoring GI tolerance*: Patients should be monitored continually for evidence of ischemic bowel. Early indicators are those of feeding intolerance: nausea, diarrhea, bloating, and abdominal distention (repeated measurements taken at the umbilicus provide an objective indication of distention). Other signs and symptoms include cramping abdominal pain, ileus, and reduced passage of stool and flatus. These signs signal a need to reevaluate the patient, who may require a cessation of enteral feedings. Late signs, associated with significant injury, include high nasogastric output volumes, oliguria, metabolic acidosis, shock, and development of an acute abdomen. The abdominal radiographs may initially show dilated thickened loops of bowel; later, air in the wall of the intestine, the portal vein, or the peritoneal cavity may occur.

■ *Signs of need to stop enteral feedings*: In addition to increasing GI intolerance, other indicators of a need to withhold enteral feeding are a sustained mean arterial blood pressure of 70 mm Hg or less, a need for increasing doses of pressor agents, or a requirement for increased ventilatory support.

■ *Contraindications to enteral feedings*: Contraindications include ileus or bowel obstruction that cannot be bypassed (e.g., with a jejunostomy tube), severe shock, or intestinal ischemia (Weimann et al., 2006).

Improved understanding of the nutrient needs in metabolic stress, as well as better tools for monitoring GI tract perfusion in acutely ill patients, will undoubtedly improve care of these patients in the future. TPN is appropriate for those patients who do not tolerate enteral feedings and are at high nutritional risk. Overfeeding should be avoided in all patients, whether nutrients are delivered by enteral or parenteral route, to reduce hyperglycemia, metabolic demands, and the risk of infection.

Superior mesenteric artery syndrome. Superior mesenteric artery syndrome (SMA) is an uncommon condition in which the third part of the duodenum is compressed between the aorta and the mesenteric artery. The disorder is most commonly seen in very thin, cachectic individuals, but patients in body casts and those with spinal cord injury are also at risk. The symptoms of SMA include anorexia, post-prandial epigastric pain, vomiting, and weight loss. Because the symptoms are nonspecific, clinicians need to be aware of the possibility of SMA. Optimal nutrition support can relieve the condition, presumably by increasing the size of the fat pad around the mesenteric artery (Adams et al., 2007).

Organ Transplantation

Individuals undergoing organ transplantation (kidney, liver, heart, lung, small bowel, or pancreas) experience many of the same clinical problems as other critically ill and injured patients. However, the patient who experiences acute trauma or illness is likely to have been in good nutritional state before the illness or injury. In contrast, the organ transplant patient often has a variety of nutrition problems related to the underlying disease and its treatment (Box 10-2). Correction or control of these problems (to the extent possible) during the period of waiting for transplant improves graft survival and reduces morbidity and mortality.

Drug-Nutrient Interactions

After successful transplantation, most patients have improved quality of life, exercise tolerance, and nutritional status. However, they require long-term immunosuppressive therapy, with the potential for significant drug-nutrient interactions (Table 10-2). Corticosteroids are usually used in the early postoperative period and are especially likely to cause significant nutritional impact, including impaired glucose tolerance, hypercholesterolemia, and, with long-term use, osteoporosis. The current practice is to wean corticosteroid dosages as rapidly as possible to reduce the adverse effects. Episodes of organ rejection may require increased drug dosages or additional drugs in the treatment regimen. Since many side effects of immunosuppressant drugs are dose related, this can seriously impact nutritional status.

Medical Nutrition Therapy After Transplant

The following are suggested guidelines for medical nutrition therapy after transplantation (Hasse and Roberts, 2001; Stickel et al., 2008; Weimann et al., 2006); these must be modified to fit the need of the individual patient.

Box 10-2   Factors Contributing to Malnutrition in Organ Transplant Candidates

All Solid Organs

Anorexia
Nausea, vomiting
Depression, fatigue
Hypermetabolism and chronic inflammation
Diet restrictions reducing palatability
Drug-nutrient interactions

Heart

Impaired absorption caused by poor GI circulation
↑ Cardiac and pulmonary energy expenditure
Poor nutrient delivery to tissues caused by impaired circulation
Ascites and early satiety when hepatic congestion is present

Lung

↑ Work of breathing and resting energy expenditure
Complications related to cystic fibrosis: chronic infections, impaired absorption and steatorrhea, glucose intolerance and diabetes

Intestine

Complications of long-term TPN: cholestasis, cholelithiasis, hepatic dysfunction, portal hypertension, micronutrient deficiencies, metabolic bone disease

Liver

Protein intolerance
Fluid and electrolyte imbalances
Nutrient malabsorption and steatorrhea
Esophageal strictures and dysphasia
Mental alteration
Early satiety caused by ascites
Impaired hepatic protein synthesis
Malabsorption caused by ↓ bile salt concentrations
Small bowel dysfunction caused by portal hypertension or lymphostasis
Glucose intolerance and diabetes
Essential fatty acid deficiency

Box 10-2   Factors Contributing to Malnutrition in Organ Transplant Candidates—cont'd

Pancreas

Complications of diabetes: cardiovascular disease, nephropathy and albuminuria, gastroparesis

Kidney

Glucose intolerance
Hypertriglyceridemia and hypercholesterolemia
Abnormal metabolism of calcium, phosphorus, vitamin D
Anemia
↑ Protein degradation and loss

Adapted from Hasse JM, Roberts S: Transplantation. In Rombeau JL, Rolandelli RH: *Clinical nutrition-parenteral nutrition*, ed 3, Philadelphia, 2001, Saunders. Used with permission.
GI, Gastrointestinal; *TPN,* total parenteral nutrition.

- Protein intake of 1.2 to 1.5 g/kg/day for the first few weeks after surgery and 1 to 1.5 g/kg/day after the initial postoperative period is usually sufficient to allow for healing. This protein allowance must be tailored to the patient's needs (e.g., reduced if renal failure develops).

- Hyperphagia stimulated by immunosuppressant drugs and by improved well-being, along with improved absorption, contributes to weight gain after transplant. An increase in activity, behavioral measures to control eating behaviors, and instruction in healthy food choices are approaches to preventing or correcting unwanted weight gain. A modest reduction in energy intake is accomplished by limiting fried foods and high-fat foods, such as pastries, whole milk and products made with whole milk, butter, margarine, oils, nuts, chips, and other snack foods. Limiting intake of meats to no more than 5 or 6 ounces daily also reduces fat and energy intake (see Chapter 7).

- If hypertriglyceridemia is present, avoid alcohol intake; restricting intake of simple sugars (sugar, candies, desserts) helps to control both hypertriglyceridemia and hyperglycemia.

- The lifestyle changes described in Chapter 14 help to reduce cardiovascular risk if hypercholesterolemia and elevated low-density lipoprotein (LDL)–cholesterol are present.

Table 10-2   Nutritional Impacts of Immunosuppressant Therapy

Drug	GI Side Effects	Electrolyte, Metabolic, or Hematologic Alterations
Azathioprine	Oral lesions, diarrhea, steatorrhea, nausea, vomiting, anorexia, ↓ taste acuity, pancreatitis (long-term therapy)	↓ Albumin; macrocytic anemia; negative nitrogen balance
Basiliximab	Constipation, diarrhea, nausea, vomiting, abdominal pain, dyspepsia, oral candidiasis	↓ or ↑ K, ↓ Mg, ↓ P, ↓ cholesterol, ↑ glucose, anemia, ↑ uric acid, weight gain
Cyclosporine, modified	Nausea, vomiting, diarrhea, hepatotoxicity, oral candidiasis	↑ Glucose, anemia
Daclizumab	Diarrhea, nausea, vomiting, abdominal pain, pyrosis, dyspepsia, abdominal distention, epigastric pain, flatulence	
Muromonab-CD3	Diarrhea, vomiting, nausea	
Mycophenolate mofetil	Diarrhea, constipation, nausea, vomiting, dyspepsia, oral candidiasis	↑ Cholesterol, ↓ P, ↓ or ↑ K, ↑ glucose, anemia

Prednisone, other corticosteroids	Peptic ulceration, nausea, vomiting	↑ Glucose, ↑ cholesterol, ↓ K, weight gain, osteoporosis
Sirolimus	Diarrhea, constipation, nausea, vomiting, dyspepsia, abdominal pain, mouth ulceration or infection NOTE: take consistently with or without food (food alters bioavailability of drug); avoid grapefruit juice	↑ Cholesterol, ↑ triglycerides, ↓ K, anemia
Tacrolimus	Diarrhea, constipation, nausea, vomiting, anorexia, abdominal pain NOTE: take without food; grapefruit juice may raise drug concentrations	↓ or ↑ K, ↓ Mg, ↑ glucose

GI, Gastrointestinal; *K,* potassium; *Mg,* magnesium; *P,* phosphate.

- Supplements of vitamin D and calcium reduce the risk of developing osteoporosis related to disease complications (e.g., steatorrhea caused by impaired liver or small bowel function) or corticosteroid therapy. Other measures to reduce the risk of osteoporosis include limiting alcohol intake, avoiding smoking, and increasing weight-bearing exercise to at least 30 minutes most days of the week.

Conclusion

Metabolic stress—trauma, burns, major surgery, and serious infection or other critical illness—is initially characterized by a hypermetabolism, insulin resistance, and hyperglycemia. The individual who survives the initial period of stress then enters a healing phase that necessitates sufficient energy, protein, fluids, electrolytes, vitamins, and minerals to rebuild damaged tissues and restore function. People experiencing acute trauma are often in a good nutritional state before the metabolic stress begins, but those requiring organ transplantation may have some degree of impaired nutrition before surgery. The underlying nutritional status, extent of the injury or surgical procedure, and the patient's age and preexisting health status are factors that the health care team needs to consider in planning and delivering nutrition care.

REFERENCES

Adams JB et al: Superior mesenteric artery syndrome in the modern trauma patient, *Am Surg* 73:803, 2007.

Berger MM, Shenkin A: Update on clinical micronutrient supplementation studies in the critically ill, *Curr Opin Clin Nutr Metab Care* 9(6):711, 2006.

Berger MM et al: Reduction of nosocomial pneumonia after major burns by trace element supplementation: aggregation of two randomised trials, *Crit Care* 10(6):R153, 2006.

Debaveye Y, Van den Berghe G: Risks and benefits of nutritional support during critical illness, *Annu Rev Nutr* 26:513, 2006.

Devoto G et al: Prealbumin serum concentrations as a useful tool in the assessment of malnutrition in hospitalized patients, *Clin Chem* 52(12):2281, 2006.

Dickerson RN et al: Accuracy of predictive methods to estimate resting energy expenditure of thermally-injured patients, *JPEN J Parenter Enteral Nutr* 26(1):17, 2002.

Frankenfield D: Energy expenditure and protein requirements after traumatic injury, *Nutr Clin Pract* 21(5):430, 2006.

Gramlich L et al: Does enteral nutrition compared to parenteral nutrition result in better outcomes in critically ill adult patients? A systematic review of the literature, *Nutrition* 20(10):843, 2004.

Hasse JM, Roberts S: Transplantation. In Rombeau JL, Rolandelli RH: *Clinical nutrition-parenteral nutrition,* ed 3, Philadelphia, 2001, Saunders. Used with permission.

Heyland D, Dhaliwal R: Immunonutrition in the critically ill: from old approaches to new paradigms, *Intensive Care Med* 31(4):501, 2005.

Heyland DK et al: Antioxidant nutrients: a systematic review of trace elements and vitamins in the critically ill patient, *Intensive Care Med* 31(3):327, 2005.

Jacobs DG et al: Practice management guidelines for nutritional support of the trauma patient, *J Trauma* 57(3):660, 2004.

Johnson AM et al: Clinical indications for plasma protein assays: transthyretin (prealbumin) in inflammation and malnutrition. International Federation of Clinical Chemistry and Laboratory Medicine (IFCC) Scientific Division Committee on Plasma Proteins (C-PP), *Clin Chem Lab Med* 45(3):419, 2007.

Koretz RL et al: Does enteral nutrition affect clinical outcome? A systematic review of the randomized trials, *Am J Gastroenterol* 102(2):412, 2007.

Kutayli ZN, Domingo CB, Steinberg SM: Intestinal failure, *Curr Opin Anaesthesiol* 18(2):123, 2005.

Lenz A, Franklin GA, Cheadle WG: Systemic inflammation after trauma, *Injury* 38(12):1336, 2007.

McClave SA, Chang WK: Feeding the hypotensive patient: does enteral feeding precipitate or protect against ischemic bowel? *Nutr Clin Pract* 18(4):279, 2003.

Peter JV, Moran JL, Phillips-Hughes J: A metaanalysis of treatment outcomes of early enteral versus early parenteral nutrition in hospitalized patients, *Crit Care Med* 33(1):213, 2005.

Powell-Tuck J: Nutritional interventions in critical illness, *Proc Nutr Soc* 66(1):16, 2007.

Raguso CA, Dupertuis YM, Pichard C: The role of visceral proteins in the nutritional assessment of intensive care unit patients, *Curr Opin Clin Nutr Metab Care* 6(2):211, 2003.

Stickel F, Inderbitzin D, Candinas D: Role of nutrition in liver transplantation for end-stage chronic liver disease, *Nutr Rev* 66(1):47, 2008.

Weimann A et al: ESPEN Guidelines on Enteral Nutrition: Surgery including organ transplantation, *Clin Nutr* 25(2):224, 2006.

GASTROINTESTINAL, PANCREATIC, AND LIVER DYSFUNCTION

A variety of disorders that affect the gastrointestinal (GI) tract and its accessory organs—the liver, gallbladder, and pancreas—can impair nutritional status. Effects of these disorders include malabsorption, maldigestion, discomfort associated with eating, anorexia, impaired intake, and food intolerances. Disorders that often have an unfavorable impact on nutritional status and require medical nutrition therapy are discussed in this chapter. The chapter reviews motility disorders and gastric, intestinal, pancreatic, and hepatic disorders. Each section will present an overview of a specific GI disorder, its treatment, suggestions for nutrition assessment and care, and intervention and teaching strategies for the clinician. Cystic fibrosis, which affects both pancreatic and pulmonary function, is included in Chapter 15, "Pulmonary Disease."

Motility Disorders
Reflux, Gastroparesis, Achalasia, and Scleroderma

Among the problems that can interfere with normal esophageal and gastric function are gastroesophageal reflux and motor dysfunction. In **gastroesophageal reflux disease (GERD)**, reflux of stomach contents into the esophagus causes esophagitis and heartburn. Ulcer and stricture formation are two possible complications, and GERD is a major risk factor for development of Barrett esophagus (a precancerous condition) and adenocarcinoma of the esophagus. Reduced lower esophageal sphincter (LES) pressure contributes to GERD. GERD is especially common in individuals with hiatal hernia, with the likelihood of reflux being related to the size of the herniation. Other contributing factors include impairments of gastric emptying or esophageal peristalsis. Gastroparesis is associated with delayed gastric emptying of solids but not liquids. It occurs in people with neurologic deficits in the gastric region, including those who have had diabetes for a number of years and surgical damage to the gastric nerve supply, but a large number of cases are idiopathic.

Two motor disorders affecting the esophagus are **achalasia**, a complex neurologic condition that causes incomplete relaxation of the LES after swallowing, and *scleroderma*, a collagen-vascular disease causing proliferation of connective tissue and fibrosis in many organs. Achalasia obstructs the passage of food into the stomach, and **dysphagia** and regurgitation of food are common symptoms. Carcinoma of the esophagus is a potential long-term sequela. Scleroderma impairs peristalsis and LES closure; symptoms are the same as those of GERD.

Esophageal dysfunction places the patient at risk for pulmonary aspiration and subsequent pneumonia.

Treatment

Antireflux measures include elevation of the head of the bed; cessation of smoking, which reduces LES pressure; avoidance of medications that reduce LES pressure (e.g., anticholinergics, α-adrenergic antagonists, β-adrenergic agonists, calcium channel blockers, opiates, progesterone, theophylline) if possible; use of antacids; and dietary modification (see the following discussion on nutrition care). Medications to reduce gastric acidity include histamine-H_2 receptor antagonists, such as cimetidine and ranitidine, and proton pump inhibitors, such as omeprazole. Prokinetic medications, such as metoclopramide, increase LES pressure and promote gastric emptying. Antireflux surgery is a consideration for the patient who does not benefit from medical therapy.

Treatments for achalasia include drugs that relax the LES such as sublingual isosorbide dinitrate (Isordil), injection of the LES with botulinum toxin, mechanical dilation of the LES, or esophagomyotomy.

Nutrition assessment and care

A thorough nutrition assessment should be performed as described in Chapter 2. Box 11-1 highlights common or especially serious findings in GI disorders.

Intervention and education
Preventing or reducing reflux. Dietary measures should be individualized, because no one type of food stimulates reflux in all

Text continued on p. 308.

Box 11-1   Assessment in Gastrointestinal Disorders

Protein-Energy Malnutrition (PEM) or Protein-Calorie Malnutrition (PCM)

History

Decreased food intake caused by pain associated with eating (e.g., GER, cholecystitis, pancreatitis), alcohol abuse, anticipation of dumping syndrome, nausea and vomiting, or anorexia; dysphagia; increased losses from malabsorption related to persistent diarrhea or steatorrhea, pancreatic insufficiency, decreased bowel surface area in short bowel syndrome, or dumping syndrome; increased energy/protein needs in healing, infection, fever; catabolism resulting from corticosteroids

Physical examination

Muscle wasting; edema; triceps skinfold <5th percentile; weight <90% of that expected for height or BMI <18.5; for children, failure to follow individual established pattern on growth charts or height and/or weight <5th percentile on charts (see Appendix D on Evolve)

Laboratory analysis

↓ Serum albumin, transferrin, or prealbumin; ↓ creatinine-height index

Fluid Deficit

History

Excessive losses caused by severe vomiting or diarrhea

Physical examination

Poor skin turgor; dry, sticky mucous membranes; feeling of thirst; acute loss of >3%-5% of body weight; hypotension

Laboratory analysis

↑ BUN; ↑ Hct; ↑ serum sodium

Vitamin Deficiencies

A

History

Decreased absorption related to steatorrhea or pancreatic insufficiency

---

Box 11-1   Assessment in Gastrointestinal Disorders—cont'd

Physical examination

Drying of skin and cornea; papular eruption around hair follicles (follicular hyperkeratosis)

Laboratory analysis

↓ Serum retinol; ↓ Retinol binding protein (indicating PEM, with inadequate protein to manufacture carrier for vitamin A)

D

History

Decreased absorption related to steatorrhea or pancreatic insufficiency

Physical examination

Bone pain, ↓ bone density

E

History

Decreased absorption related to steatorrhea or pancreatic insufficiency

Physical examination

Neuromuscular dysfunction causing weakness

Laboratory analysis

↓ Serum tocopherol; ↑ fragility of red blood cells

K

History

Decreased absorption related to steatorrhea or pancreatic insufficiency; decreased production related to alteration of intestinal flora by antibiotic usage

Physical examination

Petechiae, ecchymoses

Laboratory analysis

Prolonged PT

Continued

Box 11-1   Assessment in Gastrointestinal Disorders—cont'd

B_{12}

History

Decreased absorption related to gastrectomy (loss of intrinsic factor necessary for absorption), inadequate acid production in stomach (frequently occurs with aging), distal ileal disease or resection (loss of absorptive sites); bacterial overgrowth in the bowel competing for vitamin B_{12} (occurs in short bowel syndrome or gastric resection)

Physical examination

Pallor; sore, inflamed tongue; neuropathy; psychiatric symptoms

Laboratory analysis

$\downarrow$ Serum vitamin B_{12}; $\downarrow$ Hct, $\uparrow$ MCV

Mineral/Electolyte Deficiencies

Calcium

History

Decreased intake of milk products because of lactose intolerance; increased losses related to steatorrhea or corticosteroid use; hip or vertebrae fractures related to osteoporosis

Physical examination

Tingling of fingers; muscular tetany and cramps, carpopedal spasm; convulsion

Laboratory analysis

$\downarrow$ Serum calcium (severe deficits only); $\downarrow$ bone mineral density (chronic calcium deficit)

Magnesium

History

Inadequate intake related to alcoholism; increased losses related to steatorrhea or diarrhea, vomiting, loss of small bowel fluid in short bowel syndrome or fistula

Physical examination

Tremor, hyperactive deep reflexes; convulsions

Box 11-1   Assessment in Gastrointestinal Disorders—cont'd

Laboratory analysis

↓ Serum magnesium

Iron

History

Blood loss; impaired absorption related to decreased acid within upper GI tract, resulting from chronic antacid or proton pump inhibitor use, aging, gastrectomy; decreased intake related to restriction of protein foods in liver disease

Physical examination

Spoon-shaped nails; pallor, blue sclerae; fatigue

Laboratory analysis

↓ Hct, Hgb, MCV; ↓ serum iron; ↓ ferritin

Zinc

History

Increased losses related to diarrhea/steatorrhea, loss of intestinal fluid in short bowel syndrome, high output ileostomy, fistula drainage; decreased intake during protein restriction

Physical examination

Anorexia; poor sense of taste, distorted taste; alopecia; poor wound healing; diarrhea; dermatitis

Laboratory analysis

↓ Serum zinc

Potassium

History

Increased losses related to diarrhea or intestinal fluid loss

Physical examination

Muscle weakness, ileus; diminished reflexes

Laboratory analysis

↓ Serum potassium; inverted T wave on ECG

Continued

Box 11-1   Assessment in Gastrointestinal Disorders—cont'd

Nutrient Excess of Iron

History

Family history of hemochromatosis

Physical examination

No abnormalities if diagnosed early; later: bronze skin (in areas not exposed to sun)

Laboratory analysis

↑ Serum iron, ↑ ferritin, ↑ transferrin saturation

BMI, Body mass index; *BUN,* blood urea nitrogen; *ECG,* electrocardiogram; *GER,* gastroesophageal reflux; *GI,* gastrointestinal; *Hct,* hematocrit; *Hgb,* hemoglobin; *MCV,* mean corpuscular volume; *PT,* prothrombin time.

individuals with GERD. In general, these guidelines are associated with the least risk of reflux (Karamanolis and Tack, 2006):

- Reduce weight if overweight or obese, and avoid tight clothing.
- Consume small, frequent meals. High-volume meals are more likely to cause reflux.
- Wine and other alcoholic beverages, chocolate, chili, and onions reduce LES pressure and may contribute to reflux. Salty foods and addition of table salt seem to increase GERD symptoms in a dose-dependent manner.
- Carbonated beverages and acidic juices may contribute to reflux. Coffee does not appear to be related to reflux.
- Do not lie down within 2 hours of a meal. Eat the last meal of the day several hours before bedtime, and avoid late-night snacking. Keep the head of the bed elevated at least 15 cm (6 in).
- Avoid smoking, because nicotine reduces LES pressure.

Promoting gastric emptying. The severity of gastroparesis varies greatly among individuals. Some measures that may be beneficial include the following:

- Increase liquid intake, and puree foods if necessary.
- Consume small, frequent meals.

- Limit carbonated beverages because they expand the stomach. Avoid alcoholic beverages and smoking because they delay gastric emptying.
- If vomiting is a problem, ensure that fluid and electrolyte intake is sufficient to replace losses; fluid intake should be at least 1 to 1.5 L/day.

Coping with dysphagia. Solid foods and thin liquids usually cause the most difficulty. Foods that create a semisolid bolus when chewed are generally best tolerated.

- Liquids can be thickened with dry infant cereals, mashed potatoes or potato flakes, cornstarch, or yogurt.
- Commercial thickened fluids are available for individuals with dysphagia. Water, tea, a variety of juices, and milk are among the thickened fluids that can be purchased.
- Fluids in frozen form (e.g., sherbet or fruit ices) can be used.
- A speech therapist may be able to assist dysphagic individuals in improving their swallowing techniques.

Providing nutrition support as needed. Where esophageal obstruction exists or reflux or dysphagia is severe, impairing intake so much that weight loss occurs or placing the individual at high risk of pulmonary aspiration, tube feedings (by means of gastrostomy or jejunostomy if esophageal obstruction is present) may be needed. Special care must be taken to reduce the risk of pulmonary aspiration (e.g., elevation of the head of the bed and avoiding excessive volumes of feeding at any one time).

Gastric Disorders
Gastrectomy

Partial or total resection of the stomach is sometimes required for treatment of gastric cancer. Fat malabsorption and dumping syndrome are common after gastrectomy. Fat malabsorption results from the bypass of the duodenum by the Roux-en-Y esophagojejunostomy and other common gastrectomy procedures. Bacteria multiply within the bypassed duodenum, and the bacteria deconjugate bile salts, making micelle formation and fat absorption inadequate (see Chapter 8 for a discussion of fat absorption). Dumping syndrome results from the rapid passage of foods into the small bowel, caused by the loss or bypass of the pyloric sphincter. Rapid digestion of nutrients increases the osmolality (concentrations of solutes) within the upper small bowel. Fluid from the plasma and extracellular space is drawn into the bowel to dilute the hypertonic intestinal contents (DeLegge, 2006). Symptoms include nausea, abdominal pain, weakness, diaphoresis (sweating), diarrhea, and weight loss.

Nutrition assessment and care

Assessment is summarized in Box 11-1 and described more fully in Chapter 2.

Intervention and education

Nutrition support. Individuals recovering from surgery for cancer of the stomach or gastroesophageal junction frequently require enteral tube feedings while the surgical area heals. A jejunostomy is often placed at the time of surgery.

Dietary modifications and their rationale. Reduce the likelihood of dumping syndrome with the following measures (DeLegge, 2006):

- Eat small meals and snacks often; 6 meals per day may be needed.
- Avoid beverages at mealtime. Drink fluids at least 1 hour before or after meals.
- Although fresh fruits are high in simple carbohydrates, they are often well tolerated because of their content of soluble fibers, such as pectin. They can be used as desserts and snacks.
- Avoid concentrated sweets (e.g., candy, cookies, pies, cakes, jam, jelly, soft drinks, sugared beverages or foods).
- Maintain nonstressful eating practices. Eat slowly in a relaxed setting. Lying down for about 1 hour after meals can also help prevent dumping syndrome.

Supplementation. Calcium and iron, which are best absorbed in an acidic environment, may be poorly absorbed postoperatively. Normally, much of their absorption takes place in the duodenum, which is acidified by the entry of the stomach contents that have not yet been alkalinized by the pancreatic secretions. Calcium and iron supplements help to reduce the risk of osteoporosis or osteopenia and iron deficiency anemia.

Intrinsic factor and hydrochloric acid, both produced in the stomach, are required for absorption of vitamin B_{12}. Therefore supplemental vitamin B_{12} (regular injections or high-dose oral supplements) is usually necessary for the remainder of the person's life. Some individuals may be able to absorb sufficient vitamin B_{12} if given very–high-dose oral supplements (1000 mcg or more) daily.

Intestinal Disorders

Nutrients are absorbed at specific sites in the small intestine (see Figure 1-5); therefore the location and the extent of small intestinal disease or resection determine which nutrients will be affected. Generally, the proximal small intestine is more effective in increasing its absorptive capacity following resection of the distal bowel than the distal bowel is in adapting to the loss of the proximal intestine. However, the proximal small intestine cannot take on the absorption of vitamin B_{12}.

Osteoporosis is especially common among individuals with diseases causing malabsorption of fat (DeLegge, 2006). The etiology and nutritional treatment of osteoporosis are summarized in Box 11-2.

Short Bowel Syndrome

Massive resection of the small bowel, creating **short bowel syndrome**, severely reduces the area available for the absorption of nutrients. Small bowel resection is sometimes required in Crohn disease, necrotizing enterocolitis (see Chapter 20), congenital atresias, acute volvulus, strangulated hernias, mesenteric artery occlusion, and similar disorders. The adaptive response takes place in phases (Keller et al., 2004):

Acute phase: In the immediate postoperative period, enormous losses of fluids, electrolytes, magnesium, calcium, zinc, and amino acids occur. In addition to the loss of absorptive area, temporary gastric hypersecretion contributes to fluid and electrolyte losses. This phase usually lasts less than 1 month.

Adaptation phase: The bowel surface area increases as a result of hypertrophy. Diarrhea diminishes, along with fluid and electrolyte problems. This phase lasts up to 2 years.

Maintenance phase: The patient requires individualized dietary modifications for the remainder of the life span. Adequate treatment of preexisting disease (e.g., Crohn) is essential to allow stable GI function.

Box 11-2   Osteoporosis and Osteopenia Related
to Gastrointestinal Disorders

Possible Etiologies

- Malabsorption of vitamin D and calcium because of steatorrhea
- Impaired absorption of calcium because of decreased acidity in proximal small intestine (e.g., gastrectomy)
- Chronic (3 months or longer) or repeated treatment with corticosteroids
- Inflammatory processes (bone resorption is stimulated by the inflammatory cytokines)
- Lactose intolerance
- Alcohol abuse (increased excretion of calcium, possibly poor dietary intake)

Nutrition and Lifestyle Measures to Reduce the Risk of Osteoporosis

- Adequate calcium intake: At least 1000 mg daily in young men and premenopausal women and 1200 mg daily for men older than 50 years and postmenopausal women; individuals with malabsorption may need increased amounts.
  - Dietary sources include milk and milk products, calcium-fortified juices, sardines and other canned fish, and most dark green, leafy vegetables.
  - Supplements of calcium carbonate (40% calcium) or calcium citrate (24% calcium) may be needed to achieve adequate intakes. Calcium citrate has higher bioavailability and may cause less bloating and constipation.
  - If renal calcium loss is high, kidney stones may occur. Individuals excreting more than 4 mg/kg/day are at risk of stone formation. Thiazide diuretics can be used to decrease calcium excretion.
- Adequate vitamin D intake: Healthy adults need 5 to 10 mcg/day (200 to 400 international units/day), and those with malabsorption may need several times more.
  - Vitamin D may cause toxicity, including hypercalcemia and hypercalciuria, at high doses, and therefore vitamin D intake should be carefully evaluated.
- Avoid smoking.
- Avoid excessive alcohol intake.
- Engage in weight-bearing exercise most days of the week.

Treatment

Antidiarrheal and anticholinergic drugs, such as codeine, loperamide (Imodium), diphenoxylate with atropine (Lomotil), or glycopyrrolate (Robinul), may be helpful in controlling diarrhea during phases 1 and 2. If the ileum is removed, large amounts of bile salts can enter the colon and cause diarrhea by stimulating colonic water secretion. At least 100 cm of ileum is required for complete absorption of bile salts. Cholestyramine is sometimes used to bind the bile salts and reduce diarrhea. Some patients with short bowel syndrome who depend on total parenteral nutrition (TPN) for survival have undergone small bowel transplantation. The patients most commonly undergoing transplantation are those with TPN-related complications or inadequate vascular access for continued TPN. Growth hormone and glucagon-like peptide 2 have been used to enhance mucosal growth and improve absorption, in an effort to free patients from reliance on TPN (Keller et al., 2004; Jeppesen, 2007).

Nutrition assessment and care

Assessment is summarized in Box 11-1 and described in more detail in Chapter 2. Massive small bowel resection can be expected to affect absorption of almost every nutrient and to have great potential for causing malnutrition.

Intervention and education
Replacing losses and maintaining nutritional status. The patient who successfully adapts to the loss of a significant portion of the bowel moves through several stages, as follows (Keller et al., 2004):

Acute phase: Intravenous (IV) support is essential to replace fluids, electrolytes, and other nutrient losses. Most individuals require TPN for at least a few weeks after surgery. It is especially important to replace zinc losses (12 to 17 mg of zinc is lost per kilogram of feces or ileostomy drainage) because wound healing is impaired without zinc, and standard TPN solutions do not contain enough zinc to replace losses from profuse diarrhea.

Adaptation phase: The presence of nutrients within the GI tract is necessary for bowel adaptation to occur. Enteral feedings are often started as soon as the volume of fecal losses decreases to less than 1 L/day. An elemental diet with hydrolyzed protein and medium-chain triglycerides (MCTs) is usually better absorbed than a polymeric diet (see Chapter 8). Typically, TPN continues as continuous tube feedings are begun. Small oral feedings may also be started. They are generally low in fat (<10 g/day) and fiber and high in starch. White rice, enriched white bread and toast, noodles, macaroni, and peeled boiled or baked potato (all without added milk, cheese, margarine, butter, or other fat) are examples of possible foods. The diet is liberalized if the patient tolerates feeding without excessive losses. Dietary restrictions are avoided if possible, because they tend to limit energy intake.

Maintenance phase: An individualized diet plan should be followed, with consultation by a registered dietitian. Feedings should be small and frequent. Fat intake can be increased unless **steatorrhea** worsens. Concentrated sugars, excessive fat, or alcohol consumption may worsen malabsorption. MCTs (see Chapter 8) can be used in cooking or added to foods such as applesauce or hot cereals for caloric supplementation, but excessive amounts can worsen diarrhea. TPN will continue to be required if the individual is unable to maintain adequate nutritional status with oral or oral plus enteral tube feedings.

The individual who enters the adaptation and maintenance phases will need instruction in a high-energy diet with small, frequent feedings. Severe steatorrhea may improve with a low-fat diet (Table 11-1), but the need for such a diet should be determined on an individual basis since it also tends to reduce total energy intake. Fat restriction appears to be most effective in individuals who still have the colon (Lochs et al., 2006). Lactose intolerance is common, but yogurt, hard cheeses, milk accompanied by intake of lactase enzyme, and calcium-fortified juices provide well-tolerated calcium sources. Adequate vitamin D and calcium are needed to replace fecal losses and reduce the risk of osteopenia or osteoporosis (see Box 11-2).

Patients with a proximal jejunostomy (in the upper portion of the jejunum) should be encouraged to consume electrolyte-containing drinks rather than plain water as fluid replacement. Fluid and electrolyte losses are so great that plain water results in more losses than it replaces (O'Keefe, 2007). Oral rehydration solutions (e.g., Pedialyte, Enfalyte, WHO/UNICEF oral rehydration salts [http://rehydrate.org/ors/low-osmolarity-ors.htm]) are suited to replacement of fluid losses. Small amounts of fluid taken at frequent intervals are usually better tolerated than larger amounts taken less often.

Table 11-1   Fat-Restricted Diet

Foods to Include	Foods to Avoid
Milk Products	
Milk products made with skim milk; fat-free ice cream, cottage cheese, cheese, and yogurt	Milk products made with 2% or whole milk
Meat and Meat Substitutes	
Lean meat, fish (water packed, if canned), poultry without skin, egg whites	Fried meats, sausage, frank-furters, poultry skins, duck, goose, salt pork, luncheon meats, peanut butter, egg yolk except as allowed*
Breads and Cereals	
Plain pasta, cereals, whole-grain or en-riched bread or rolls	Biscuits, doughnuts, pancakes, sweet rolls, waffles, muffins, high-fat rolls, such as croissants
Fruits	
All except avocado	Avocado except as allowed as a fat serving*
Vegetables	
All if plainly prepared	Fried, au gratin, creamed, or buttered
Desserts	
Sherbet made with skim milk, sorbet, angel food cake, gelatin, pudding made with skim milk, fruit ice	Cake, pie, pastry, ice cream (except fat free or light, as allowed*), or any dessert con-taining fat or chocolate (other than cocoa powder)
Sweets	
Jelly, jam, syrup, sugar, hard sugar candies, jelly beans, gum drops	Any candy made with chocolate, nuts, butter, margarine, or cream

Continued

Table 11-1   Fat-Restricted Diet—cont'd

Foods to Include	Foods to Avoid
Fats and Related Foods	
Nonstick cooking spray, nonfat salad dressings	Limit fatty foods to 3 to 6 servings daily; 1 serving = 1 tsp butter, margarine, oil, or regular mayonnaise; 1 tbsp regular salad dressing or cream; 1 strip crisp bacon; ⅛ avocado; 6 small nuts; 10 peanuts; 5 small olives; ½ C "light" ice cream; 1 egg yolk or whole egg

*See "Fats and Related Foods."

Hyperoxaluria (excessive urinary excretion of oxalates), which may result in formation of urinary stones, occurs in some individuals with steatorrhea. Normally, calcium binds oxalate in the gut to inhibit oxalate absorption, but calcium forms natural soaps with the unabsorbed fat and is lost in the feces. Excessive fecal calcium losses allow increased absorption of oxalate. A low-oxalate diet can be used if a calcium supplement is not sufficient to correct the hyperoxaluria. Foods high in oxalate include nuts, chocolate, spinach, chard, beets, rhubarb, chocolate soy milk, miso, sesame seeds, buckwheat, wheat bran, and whole grains. A detailed listing of the oxalate content of foods is available at http://www.ohf.org/docs/Oxalate2008.pdf.

Supplementation

Individuals not receiving TPN: Daily supplements are often necessary, particularly water-miscible forms of the fat-soluble vitamins A and E; vitamins D and K; iron; calcium; magnesium; and zinc.

Severe steatorrhea: Water-miscible forms of vitamins A, D, E, and K may be better absorbed than standard fat-soluble forms. Hypomagnesemia and hypocalcemia are common; a low-fat diet combined with supplements of these minerals helps to correct deficiencies. Zinc supplements may also be needed.

Absence of the terminal ileum: Vitamin B$_{12}$ supplements are needed, usually in regularly scheduled injections.

Emotional support. The effects of massive bowel resection are catastrophic and are likely to be permanent. The individual and family need encouragement and reinforcement, particularly if home TPN or tube feedings are required.

Home nutrition support. Most individuals will need instruction in home TPN or tube feedings because these may need to continue at least until maximal adaptation occurs (see Chapters 8 and 9). TPN is especially likely to be necessary for a prolonged period, or permanently, if (1) more than 80% of the small bowel is resected, (2) less than 100 cm of jejunum remains and there is no colon, or (3) the unresected bowel is damaged or diseased (Keller et al., 2004; Buchman, 2006; Parekh and Steiger, 2007).

Celiac Disease (Nontropical Sprue or Gluten-Sensitive Enteropathy)

Celiac disease is a genetic disorder that results from an immune reaction to the **gliadin** portion of **gluten** (a protein found in wheat) and to closely related proteins in rye and barley. The immune response brings about a marked decrease in the length of the villi and in the surface area of the bowel, and the capacity for digesting disaccharides such as sucrose and lactose and peptides is low because the enzymes required are found in the intestinal mucosal cells. Diarrhea, steatorrhea, impaired absorption of all nutrients, muscle wasting, weight loss or failure to gain weight (in children), and anemia are common signs and symptoms. Dermatitis herpetiformis is a severe, itchy, blistering skin disease caused by gluten intolerance. Although dermatitis herpetiformis is a separate disease, affected individuals are likely to have intestinal damage similar to those with celiac disease.

Measurement of tissue transglutaminase antibody is the best single blood test for celiac disease, but a small bowel biopsy to look for microscopic evidence of blunting of the villi is currently the definitive diagnosis. Improvement of symptoms in response to a trial of a gluten-restricted diet is further evidence of celiac disease (AGA Institute, 2006).

Nutrition assessment and care

A thorough nutrition assessment should be carried out as described in Chapter 2. Especially common or significant findings are summarized in Box 11-1.

Intervention and education

Gluten-free diet. Permanent removal of gluten and related proteins from the diet is the only treatment for celiac disease. Following the diet is especially important because GI lymphoma appears to be more common in individuals who fail to do so (AGA Institute, 2006). This diet is difficult to follow because grain products are so widely used in processed foods and because they form the basis of many common dishes. The individual and family need extensive encouragement and reinforcement.

Recommendations for restricting gluten include the following:

- Avoid wheat, barley, rye, and all products made with these grains. Buckwheat is a grass not related to wheat, and it is acceptable for use. Table 11-2 lists foods to include and to avoid in gluten sensitivity. Alternative names for wheat products, such as graham (whole wheat), durum, and semolina, are frequently used on food packaging. Some products that are naturally gluten free are processed in plants where gluten-containing grains are also processed and can become contaminated with gluten as a result. Check the label of all grain products for the "gluten-free" health claim.
- The use of oats in celiac disease is controversial. Some evidence suggests that oats (at least up to 60 g daily) may be tolerated by most adults with celiac disease, but data regarding the safety of oats in celiac disease are not yet conclusive (NIDDK, 2007). If oats are included in the diet, it is necessary to be sure that they come from a source where there is no chance of contamination with wheat, barley, and rye during harvesting, storage, or processing.
- Read labels carefully because gluten and gluten-containing grains are added to many products. When it is unclear whether a product contains gluten, contact the manufacturer or distributor (whose address must appear on the food label) or consult their website to obtain further information. Look for the term *gluten free* on food labels; some manufacturers are adding this information voluntarily. In restaurants, ask whether unfamiliar foods contain restricted grains.
- Cornmeal; cornstarch; flour made from rice, peas, beans, or potatoes; amaranth; and tapioca are examples of products that can be used instead of wheat flour for thickening foods and preparing bread products.

Table 11-2   Diet for Gluten Intolerance

Foods to Include	Foods to Avoid*
Milk Products and Cheeses	
All except those with gluten additives	Malted milk, some milk drinks, and some flavored or frozen yogurt; any cheese containing oat gum†; some pasteurized process cheese
Meat, Poultry, Fish, Eggs, Dry Beans and Peas, Nuts	
All fresh, unprocessed meat, poultry, and fish; dried beans and peas; soybeans; nuts; peanut butter; cold cuts, frankfurters, and sausage without fillers	Breaded products; some sausages, frankfurters, luncheon meats, and sandwich spreads (with fillers); some imitation seafood and bacon bits; self-basting turkey; some egg substitutes
Breads and Starches	
Potatoes, potato flour, rice, rice flour, wild rice, corn, cornstarch, hominy, grits, buckwheat, amaranth, bean or pea flour, quinoa, flax, sago, teff, tapioca, arrowroot, soy and soy flour, millet, sorghum, cassava, yucca, gluten-free pasta and breads	All products containing wheat, rye, barley, triticale (wheat-rye hybrid); cracked wheat; wheat starch; wheat bran; wheat germ; graham, durum, bromated, enriched, self-rising, white, or phosphorated flour; bulgur; farina; spelt; kamut; wheat-based semolina; cereals with malt flavoring or extracts; hydrolyzed wheat protein; some rice mixes; communion wafers; possibly oats†
Vegetables	
All plain varieties—fresh, frozen, or canned	Creamed, au gratin, breaded, or in sauce (unless made with gluten-free starch); canned baked beans; some French fries

Continued

Table 11-2 Diet for Gluten Intolerance—cont'd

Foods to Include	Foods to Avoid*
Fruits	
All plain varieties—fresh, frozen, or canned	Some commercial fruit pie fillings
Beverages	
Pure instant and ground coffee; tea; carbonated drinks; wine; tequila; sake; rum; distilled grain alcohol including whiskey, bourbon, and gin	Flavored instant coffee, hot cocoa mixes, herbal tea, beer, ale, malted beverages, some vodka
Miscellaneous	
Most seasonings and flavorings; sauces, soups, and condiments prepared with allowed ingredients; butter, margarine, oils; sugar, honey, plain chocolate, coconut, molasses, meringue, marshmallows; acacia, xanthan and guar gums; distilled vinegar	Some nondairy creamers; commercial salad dressings; prepared soups; condiments, sauces, and seasonings prepared with grains that are not allowed; gravy; some bouillon cubes; some types of snack chips; seasoned tortilla chips; some soups; licorice; malt vinegar; chocolate bars

*Some of these products are available in gluten-free varieties that can be included in the gluten-free diet. Consult the label.

†Evidence suggests that some individuals with celiac disease tolerate oats, but oats have also been found to cause intestinal inflammation in some people with the disorder. Thus it is not possible at this time to make a firm statement about the place of oats in a gluten-free diet (NIDDK, 2007). It is likely that many oat products are contaminated by other grains harvested, stored, or processed with the oats, and this may be the cause of gastrointestinal symptoms after oat consumption. Pure oats are available in Canada; these are grown, processed, and tested under the guidance of the Canadian Food Inspection Agency and Health Canada. The Canadian Celiac Association advises that adults can safely consume up to 70 g (½ to ¾ C) of pure oats per day and children can consume up to 25 g (¼ C) (Rashid et al., 2007).

- Some individuals with celiac disease are nonresponsive to treatment. In some instances this reflects failure to diagnose other disorders, such as pancreatic insufficiency or intestinal lymphomas (ADA Institute, 2006), but in most cases it results from inadvertent or deliberate consumption of gluten-containing foods. A dietitian familiar with celiac disease and its treatment is the professional best prepared to educate and advise the person with celiac disease. Celiac disease support groups can provide recipes, practical information, and support for the affected individual and the family. Local groups can be located through the national Celiac Sprue Association (see Appendix H on Evolve).

Supplementation. A complete blood count and measurement of serum ferritin, folate, and vitamin B_{12} provide a guide to the need for supplementation.

- Supplements of iron, folic acid, and vitamin B_{12} may be needed if deficiency is indicated, although levels of these nutrients often normalize as the person follows the gluten-free diet and absorption improves.
- Severe hypokalemia and hypomagnesemia might be present because of losses in steatorrhea. Immediate correction of these deficits should be carried out; as the patient responds to the change in diet, these problems will not recur.
- Osteoporosis and osteopenia are common among individuals with celiac disease (ADA Institute, 2006). See Box 11-2 for nutrition interventions.

Inflammatory Bowel Disease (Crohn Disease and Ulcerative Colitis)

Inflammatory bowel disease (IBD) can affect individuals of all ages. In **Crohn disease** (regional ileitis), inflammation extends through all layers of the bowel wall. It can affect any part of the GI tract but most often affects the terminal ileum. In acute exacerbations, abdominal pain, fever, nausea, and diarrhea occur. In chronic disease, weight loss, anorexia, anemia, and steatorrhea are common.

In **ulcerative colitis**, congestion, edema, and ulcerations affect the mucosal and submucosal layers of the bowel. It usually involves the rectum and colon and sometimes extends to the ileum. Bloody diarrhea, abdominal and rectal pain, weight loss, and anorexia are common.

Diagnosis is made by barium enema, endoscopy (sigmoidoscopy, colonoscopy, or esophagoscopy), and intestinal biopsy.

Treatment

Drugs that are often used include corticosteroids to decrease inflammation; antidiarrheals, such as diphenoxylate (Lomotil); and antispasmodics to decrease discomfort. Aminosalicylates such as sulfasalazine and mesalamine are for their antiinflammatory effects. Antibiotics, including ciprofloxacin and metronidazole, are used especially in patients with GI fistulas or perianal disease. Immune response modulators such as 6-mercaptopurine and azathioprine may be used as adjuncts to treatment. Infliximab reduces inflammation in Crohn disease by blocking the effects of tumor necrosis factor–α. See Appendix G on Evolve for drug-nutrient interactions). Surgery may be necessary if fistulas, hemorrhage, perforation, or intestinal obstruction occurs. Resection of the colon is often performed after several acute exacerbations of ulcerative colitis because of the risk of developing colon cancer.

Nutrition assessment and care

A thorough nutrition assessment should be carried out as described in Chapter 2. Especially common or significant findings are summarized in Box 11-1.

Intervention and education
Diet and other lifestyle modifications

Acute disease: For adults, enteral nutrition support combined with corticosteroid therapy has been effective in producing a remission of disease. For children, where long-term corticosteroid therapy is undesirable because it impairs growth, enteral nutrition support alone may be effective in bringing about remission (Lochs et al., 2006).

Remission: A low-fat diet (see Table 11-1) may be prescribed to decrease steatorrhea, which is common with ileal involvement. A high-protein diet (1.5 to 2 g/kg/day) helps promote bowel regeneration and replace losses. Enteral nutrition support may be used to correct nutritional deficits (Lochs et al., 2006). Additional measures to consider include the following:

■ If areas of intestinal inflammatory stenosis are present, enteral nutrition support may be of benefit but must be used with caution (Lochs et al, 2006).

■ Lactose intolerance is common in Crohn disease. Some lactose-intolerant individuals can tolerate yogurt, buttermilk, and hard cheeses. Lactase enzyme can be consumed with milk to hydrolyze the lactose.

Supplementation. The following supplements may be needed:

■ Iron if blood loss is sufficient to cause anemia.
■ Vitamins A and E in water-miscible forms, vitamin D, vitamin K, calcium, magnesium, and zinc if steatorrhea is present (DeLegge, 2006). Osteoporosis and osteopenia are common among individuals with IBD. See Box 11-2 for nutrition intervention to reduce the risk of osteoporosis. Adequate vitamin D and calcium intakes are key dietary measures for reducing the risk of osteoporosis (O'Sullivan and O'Morain, 2006).
■ Vitamin B_{12} if the terminal ileum is involved. Delivery by injection or nasal gel or spray may be necessary if there is severe damage to the ileum.

Irritable Bowel Syndrome

Irritable bowel syndrome (IBS) is a relatively common functional disorder characterized by symptoms related to the colon, including pain relieved by defecation or associated with change in stool frequency or consistency. The disorder can be diarrhea predominant, constipation predominant, or pain/bloating predominant (Karamanolis and Tack, 2006). The cause is unclear but could include allergic/hypersensitivity reactions, psychosocial factors, or altered GI motility. The pain/bloating–predominant form is associated with increased intestinal gas production. The disease is not life threatening, but in its severe form, it can interfere with being able to work, participate in social activities, and carry out many activities of daily living.

Treatment

Keeping a diary of symptoms can help to reveal precipitating causes of bouts of IBS. The treatment often includes medications acting at the serotonin receptor, e.g., alosetron for diarrhea or tegaserod for constipation, antidepressants, and psychologic support and intervention. Tegaserod is currently available only under an investigational new drug protocol for women younger than 55 years of age with no evidence of heart disease who give their informed consent for use of the drug and for whom the benefits of tegaserod outweigh the risks (U.S. Food and Drug Administration, 2007).

Nutrition assessment and care

Most patients with IBS believe that diet components either cause or worsen their symptoms. Nutrition intervention should be based only on a thorough assessment with a diet history and food record (see Box 11-1).

Intervention and education
Diet and other lifestyle modifications. Diet intolerances are unlikely to cause most cases of IBS, but individualized diet modifications can improve symptoms for many patients. Some measures that reduce symptoms in certain individuals with IBS are as follows (AGA 2002a; Karamanolis and Tack, 2006):

- *Dietary fiber*: Some individuals with constipation-predominant IBS improve when they increase their fiber intake to at least 20 to 30 g/day. Soluble fiber (found in food products such as oats, vegetables, and guar gum and in guar and psyllium seed fiber supplements) seems to be especially beneficial.
- *Lactose*: Some individuals with IBS report improvement with a decrease in lactose intake.
- *Caffeine and monosaccharides, such as fructose, sorbitol, xylitol, and mannitol*: The effects of these diet components are controversial, but their use should be evaluated, especially in people with diarrhea-predominant IBS. Fructose and sorbitol are found in fruits and other foods, but they can also be added as sweeteners in food manufacturing. Xylitol is used primarily as a sweetener in chewing gum.

Pancreatic Dysfunction
Pancreatitis

Pancreatitis refers to inflammation, edema, and necrosis of the pancreas as a result of digestion of the pancreas by enzymes normally secreted by the pancreas. Alcoholism, biliary tract disease, trauma, obstruction of the pancreatic duct, peptic ulcer disease, hyperlipidemia, and the use of certain drugs, including glucocorticoids, sulfonamides, chlorothiazides, and azathioprine, may cause pancreatitis.

Symptoms include pain in the epigastric region, persistent vomiting, abdominal rigidity, and elevated serum amylase. Malabsorption and decreased glucose tolerance are common in chronic pancreatitis (Forsmark, 2006).

Treatment

Abstinence from alcohol is one of the most important measures in treatment. In addition, analgesics are used as needed for pain relief. Taking pancreatic enzymes with meals and snacks can reduce the stimulus for the pancreas to release enzymes and therefore reduce pancreatic damage and pain. Endoscopic removal of stones in the pancreatic duct or placement of a stent to bypass an obstruction of the duct may relieve the pain (Forsmark, 2006).

Nutrition assessment and care

A thorough assessment should be carried out as described in Chapter 2. Especially common or significant findings are summarized in Box 11-1.

Intervention and education

Acute pancreatitis. The goal of treatment is to avoid pain and reduce inflammation caused by pancreatic stimulation (Meier and Beglinger, 2006).

- All oral feedings may be withheld during the first 2 to 5 days. IV fluids and electrolytes are given to replace the massive losses that occur during inflammation. For patients with mild acute pancreatitis, a high-carbohydrate diet with moderate protein and fat usually causes less pain than an unrestricted diet. The diet is gradually liberalized as tolerated.
- For patients with severe acute pancreatitis, whose symptoms are worsened even with low fat oral intake, jejunal tube feedings can be given, since these seem to stimulate pancreatic secretion very little. Some clinicians use a low-fat elemental diet, but others use a standard formula. If enteral feedings are not tolerated, supplemental TPN may be needed. Oral feedings of a high carbohydrate, moderate fat and protein diet can begin when pain has subsided and serum amylase and lipase concentrations are decreasing.
- Alcohol is contraindicated because it increases pancreatic damage and pain.

Chronic pancreatitis. The goal of treatment is to promote healing and compensate for the decrease in pancreatic secretion (Meier and Beglinger, 2006).

- Alcohol intake is contraindicated.
- A high-protein, high-carbohydrate diet with as much fat as can be tolerated promotes healing. Skinned, baked, or broiled poultry; lean meats; low-fat cheeses; and vegetable proteins, such as dried beans and peas, provide protein with a low to moderate fat intake.
- The individual may find that limiting fat in the diet reduces steatorrhea and pain (see Table 11-1). If additional food energy is needed, MCT oil can be used to replace the usual dietary fats in cooking, combined into a shake with milk and ice milk, or served in cooked cereals or juice.
- Pancreatic enzyme replacement may be administered with each meal to improve digestion.
- If fat malabsorption is severe, water-miscible forms of vitamins A, D, E, and K, as well as supplements of zinc and calcium, may be needed.
- Insulin secretion is likely to be impaired. If glucose intolerance is present, then the patient is treated as having diabetes (see Chapter 17).
- If the diet is inadequate even with thorough diet counseling and use of supplements, enteral nutrition support may be needed.

Hepatic Diseases
Hepatitis

Hepatitis is an inflammation of the liver caused by a virus, toxin, obstruction, parasite, or drug (alcohol, chloroform, or carbon tetrachloride). Symptoms include jaundice, abdominal pain, hepatomegaly, nausea, vomiting, and anorexia. Elevated serum levels of bilirubin, aspartate aminotransferase (AST, or serum glutamic-oxaloacetic transaminase [SGOT]), alanine aminotransferase (ALT, or serum glutamic-pyruvic transaminase [SGPT]), and lactic dehydrogenase (LDH) are commonly present.

Treatment

If the cause of hepatitis is known, then it should be removed. Antiviral treatments, if applicable, are the primary treatments.

Nutrition assessment and care

A thorough assessment should be carried out as described in Chapter 2. Especially common or significant findings are summarized in Box 11-1.

Intervention and education

- Alcohol is toxic to the liver and should be avoided during convalescence. Individuals with hepatitis C should be especially careful to abstain from alcohol intake because of the likelihood of the disease progressing to cirrhosis.
- A high-energy, high-protein (70 to 100 g), moderate-fat diet promotes liver regeneration.
- Lean meats, poultry, legumes, and cheese or cottage cheese made with skim or low-fat milk are good protein sources that are low to moderate in fat. Starches, such as pasta, rice, potatoes, cereals, and breads, are good energy sources.
- Frequent, small feedings are better tolerated than large feedings.
- If steatorrhea is present, then supplemental water-miscible vitamins A, D, E and K; calcium; iron and zinc may be needed.

Nonalcoholic Fatty Liver Disease

Nonalcoholic fatty liver disease (NAFLD) is an increasingly common cause of liver dysfunction. Liver function tests are elevated in NAFLD, as in hepatitis, and prothombin time may be prolonged. After ruling out other causes of liver disease (e.g., consumption of more than 20 to 30 g [1 or 2 drinks] of alcohol per day), NAFLD may be diagnosed by liver biopsy. Fatty infiltration of the liver (steatosis) is present, and there may be necrosis of the hepatocytes and fibrosis, a form of NAFLD referred to as nonalcoholic steatohepatitis (NASH). The disorder may progress to cirrhosis and liver failure. NAFLD is present in all age-groups, with the prevalence rising among obese people (Cave et al., 2007). The disorder is often associated with the metabolic syndrome (described in Chapter 5), which includes abdominal obesity, insulin resistance, diabetes, hypertriglyceridemia, and hypertension.

Treatment

No specific drug therapy exists for NAFLD. Antioxidant supplements such as vitamin E have been used in some clinical trials, but data regarding their effectiveness are inconclusive (Lirussi et al., 2007).

Good control of disorders associated with NASH, such as diabetes and hyperlipidemia, is recommended (Cave et al., 2007). Insulin-sensitizing/antidiabetic agents, such as pioglitazone and metformin, can be used in treatment of the insulin resistance of the metabolic syndrome.

Nutrition assessment and care

A thorough assessment should be carried out as described in Chapter 2. Especially common or significant findings are summarized in Box 11-1.

Intervention and education. Weight loss is recommended for individuals with NAFLD who have a body mass index (BMI) greater than 25, with the initial goal being a loss of 10% of body weight, at a rate of 0.5 to 1 kg (1 to 2 lb)/wk. Lifestyle changes to bring about gradual weight loss are described in Chapter 7. Surgery for weight reduction is a consideration for morbidly obese individuals (BMI of 35 or greater), but these patients must be carefully evaluated to ensure that rapid weight loss is unlikely to precipitate hepatic failure (AGA, 2002b).

Cirrhosis and Hepatic Encephalopathy or Coma

Cirrhosis occurs following hepatic damage. Causes of damage include alcoholism, biliary tract obstruction, and viral infection. Although the liver is able to regenerate much of the damaged tissue, some fibrous tissue develops, impairing the normal flow of blood, bile, and hepatic metabolites. Portal vein hypertension occurs, with esophageal and gastric varices, GI bleeding, hypoalbuminemia, ascites, and jaundice. Severe liver dysfunction results in intolerance to protein and **hepatic encephalopathy**. Signs of encephalopathy include confusion, increased serum ammonia levels (worsened by high-protein intake), and a flapping hand tremor, with progression to somnolence and coma. The underlying cause of hepatic encephalopathy remains undetermined, but at least three possible explanations are available. One possibility is that an increase in the ratio of aromatic amino acids (phenylalanine and tyrosine) to branched-chain amino acids (BCAAs) occurs in liver disease and may contribute to the problem, by formation of false neurotransmitters in the central nervous system. The second possible explanation is that intestinal bacteria digest nitrogen-containing compounds (from food and urea) in the GI tract, and resulting toxins such as ammonia and mercaptans released by this process are absorbed into the body; the toxin levels increase in the blood and the brain when the diseased liver is unable to remove them adequately. The third possible explanation is that increased levels of the neurotransmitter γ-aminobutyric acid build up and cause abnormal nerve transmission (Fitz, 2006).

Treatment

Drug therapy includes use of lactulose, which reduces absorption of ammonia from the GI tract, and poorly absorbed antibiotics such as neomycin, which are given orally to destroy intestinal bacteria that produce ammonia.

Nutrition assessment and care

A thorough assessment should be carried out as described in Chapter 2. Especially common or significant findings are summarized in Box 11-1.

Intervention and education. The goal is to avoid inducing encephalopathy or worsening symptoms, while providing as nutritious a diet as possible.

- Alcohol intake must be eliminated because it increases liver damage.
- A moderately high-energy diet (25 to 40 kcal/kg) prevents breakdown of body tissues to meet energy needs (Lochs and Plauth, 1999; Wright and Jalan, 2007). Carbohydrates provide most of the energy. Moderate fat (30% of total energy intake) can be provided unless steatorrhea is present. If steatorrhea occurs, then fat can be reduced. MCTs can be used to increase energy intake where steatorrhea is present.
- Protein intake is usually limited to 1 to 1.5 g/kg desirable weight per day unless hepatic encephalopathy is impending (Lochs and Plauth, 1999; Wright and Jalan, 2007). In encephalopathy, protein is often limited to 60 g daily (Fitz, 2006). With improvement, intake can be gradually liberalized. Vegetable protein appears to be better tolerated than meat protein by some patients with chronic hepatic encephalopathy. There is some evidence that increased intakes of BCAAs are beneficial for selected patients with encephalopathy. Enteral formulas high in

BCAAs (Hepatic-Aid II and NutriHep [Nestle]) can be taken orally or delivered by tube. BCAA-enriched amino acid solutions are available for use in TPN.

■ Small, frequent feedings are better tolerated than larger, less frequent ones. Soft foods that are low in fiber help prevent bleeding from esophageal varices, which may result in elevated ammonia levels as the blood proteins are absorbed or in shock if severe acute bleeding occurs.

■ Supplements of water-soluble vitamins are often used. Many individuals with cirrhosis have alcoholism and have followed poor diets; they have poor tissue stores of vitamins. Fat-soluble vitamins may be poorly absorbed, especially if steatorrhea is present, and supplements of vitamins A, D, E, and K may be needed (Lochs and Plauth, 1999; Fitz, 2006).

Hemochromatosis

Hemochromatosis is a genetic disorder in which excessive iron is stored in various organs, especially the liver, pancreas, heart, gonads, skin, and joints, disrupting organ function. Cirrhosis of the liver, bronzing of the skin, and diabetes are likely to occur if the disorder is left untreated. The laboratory evidence of hemochromatosis includes elevated serum iron and ferritin concentrations, saturated iron-binding capacity, and excessive parenchymal iron in liver biopsy tissue.

Treatment

Regular phlebotomy is used to remove excessive iron stores, with the goal being to maintain serum ferritin at 50 mcg/L or less.

Nutrition assessment and care

Assessment is summarized in Box 11-1 and described more fully in Chapter 2.

Intervention and education. The goal of medical nutrition therapy is to limit dietary iron and its absorption. To decrease iron in the diet, do the following (Limdi and Crampton, 2004):

■ Avoid iron supplements and multivitamin-multimineral supplements containing iron, breakfast cereals and other foods highly fortified with iron, and food prepared in iron cookware.

■ Use red meats only in moderation.

- Avoid consuming vitamin C supplements or food sources rich in vitamin C with meals, and avoid supplements with excessive amounts of vitamin C, which can increase iron absorption.
- Choose foods rich in fiber and drink tea, coffee, or milk with meals, to reduce the absorption of iron from the meal.
- Avoid alcohol intake, or consume alcohol in very limited amounts. Alcohol potentiates liver damage from hemachromatosis and increases the likelihood of cirrhosis and death.
- Follow food safety guidelines carefully (see Appendix J on Evolve) and avoid raw shellfish because people with hemochromatosis have increased susceptibility to food-borne illness caused by organisms such as *Vibrio vulnificus, Listeria monocytogenes, Klebsiella* sp., and *Yersinia* sp.

Conclusion

Many GI disorders have substantial nutritional impacts and require complex dietary changes. A registered dietitian can make an invaluable contribution to their care and instruction.

REFERENCES

American Gastroenterological Association (AGA) Institute: Medical position statement on the diagnosis and management of celiac disease, *Gastroenterology* 131:1977, 2006.

American Gastroenterological Association (AGA): Medical position statement: irritable bowel syndrome, *Gastroenterology* 123(6):2105, 2002a.

American Gastroenterological Association (AGA): Medical position statement: nonalcoholic fatty liver disease, *Gastroenterology* 123(5): 1702, 2002b.

Buchman AL: Short bowel syndrome. In Feldman M, Friedman LS, and Brandt LJ, editors: *Sleisenger & Fordtran's gastrointestinal and liver disease: pathophysiology, diagnosis, management*, ed 8, Philadelphia, 2006, Saunders.

Cave M et al: Nonalcoholic fatty liver disease: predisposing factors and the role of nutrition, *J Nutr Biochem* 18(3):184, 2007.

DeLegge MH: Nutrition in gastrointestinal diseases. In Feldman M, Friedman LS, and Brandt LJ, editors: *Sleisenger & Fordtran's gastrointestinal and liver disease: pathophysiology, diagnosis, management*, ed 8, Philadelphia, 2006, Saunders.

Fitz JG: Hepatic encephalopathy, hepatopulmonary syndromes, hepatorenal syndrome, and other complications of liver disease. In Feldman M,

Friedman LS, and Brandt LJ, editors: *Sleisenger & Fordtran's gastro-intestinal and liver disease: pathophysiology, diagnosis, management*, ed 8, Philadelphia, 2006, Saunders.

Forsmark CE: Chronic pancreatitis. In Feldman M, Friedman LS, and Brandt LJ, editors: *Sleisenger & Fordtran's gastrointestinal and liver disease: pathophysiology, diagnosis, management*, ed 8, Philadelphia, 2006, Saunders.

Jeppesen PB: Growth factors in short-bowel syndrome patients, *Gastroenterol Clin North Am* 36(1):109, 2007.

Karamanolis G, Tack J: Nutrition and motility disorders, *Best Pract Res Clin Gastroenterol* 20(3):485, 2006.

Keller J, Panter H, Layer P: Management of the short bowel syndrome after extensive small bowel resection, *Best Pract Res Clin Gastroenterol* 18(5): 977, 2004.

Limdi JK, Crampton JR: Hereditary haemochromatosis, *QJM* 97(6):315, 2004

Lirussi F et al: Antioxidant supplements for non-alcoholic fatty liver disease and/or steatohepatitis, *Cochrane Database Syst Rev* (1): CD004996, 2007.

Lochs H, Plauth M: Liver cirrhosis: rationale and modalities for nutritional support—the European Society of Parenteral and Enteral Nutrition consensus and beyond, *Curr Opin Clin Nutr Metab Care* 2(4):345, 1999.

Lochs H et al: ESPEN guidelines on enteral nutrition: gastroenterology, *Clin Nutr* 25(2):260, 2006.

Meier RF, Beglinger C: Nutrition in pancreatic diseases, *Best Pract Res Clin Gastroenterol* 20(3):507, 2006.

National Institute of Diabetes and Digestive and Kidney Diseases (NIDDK): Celiac disease. Available at http://digestive.niddk.nih.gov/ddiseases/pubs/celiac/index.htm#5.2007. Accessed November 11, 2007.

O'Keefe SJD: Nutritional management and gut adaptation, American College of Surgeons 92nd Annual Clinical Congress. Available at http://www.facs.org/education/gs2006/gs40okeefe.pdf. Accessed November 10, 2007.

O'Sullivan M, O'Morain C: Nutrition in inflammatory bowel disease, *Best Pract Res Clin Gastroenterol* 20(3):561, 2006.

Parekh NR, Steiger E: Short bowel syndrome, *Curr Treat Options Gastroenterol* 10(1):10, 2007.

Rashid M et al: Consumption of pure oats by individuals with celiac disease: a position statement by the Canadian Celiac Association, *Can J Gastroenterol* 21(10):649, 2007.

U.S. Food and Drug Administration: FDA permits restricted use of zelnorm for qualifying patients. Available at http://www.fda.gov/bbs/topics/NEWS/2007/NEW01673.html. Accessed November 9, 2007.

Wright G, Jalan R: Management of hepatic encephalopathy in patients with cirrhosis, *Best Pract Res Clin Gastroenterol* 21(1):95, 2007.

CANCER

Cancer and nutrition are closely related. Evidence suggests that nutritional factors have a role in development of many types of tumors. Once cancer has developed, it can have severe adverse effects on nutritional status. Not only does the cancerous tumor draw nutrients from the host, but also the treatment modalities and the psychologic impact of cancer can interfere with maintenance of adequate nutrition.

Cancer Prevention

Approximately one third of all cancer deaths in the United States are estimated to be related to diet and nutrition, physical inactivity, overweight, and obesity (ACS, 2007), and thus healthy habits in these areas are an important part of primary prevention. Box 12-1 summarizes the recommendations of the American Cancer Society (ACS) regarding nutrition and physical activity as measures for cancer prevention. These guidelines are consistent with those of the American Heart Association and American Diabetes Association for primary prevention of cardiovascular disease and diabetes.

Cancer's Nutritional Effects

Cancerous tumors differ according to their site, size, cellular types, and metabolic effects. Some tumors are associated with **cancer cachexia**, a condition of involuntary weight loss, muscle wasting, and weakness or diminished performance that can occur in patients with cancer, acquired immunodeficiency syndrome (AIDS), and other chronic diseases (Winkler, 2004). Oxidative stress and cytokines, such as tumor necrosis factor–α, are involved in these metabolic changes (Fortunati et al., 2007). The fatigue and anorexia many patients experience may be related, at least in part, to cachexia. Cachexia is most common in solid tumors such as lung

---

Box 12-1   American Cancer Society Guidelines on Nutrition and Physical Activity for Cancer Prevention

---

ACS Recommendations for Individual Choices

Maintain a healthy weight throughout life.

- Balance caloric intake with physical activity.
- Avoid excessive weight gain throughout the life cycle.
- Achieve and maintain a healthy weight if currently overweight or obese.

Adopt a physically active lifestyle.

- Adults: Engage in at least 30 minutes of moderate to vigorous physical activity, above usual activities, on 5 or more days of the week; 45 to 60 minutes of intentional physical activity are preferable.
- Children and adolescents: Engage in at least 60 minutes per day of moderate to vigorous physical activity at least 5 days per week.

Consume a healthy diet, with an emphasis on plant sources.

- Choose foods and beverages in amounts that help achieve and maintain a healthy weight.
- Eat 5 or more servings of a variety of vegetables and fruits each day.
- Choose whole grains in preference to processed (refined) grains.
- Limit consumption of processed and red meats.

If you drink alcoholic beverages, limit consumption.

- Drink no more than 1 drink per day for women or 2 per day for men.

ACS Recommendations for Community Action

Public, private, and community organizations should work to create social and physical environments that support the adoption and maintenance of healthful nutrition and physical activity behaviors.

- Increase access to healthful foods in schools, worksites, and communities.
- Provide safe, enjoyable, and accessible environments for physical activity in schools and for transportation and recreation in communities.

From the American Cancer Society: Nutrition and physical activity guidelines for cancer prevention: summary. Available at http://www.cancer.org/docroot/PED/content/PED_3_2X_Diet_and_Activity_Factors_That_Affect_Risks.asp?sitearea=PED. Accessed March 14, 2008. Used with permission.
ACS, American Cancer Society.

cancer and upper gastrointestinal (GI) cancers; it occurs less often in tumors of the breast and lower GI tract. In general, an unexplained weight loss of 5% or more within 6 months should be suspected as a sign of cachexia (Winkler, 2004). Psychologic stress associated with the cancer diagnosis and treatment can also contribute to deterioration of nutritional status. In addition, side effects of cancer therapies, including mucositis, impaired salivation, nausea, vomiting, loss of the senses of taste and smell, aversions to specific foods, and diarrhea, negatively impact nutrition.

Cancer Treatment—Interaction with Nutrition

Surgery, radiation therapy, and chemotherapy are used alone or in combination in cancer treatment. Table 12-1 summarizes some of the nutritional impacts of cancer therapies. Poor nutritional status can interfere with cancer treatment; e.g., a significant amount of weight loss may make it necessary to reduce the chemotherapy dosages.

Nutrition Assessment and Care

The goals of nutrition care are to identify and prevent or correct nutritional deficiencies resulting from cancer or its therapies and to maintain or improve functional capacity and quality of life.

The subjective global assessment (SGA) has been validated as a method of assessing the nutritional status of cancer patients and is widely used among other groups of patients, including those in renal failure. The SGA (Figure 12-1) provides an estimate of nutritional risk that can be quickly carried out in a variety of settings. Cancer patients should be screened at diagnosis and reassessed regularly to identify those who are at nutritional risk. Those at nutritional risk should receive a thorough nutrition assessment, as described in Chapter 2. Based on the assessment, an individualized nutrition care plan can be designed. The clinical dietitian is the health team member best suited to creating a nutrition care plan for patients at risk.

Intervention and education
Diet and lifestyle during and after treatment. The ACS has established guidelines for nutrition and physical activity during and after cancer treatment (Doyle et al., 2006), and the guidelines are summarized here. The goals are to correct or prevent nutritional

Text continued on p. 342

Table 12-1   Nutritional Implications of Cancer Therapy

Procedure	Surgery Nutritional Implications
Radical resection of the head and neck	Oral intake usually impossible, at least temporarily; enteral feeding necessary until oral intake adequate; may have permanent difficulty chewing and swallowing
Esophagectomy	Enteral feeding usually necessary until oral intake adequate; long-term effect: gastric stasis and fat malabsorption as a result of vagotomy
Gastrectomy	Dumping syndrome (cramps, diarrhea after eating); impaired absorption of energy, vitamin B_{12}, iron, and calcium; early satiety caused by decreased size of the reservoir
Pancreatoduodenectomy (pancreatic cancer)	Diabetes mellitus; loss of pancreatic digestive enzymes with potential for impaired absorption of fat and fat-soluble vitamins, calcium, zinc, magnesium, and protein
Small bowel resection	Depends on extent of resection and portion of bowel involved (see Figure 1-5); lactose intolerance possible; ileal resection: impaired absorption of fat and fat-soluble vitamins, calcium, zinc, magnesium, and vitamin B_{12}, impaired absorption of bile salts with resulting diarrhea and loss of fluid and electrolytes; with massive resection, loss of all nutrients, weight loss, and dehydration occur unless adequate nutrition support is given for a prolonged period of time; potential for adaptation of remaining small bowel so that enteral tube feedings or TPN can be discontinued if >70-100 cm of small bowel, the ileocecal valve, and the large bowel remain (Keller et al., 2004)
Colon resection	Impaired absorption of water and electrolytes

	Radiation Therapy	
Site of Treatment	Acute Effect	Long-Term Effect[*]
Central nervous system	Anorexia, nausea, vomiting (occasionally)	
Head and neck	Xerostomia (dry mouth),[†] mucositis, anorexia, hypogeusia (diminished sense of taste), dysphagia	Xerostomia, bony necrosis, dental caries, altered taste, dysphagia
Esophagus, lung	Dysphagia, odynophagia, gastroesophageal reflux; anorexia, shortness of breath, sore throat	Esophageal stenosis and/or stricture, fistula
Upper abdomen	Anorexia, nausea, vomiting	GI ulcer
Whole abdomen	Nausea, vomiting, diarrhea, cramping	GI ulcer, diarrhea, maldigestion and malabsorption; chronic enteritis or colitis
Pelvis	Diarrhea	Diarrhea; chronic enteritis or colitis
Whole body (bone marrow transplant)	Immunosuppression and vulnerability to infection	

Continued

Table 12-1   Nutritional Implications of Cancer Therapy—cont'd

Chemotherapy	
Chemotherapeutic Agent	Nutritional Implications
Anastrozole, bleomycin, carboplatin, carmustine, cisplatin,[†] cyclophosphamide,[†] cytarabine, dacarbazine, dactinomycin,[†] doxorubicin, epirubicin, estramustine, etoposide, floxuridine, fludarabine, fluorouracil,[†] fulvestrant, gemcitabine, hydroxyurea,[†] ifosfamide, imatinib, lomustine, mechlorethamine,[†] mesna, methotrexate,[†] mitotane, mitoxantrone, octreotide, oxaliplatin, paclitaxel, procarbazine, thiotepa, topotecan, vinblastine, vincristine, vinorelbine	Anorexia, nausea, vomiting
Bleomycin, cytarabine, dactinomycin,[†] docetaxel, doxorubicin,[†] epirubicin,[†] floxuridine, fluorouracil,[†] gemcitabine, methotrexate,[†] mitoxantrone, oxaliplatin, paclitaxel, topotecan, vinblastine,[†] vincristine[†]	Mucositis (stomatitis, esophagitis, intestinal ulcerations)
Bortezomib, capecitabine, cytarabine, erlotinib, estramustine, fluorouracil,[†] gefitinib, gemcitabine, hydroxyurea,[†] imatinib, irinotecan,[†] mesna, methotrexate,[†] mitotane, mitoxantrone, octreotide, paclitaxel, topotecan, vinblastine	Diarrhea

Gemcitabine, topotecan, vinblastine, vincristine	Constipation/paralytic ileus
Asparaginase, estramustine, megestrol acetate, streptozocin	Hyperglycemia
Fludarabine, topotecan	Fatigue
Megestrol acetate	Unwanted weight gain/increased appetite

Biologic Response Modifiers

Agent	Nutritional Implications
Alemtuzumab, bevacizumab, bortezomib, cetuximab, interleukin-2 (IL-2, aldesleukin)	Anorexia
Alemtuzumab, cetuximab, thalidomide	Constipation
IL-2, tositumomab, trastuzumab	Diarrhea
Alemtuzumab, IL-2	Fatigue
Alemtuzumab, bevacizumab, cetuximab	Mucositis, stomatitis
Alemtuzumab, bortexomib, cetuximab, etanercept, ibritumomab tiuxetan, IL-2, rituximab, tositumomab	Nausea, vomiting

GI, Gastrointestinal; *TPN,* total parenteral nutrition.
*May occur within a few months of therapy or appear years later.
†Side effect is especially common.

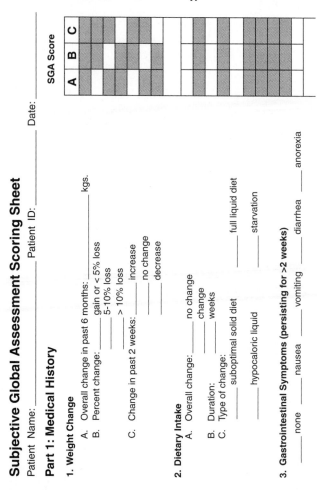

Figure 12-1
Subjective Global Assessment. Modified from Detsky,
J. McLaughlin, J. Baker et al.: What is subjective global
assessment of nutritional status? *JPEN* 11 (1987), pp. 8–13.

The subjective global assessment allows the health care provider to estimate the patient's nutritional risk. For each category, the patient is classified as: A. Well-nourished, B. Mildly malnourished or suspected of malnutrition, or C. Severely malnourished. Clinicians place the patient into one of these categories based upon their subjective rating of the patient's medical history and physical examination. In scoring the form, if there seem to be more B and C ratings, the patient is more likely to be malnourished.

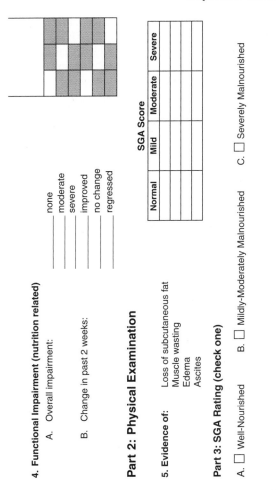

4. Functional Impairment (nutrition related)

A. Overall impairment:

_____ none
_____ moderate
_____ severe

B. Change in past 2 weeks:

_____ improved
_____ no change
_____ regressed

Part 2: Physical Examination

5. Evidence of: Loss of subcutaneous fat
                       Muscle wasting
                       Edema
                       Ascites

	SGA Score		
Normal	Mild	Moderate	Severe

Part 3: SGA Rating (check one)

A. ☐ Well-Nourished   B. ☐ Mildly-Moderately Malnourished   C. ☐ Severely Malnourished

The severely malnourished (C) rating is given whenever a patient has physical signs of malnutrition such as severe loss of subcutaneous fat, severe muscle wasting, or edema, in the presence of a medical history suggesting risk, such as continuing weight loss with a net loss of 10% or more, or a decline in dietary intake. When weight loss is 5%-10% with no regain of weight, in conjunction with mild subcutaneous fat or muscle loss and a reduction in dietary intake, the patient is assigned the mildly/moderately malnourished (B) rating. If the patient has no physical signs of malnutrition, no significant weight loss, no dietary difficulties, no nutritionally related functional impairments, or no GI symptoms that might predispose to malnutrition, the patient should be assigned to the well-nourished (A) category.

deficiencies, preserve lean body mass, reduce the nutrition-related side effects of therapy, and improve quality of life. During therapy, individualized counseling by a nutrition professional can help meet these goals and is strongly recommended. Examples of individualized approaches to a number of nutrition-related problems are given in Box 12-2. Aerobic and strengthening exercises as tolerated can improve muscle strength and quality of life and potentially reduce long-term effects of therapy, such as loss of bone mineralization.

For cancer survivors an important goal is striving to achieve and/or maintain a healthy weight. If the patient became underweight during the initial treatment, this deficit can be gradually corrected. On the other hand, overweight and obesity make the person more likely to develop other chronic diseases, such as diabetes and cardiovascular disease. Moderate weight loss (no more than 2 lb/wk) can be encouraged for the stable patient. Survivors can be encouraged to maintain or achieve a more active lifestyle; again, advice should be tailored to the needs of the individual, and there are specific concerns with particular forms of therapy. For instance, the immunosuppressed patient should avoid public gyms and other public places; for the bone marrow transplant recipient, this avoidance lasts for 1 year. Consult the ACS guidelines (Doyle et al., 2006) for more extensive information.

Certain cancer sites deserve special consideration (summarized in Doyle et al., 2006):

- *Breast*: Weight reduction in overweight/obese women is especially important, because overweight is associated with a worse prognosis. A diet rich in vegetables, fruits, and whole grains and low in saturated fat (e.g., lean meats and dairy products that are skim or low fat) is recommended. Physical activity might reduce the risk of recurrence.
- *Colorectal*: Maintain a healthy weight, and eat a diet consistent with the guidelines for cancer and heart disease prevention (see Box 12-1). Physical activity improves quality of life and may reduce the risk of recurrence. Patients with chronic bowel problems or malabsorption should be referred to a dietitian for counseling.
- *Hematologic cancers and cancers treated with bone marrow transplantation or hematopoietic stem cell transplantation*: Patients usually have severe side effects with nausea, mucositis, diarrhea, and malabsorption. Their intake and nutritional status must

Text continued on p. 348

Box 12-2   Common Nutrition Problems and Dietary
Suggestions for Individuals with Cancer

Anemia

Suggestions: Diet counseling related to iron, folate, vitamin B_{12}
intake (depending on anemia etiology); micronutrient supplements as needed; erythropoietin (EPO) therapy in nonmy-
eloid malignancies if anemia is due to chemotherapy rather
than nutritional deficits (ensure adequate iron, folate, and B_{12}
intake during EPO treatment) (Schwartz, 2007).

Anorexia/Weight Loss

Diet: Regular foods served attractively, with variety in texture
and color; small frequent feedings.

Supplements and nutrition support: Modular products added
to regular foods; complete liquid supplements (allow the
individual to taste several and select the one[s] preferred);
enteral tube feedings if necessary. See Chapter 8 for modular products and supplements.

Suggestions: Avoid beverages until after a meal, since fluids can
be filling; participate in regular physical activity; involve
children with anorexia in food preparation if tolerated or
make foods special in some way (e.g., cut sandwiches into
shapes with cookie cutters). See Box 12-3 for additional tips.

Problem foods: Large meals, high-fat foods.

Constipation

Diet: High fiber (see Appendix C on Evolve); adequate hydration.

Supplements: Bran, 2 tbsp/day, or other fiber supplement (see
Table 5-3).

Suggestions: Be physically active as tolerated. Attempt to
maintain bowel habits that were previously successful, e.g.,
try to defecate at the same time every day. Warm beverages
may increase peristalsis.

Diarrhea

Diet: Low lactose, low fat; adequate fluids to replace losses. Eat
foods high in potassium (e.g., fruits, vegetables, meats). If
pelvic radiation enteritis is present, choose a low-fiber diet.

Continued

Box 12-2   Common Nutrition Problems and Dietary
Suggestions for Individuals with Cancer—cont'd

Supplements: Lactose-free liquid supplements. If steatorrhea
    is present, MCT-containing supplements may be absorbed
    better than those without MCTs.
Suggestions: Take antidiarrheal medications such as loper-
    amide or diphenoxylate/atropine as prescribed.
Problem foods: Milk and other lactose-containing foods, fatty
    or fried foods, high-fiber foods.

Dysgeusia (Altered Taste)

Diet: Regular foods; individualize to meet patient needs. If red
    meat tastes bitter or otherwise unpleasant, choose cheese,
    eggs, poultry, or vegetable sources of proteins (soy and other
    legumes, grains, etc.).
Supplements: Beverages, puddings, soups, etc. (patient should
    taste different ones to find those that taste best); modular
    supplements added to foods or beverages.
Suggestions: Try spices and flavorings to see if these enhance
    or improve flavors.
Problem foods: Coffee, chocolate, red meats, others (varies
    with the individual).

Dysphagia

Diet: Emphasize foods that form a semisolid bolus in the mouth
    (e.g., macaroni and cheese).
Supplements: Carbohydrate or protein modules added to foods,
    thickened liquid supplements (see Suggestions); pudding-
    type supplements; commercial thickened foods and thicken-
    ers to be added to foods and beverages.
Suggestions: Thicken liquids with dry infant cereals, mashed
    potatoes, potato flakes, or cornstarch; add commercial thick-
    eners (ThickenUp [Nestle], Thick & Easy [Hormel Health
    Labs], or Hydra-Aid [Links Medical]) to beverages or use
    commercial thickened liquids (Thick & Easy thickened
    juices, water, coffee, tea, and milk [Hormel Health Labs]
    and Resource thickened beverages [Nestle]); use gravies and
    sauces to moisten meats and vegetables; if dysphagia is very
    severe, consider tube feedings.

Box 12-2   Common Nutrition Problems and Dietary Suggestions for Individuals with Cancer—cont'd

Problem foods: Thin liquids such as water, tea, coffee; foods that are not uniform in consistency, such as stews; dry foods, such as overcooked meats, hard rolls, nuts; foods that stick to the palate, such as peanut butter or soft bread; slippery foods, such as gelatin.

Hypogeusia or Ageusia (Partial or Complete Loss of Sense of Taste)

Diet: Regular foods with strong flavors or seasonings and interesting textures.

Supplements: Complete liquid supplements with added flavors if necessary; fortified puddings or other fortified foods.

Problem foods: Bland foods.

Fatigue

Diet: Regular food; small, frequent meals and snacks; emphasize nutrient-dense, easy to eat foods.

Supplements: Complete liquid supplements; pudding, soup, or other supplements.

Problem foods: Tough foods, foods that are hard to chew, large meals, foods that require extensive preparation by the patient.

Mucositis (Stomatitis, Esophagitis)

Diet: Nonabrasive, soft foods served cold, cool, or at room temperature: sherbet; canned or soft, fresh, low-acid fruits; fruit ices; popsicles; custard; gelatin, ice cream; yogurt; cottage cheese; puddings; soft vegetables or vegetable casseroles; eggs; cooked cereals (warm, not hot).

Supplements: Complete liquid supplements or custard or pudding supplements.

Suggestions: Try cryotherapy, or swishing ice chips in the mouth, to reduce mucositis associated with 5-fluorouracil treatment; the ice therapy should start about 5 minutes before the treatment and continue for about 30 minutes as the treatment is administered. For treatment of mucositis, follow a stepped approach, starting with step 1 and progressing if necessary: (1) Keep mouth clean: use a soft toothbrush to clean teeth,

Continued

Box 12-2   Common Nutrition Problems and Dietary
Suggestions for Individuals with Cancer—cont'd

---

and rinse mouth often with 0.9% saline or saline/sodium
bicarbonate solution (add to saline 1 tsp baking powder per
liter); (2) use topical anesthetics, such as viscous lidocaine, but
be careful in eating because numbed tissues may inadvertently
be bitten or burned; (3) use mucosal coating agents, such as
Gelclair; and (4) take analgesics such as opioid drugs (NCI,
2007b). Palifermin (keratinocyte growth factor–1) has been
approved to decrease the incidence and duration of severe oral
mucositis in patients with hematologic cancers undergoing
high-dose chemotherapy followed by a bone marrow transplant. Allopurinol mouthwashes and granulocyte macrophage–
colony stimulating factor might be effective in treatment of
mucositis but require further study (Clarkson et al., 2007).

Problem foods: Acidic fruits and juices such as citrus (evaluate
vitamin C intake when citrus fruits are avoided); salty or
spicy foods; hard or abrasive foods, such as chips, pretzels,
nuts, seeds; foods served hot.

Nausea and Vomiting

Diet: Liquids and soft foods served cool or cold: juices, carbonated beverages, gelatin, fruits; dry, bland foods: toast, crackers, plain bagels; tart foods and fluids: lemonade; sport
drinks; serve small amounts frequently.

Supplements*: Liquid supplements served cool; clear liquid
supplements, such as Boost Breeze (Nestle), if severe nausea is present.

Suggestions: Keep environment cool, well ventilated, free of
odors from cooking, emesis, etc.; dry starchy foods (crackers,
toast) before rising can help prevent vomiting; liquids should
be sipped slowly; try complementary therapies: relaxation
techniques may reduce anticipatory nausea and vomiting, and
hypnosis may reduce both anticipatory and chemotherapy-
induced nausea and vomiting (Figueroa-Moseley et al., 2007;
Richardson et al., 2007); premedicate with antiemetics; plan
the medication schedule so that drugs with high emetic potential are not given close to mealtime, if possible; avoid serving
favorite foods during nausea to reduce the risk of developing
aversions to them.

Box 12-2   Common Nutrition Problems and Dietary
Suggestions for Individuals with Cancer—cont'd

Problem foods: Hot foods, fried or fatty foods, foods with strong odors.

Neutropenia (Immunosuppression) with Potential for Infection and Food-Borne Illness

Diet: Regular.

Suggestions: Cook eggs, meats, poultry, and fish well; thoroughly wash fruits and vegetables to be eaten raw; avoid cross-contamination (e.g., carefully clean cutting boards used for trimming raw meat before using them to prepare raw vegetables); refrigerate cooked foods immediately after meal.[†]

Supplements: Commercial ready-to-use supplements.

Problem foods: Raw or undercooked eggs, meats, poultry, fish, shellfish, sushi or sashimi, rare meats, homemade mayonnaise, Caesar salad, key lime pie, and "royal" icing or other decorative icings and glazes unless they are known not to contain raw eggs; food from salad bars or buffets.

Xerostomia (Reduced Saliva Production)

Diet: Regular, moist foods: casseroles, gravies, sauces; encourage fluids, including popsicles, fruit ices, sherbet, gelatin, soups.

Suggestions: Use good oral hygiene because dental caries is common when saliva production is insufficient to buffer acids produced by mouth bacteria; use topical 0.4% stannous fluoride gel once daily to minimize dental caries (Chambers et al., 2004; NCI, 2007b). Oral antimicrobial agents, such as chlorhexidine gluconate, can help prevent oral infection. Salivary substitutes or rinses containing hydroxyethylcellulose, hydroxypropylcellulose, or carboxymethylcellulose may be of benefit; pilocarpine can be used to stimulate salivation if there is any residual capacity to produce saliva (Chambers et al., 2004).

Problem foods: Dry foods; sweet, sticky foods; sugars in gum or candy.

MCT, Medium-chain triglyceride.

*See Chapter 8.

[†]For further food safety information, see Appendix J on Evolve and http://www.cancer.org/docroot/MBC/content/MBC_6_2X_Impact_of_Altered_Immune_Function.asp.

be carefully monitored. Specialized nutrition support (SNS), i.e., enteral tube feeding and total parenteral nutrition (TPN), is usually required. Many centers have increased their use of enteral tube feeding relative to TPN, and this may reduce complications and costs.

■ *Lung*: Many patients have nutritional deficits at diagnosis, and therapy often creates others. They should strive for a healthy weight, following a balanced diet and being physically active. A vitamin-mineral supplement may be beneficial.

■ *Prostate*: Heart disease is the leading cause of death in prostate cancer patients, and they should strive for a healthy weight and consume a diet low in saturated fat and high in vegetables, fruits, and whole grains. Some data suggest that they should decrease dairy product intake, but this is balanced by the fact that they are prone to fractures because of the osteopenia associated with antiandrogen therapy.

■ *Head and neck and upper gastrointestinal*: Follow the guidelines for cancer prevention in Box 12-1. Chewing and swallowing difficulties are common, and a registered dietitian should be available for counseling.

Nutrition problems associated with cancer therapy. Box 12-2 summarizes problems often encountered during cancer therapy and approaches to alleviating them. A marked reduction in lean body mass is associated with a poor prognosis, and therefore preventing weight loss in the malnourished or at-risk patient is of great importance. Box 12-3 includes tips for improving oral intake for the patient with difficulty maintaining an adequate nutritional status.

Most chemotherapeutic agents cause immunosuppression by reducing the bone marrow production of the white blood cells. Whole-body irradiation in preparation for bone marrow transplantation has a similar effect. Although all blood cells and platelets are affected, the problem is commonly referred to as "neutropenia" because of the important role of neutrophils in resisting infection. The immunosuppressed patient is at risk of contracting a foodborne or other infection (see Box 12-2). Some measures that reduce the risk of food-borne illness in the immunocompromised cancer patient are as follows (NCI, 2007a):

■ Wash all raw fruits and vegetables well. If a fruit or vegetable cannot be well washed (as with raspberries), avoid it.

Box 12-3   Tips for Increasing Energy Intake

Serve Small Meals Frequently

- Eat when hungry and not just when it is mealtime.
- Try to eat at least every 2 to 3 hours when awake.

Eat a Larger Meal at Breakfast or Whenever Appetite Is Best

- Appetite and energy levels may be highest in the morning.
- Eat food that is appealing, even if it is not the "right time of day" (e.g., have pizza for breakfast or waffles for dinner).

Keep Snacks Available at All Times

- Nuts, hummus, dried fruits, muffins, crackers and cheese, granola, ice cream or sherbet, yogurt or frozen yogurt, milk-shakes, fruit smoothies, and puddings are some examples.

Prepare Foods in a Manner to Make Them as Energy Dense as Possible

- Soups, hot cereals, cocoa from a mix, and instant puddings can be prepared with whole milk or half and half, rather than water. For individuals with lactose intolerance, soy or rice milk may be used in milk-based drinks and foods, or lactase enzyme can be taken with milk products.
- Sauces can be added to cooked vegetables and pastas. Alfredo sauce, prepared with cream, contains more energy than tomato-based pasta sauces.
- Add dry powdered milk to puddings, milkshakes, mashed potatoes, or any recipe using milk if lactose intolerance is not a problem.

Do Not Allow Foods of Low Energy Density to Displace More Concentrated Energy Sources

- Beverage consumption is best delayed until after, rather than before or during, meals. Low-calorie or no-calorie beverages (artificially sweetened drinks, unsweetened tea or coffee, water) should be avoided as much as possible. Glucose oligo-saccharides (also called corn syrup solids and glucose polymers) can be added to tea, coffee, or juices.
- Raw vegetables and salads should be served only at the end of the meal, or energy-dense foods (cheese, egg, poultry, meat, beans, salad dressing) should be added.

Continued

Box 12-3   Tips for Increasing Energy Intake—cont'd

Keep Mealtime Pleasant
- Eat with family or friends if possible.

Do Not Let Fatigue Interfere with Eating
- Have others cook whenever feasible.
- Keep easy-to-prepare meals and snacks available.
- Rest before meals.

Scrub rough surfaces, such as the skin of melons, before cutting.
- Carefully wash your hands and food preparation surfaces (knives, cutting boards) before and after preparing food, especially after handling raw meat.
- Thaw meat in the refrigerator, not on the kitchen counter.
- Be sure to cook meat, poultry, fish, and eggs thoroughly (internal temperature 160° F for meat and 180° F for poultry; the whites of eggs should be firm, and the yolks should not be runny).
- Avoid raw shellfish and raw vegetable sprouts, and use only pasteurized or processed ciders and juices and pasteurized milk, cheese, and yogurt.
- Avoid foods containing raw eggs, such as cookie dough, cake batter, and Caesar salad.
- Avoid cheeses with molds, such as blue and Roquefort.

Additional information is available at http://www.cancer.org/docroot/MBC/content/MBC_6_2X_Impact_of_Altered_Immune_Function.asp.

Food aversions can develop as a conditioned response in individuals experiencing nausea and vomiting caused by radiation or chemotherapy. For example, aversions to red gelatin might occur in individuals receiving doxorubicin (Adriamycin), a red drug. Individualization of the diet through a process of trial and error appears to be the most successful way of dealing with food aversions.

Specialized nutrition support. The American Society for Parenteral and Enteral Nutrition (ASPEN Board of Directors, Clinical

Guidelines Task Force, 2002) has established guidelines for the use of SNS in cancer patients. The guidelines state that SNS should be reserved for those patients who are malnourished or at risk of becoming malnourished and are not expected to be able to consume or absorb adequate nutrients for an extended time. Malnourished patients who are undergoing major surgery may benefit from 1 to 2 weeks of preoperative SNS, but the benefits must be balanced against the risks of tube feeding or TPN and of delaying the surgery. Although SNS can be invaluable in helping the patient to maintain nutritional status throughout aggressive cancer treatment, SNS does not seem to be beneficial in palliative care.

Enteral tube feedings can be given by means of nasogastric (NG), nasoduodenal or nasojejunal (ND/NJ), gastrostomy, or jejunostomy tubes. Gastrostomy or jejunostomy tubes may be inserted during surgery or placed using percutaneous endoscopic gastrostomy or jejunostomy methods (PEG or PEJ tubes).

- *Indications*: Inadequate oral intake, impaired digestion or absorption requiring an elemental diet; ND/NJ feedings are useful if delayed gastric emptying is present; requires adequate bowel motility and unobstructed lower GI tract.
- *Example of use*: Severe anorexia, oral or upper GI tumor preventing oral intake, short bowel syndrome, pancreatic resection. Jejunostomy feedings reduce the risk of vomiting in the nauseated patient.

TPN is generally reserved for those patients where enteral feeding is not possible.

- *Indications*: GI obstruction in the distal small bowel; severely impaired digestion or absorption that prevents adequate enteral intake or causes dehydration; uncontrollable vomiting.
- *Example of use*: Severe short bowel syndrome (often used in combination with enteral feeding); jejunal or ileal obstruction.

Many individuals find it impossible to maintain their weight and nutritional status without SNS. Home tube feeding or TPN is often appropriate for those receiving long-term therapy. Chapters 8 and 9 describe procedures for safe delivery of nutrition support.

Anemia. Iron deficiency anemia can result from blood loss or aversions to iron-containing foods. Patient and family education regarding iron deficiency anemia includes the following:

- Try poultry and fish if there is an aversion to red meat. Other good dietary sources of iron can be found in Appendix B on Evolve.
- Use cast iron cookware, which increases the iron content of food prepared in it.
- If an iron supplement is needed, do not take it with milk, tea, or coffee because they interfere with iron absorption. Take with foods containing vitamin C (e.g., citrus juices or fortified apple juice), which can improve iron absorption. Try taking iron supplements just before bedtime if they cause GI distress. Ferrous gluconate may be better tolerated if a ferrous sulfate supplement causes discomfort. Supplementation continues until concentrations of serum ferritin, a storage form of iron, rise to normal. Supplementation may continue to be needed for maintenance of adequate stores if intake is poor.

Folate and vitamin B_{12} deficiencies are associated with macrocytic (megaloblastic) anemia (see Chapter 2). Folate and folic acid, the form of the vitamin used in food enrichment, deficits may occur as a result of poor intake caused by problems such as anorexia, dysphagia, nausea, and vomiting. Diet counseling regarding good sources of folate/folic acid (see Appendix B on Evolve) or supplements can improve folate status. Vitamin B_{12} absorption is impaired by gastrectomy and by ileal resection or damage (e.g., abdominal radiation). Vitamin B_{12} delivered intranasally or parenterally—intramuscularly, subcutaneously, or intravenously as a TPN additive—can correct the deficit.

Some anemia in cancer patients is not related to nutritional deficiency (Schwartz, 2007). The anemia of myelosuppression can be treated with **erythropoietin** (i.e., epoetin alfa). Adequate iron stores are needed to respond effectively to these drugs, and patients who require chronic treatment almost always require iron supplementation. Anemia of chronic disease occurs in patients with some malignancies, as well as those with renal failure and other chronic illnesses. In this type of anemia, the bone marrow fails to produce adequate red blood cells, but iron stores may be normal. The anemia is often normocytic (normal-sized cells), rather than microcytic, as in iron deficiency (see Chapter 2). Iron therapy does not correct anemia of chronic disease. Serum ferritin levels help to distinguish between anemia of chronic disease and iron deficiency anemia because serum ferritin is low in iron deficiency but may be high or in the high-normal range in anemia of chronic disease. If ferritin measurements do not provide clear-cut separation between the two anemias (e.g., ferritin is low-normal), then measurement of iron stores in a bone marrow aspirate will distinguish between them.

Complementary and alternative medical therapies. Complementary and alternative medical (CAM) therapies are widely used among patients with cancer, although the exact percentages of patients using CAM therapies remain unclear. All patients with cancer should be asked about their use of CAM therapies—for example, herbs, special diets, manipulation, immune therapies, medicinal teas, and any other therapies not prescribed by their conventional health care provider. CAM therapies used by cancer patients range from treatments for symptom control (i.e., antinausea and pain treatments) to those aimed at cancer suppression. The patient and the health care provider should discuss CAM therapies before they are used. Knowledgeable health professionals can help the patient to evaluate CAM therapies and the claims made for them. Some topics to consider are (1) What types of CAM might be expected to help with stress, fatigue, and specific side effects of this type of cancer and its treatment? (2) How can reliable CAM practitioners be found? (3) How can the CAM provider and the other members of the health care team work together? (4) Will the therapy interfere with the cancer treatment? (NCI, NCCAM, 2007). A summary of objective information about specific CAM therapies and links to additional resources are available at the website of the National Cancer Institute (http://www.cancer.gov/cancertopics/treatment/cam).

Among the most common CAM therapies are vitamin and mineral supplements. In particular, patients are likely to take supplements of antioxidant nutrients such as vitamins C and E, β-carotene, and selenium. A number of clinical trials have examined the effect of various nutritional supplements, with little overall evidence of benefit in terms of improved prognosis or survival (Davies et al., 2006). Because of this, and because many foods have beneficial effects beyond their vitamin and mineral content, a diet rich in fruits and vegetables (5 to 10 servings daily) should be encouraged. During active cancer treatment, a supplement providing approximately 100% of the Recommended Dietary Allowance (RDA) for vitamins and minerals will probably be of benefit, because it may be hard to consume an adequate diet (Doyle et al., 2006). However, supplements with larger amounts of micronutrients could actually be harmful. For instance, folic acid supplements or intake of a large amount of folic acid–fortified foods (e.g., fortified cereals) during methotrexate therapy could reduce the effect of the drug, which interferes with folate metabolism. Similarly, supplements with more than the RDA of antioxidant nutrients, such as vitamins C and E and selenium, could theoretically interfere with the effects of radiation treatment and some chemotherapeutic drugs, because these therapies act through cellular oxidative damage (Doyle et al., 2006).

Conclusion

Diet and lifestyle modifications are important measures in the prevention of cancer. Achieving or maintaining a healthy weight; frequent participation in at least moderate physical activity; making good food choices with an emphasis on fruits, vegetables, and whole grains; and consuming little or no alcohol reduce the risk of a number of cancers. These include cancers of the breast, endometrium, esophagus, head and neck, and probably the colon and rectum (Kushi et al., 2006). In people diagnosed with cancer, diet and lifestyle measures improve the quality of life (Ravasco et al., 2007) and possibly the risk of disease recurrence (Doyle et al., 2006).

REFERENCES

American Cancer Society (ACS): *Cancer prevention & early detection facts & figures 2007*, Atlanta, 2007, The Society.

ASPEN Board of Directors, Clinical Guidelines Task Force: Guidelines for the use of parenteral and enteral nutrition in adult and pediatric patients, *JPEN J Parenter Enteral Nutr* 26(suppl 1):1A, 2002.

Chambers MS et al: Radiation-induced xerostomia in patients with head and neck cancer: pathogenesis, impact on quality of life, and management, *Head Neck* 26(9):796, 2004.

Clarkson J, Worthington H, Eden O: Interventions for treating oral mucositis for patients with cancer receiving treatment, *Cochrane Database Syst Rev* (2):CD001973, 2007.

Davies AA et al: Nutritional interventions and outcome in patients with cancer or preinvasive lesions: systematic review, *J Natl Cancer Inst* 98(14):961, 2006.

Doyle C et al: Nutrition and physical activity during and after cancer treatment: an American Cancer Society guide for informed choices, *CA Cancer J Clin* 56(6):323, 2006.

Figueroa-Moseley C et al: Behavioral interventions in treating anticipatory nausea and vomiting, *J Natl Compr Canc Netw* 5(1):44, 2007.

Fortunati N et al: Pro-inflammatory cytokines and oxidative stress/antioxidant parameters characterize the bio-humoral profile of early cachexia in lung cancer patients, *Oncol Rep* 18(6):1521, 2007.

Keller J, Panter H, Layer P: Management of the short bowel syndrome after extensive small bowel resection, *Best Pract Res Clin Gastroenterol* 18(5): 977, 2004.

Kushi LH et al: American Cancer Society guidelines on nutrition and physical activity for cancer prevention: reducing the risk of cancer with healthy food choices and physical activity, *CA Cancer J Clin* 56(5):254, 2006.

National Cancer Institute (NCI): Nutrition in cancer care. Available at http://www.cancer.gov/cancertopics/pdq/supportivecare/nutrition/ healthprofessional. Accessed November 18, 2007a.

National Cancer Institute (NCI): Oral complications of chemotherapy and head/neck radiation. Available at www.cancer.gov/cancertopics/pdq/ supportivecare/oralcomplications/HealthProfessional. Accessed November 18, 2007b.

National Cancer Institute (NCI), National Center for Complementary and Alternative Medicine (NCCAM): Thinking about complementary and alternative medicine. Available at http://www.cancer.gov/cancertopics/ thinking-about-CAM. Accessed November 20, 2007.

Ravasco P, Monteiro Grillo I, Camilo M: Cancer wasting and quality of life react to early individualized nutritional counselling! *Clin Nutr* 26(1):7, 2007.

Richardson J et al: Hypnosis for nausea and vomiting in cancer chemotherapy: a systematic review of the research evidence, *Eur J Cancer Care (Engl)* 16(5):402, 2007.

Schwartz RN: Anemia in patients with cancer: incidence, causes, impact, management, and use of treatment guidelines and protocols, *Am J Health Syst Pharm* 64(3 suppl 2):5, 2007.

Winkler MF: Body compositional changes in cancer cachexia: are they reversible? *Top Clin Nutr* 19(2):85, 2004.

CHAPTER 13

HIV INFECTION

Individuals infected with the human immunodeficiency virus (HIV) display a variety of responses, ranging from asymptomatic infection to acquired immunodeficiency syndrome (AIDS). The retrovirus targets lymphocytes bearing the CD4 cell marker, and as a result, the CD4 count is inversely associated with the severity of the disease. The infected individual is susceptible to opportunistic infections and cancers such as Kaposi sarcoma and non-Hodgkin lymphoma. Unintended weight loss remains common, even though improved therapies have diminished much of the wasting previously associated with HIV infection (Grinspoon and Mulligan, 2003). Weight loss is more common in individuals with the highest amount of virus in the blood (viral load), and it is associated with higher rates of morbidity and mortality (Grinspoon and Mulligan, 2003). Loss of lean body mass is a key factor diminishing survival (Ockenga et al., 2006). Multiple factors are responsible for the nutritional impairments associated with HIV infection. Respiratory infections can cause anorexia, dyspnea, fever, and increased needs for energy and nutrients. Malabsorption is a common finding, even though diarrhea may not be present (Hendricks et al., 2005; Owens and Greenson, 2007). Some possible causes of malabsorption include gastrointestinal (GI) pathogens, medications used, and enteropathy and/or GI inflammation associated with HIV infection (American Dietetic Association, Dietitians of Canada, 2004; Owens and Greenson, 2007). In addition, anorexia can be a side effect of some medications prescribed and of depression associated with the disease.

Treatment

Five types of antiretroviral agents have been approved by the U.S. Food and Drug Administration (FDA) for HIV treatment: (1) nucleotide or nucleoside reverse transcriptase inhibitors (NRTIs; abacavir, zidovudine, didanosine, zalcitabine, stavudine, tenofovir, lamivu-dine), (2) nonnucleotide reverse transcriptase inhibitors (NNRTIs; efavirenz, nevirapine, delavirdine), (3) protease inhibitors (PIs; am-prenavir, atazanavir, saquinavir, ritonavir, lopinavir, indinavir, nel-finavir, tipranavir), (4) fusion inhibitors (enfuvirtide), and (5) entry inhibitors (maraviroc). Combination therapy (highly active antiretro-viral therapy [HAART]) is common, making the patient vulnerable to a variety of medication side effects and drug-nutrient or drug-drug interactions. Secondary infections require the use of appropriate antibiotic agents, and, when applicable, patients also receive cancer therapy (see Chapter 12). The side effects of commonly used medi-cations include anorexia, nausea and vomiting, mucosal lesions, and diarrhea (Table 13-1).

Nutrition Assessment and Care

Nutrition care of the person with HIV infection focuses on identi-fying and correcting, if possible, nutritional deficits that might weaken the individual, exacerbate immune dysfunctions, or impair quality of life.

A thorough nutrition assessment should be performed as de-scribed in Chapter 2. Box 13-1 summarizes common or especially serious findings of the HIV-infected individual. Body weight, indica-tors of protein status, and micronutrient status are especially impor-tant in assessing the status of the HIV-infected individual. Assess-ment should include usual intake, current intake, food intolerances, use of micronutrient and macronutrient supplements and herbal therapies, ethnic and cultural food practices, and problems in food preparation. Potential impacts of retroviral therapy on nutrition, as well as interaction of supplements and herbal remedies with retrovi-ral agents, are essential considerations (American Dietetic Associa-tion, Dietitians of Canada, 2004).

Intervention and education
Principles of a healthful diet. Optimal nutrition will help to main-tain functional capacity, improve quality of life, and improve tolerance of treatment. Many individuals infected with HIV are extremely interested in nutrition and its potential benefits in man-aging the disease, and it is possible to build on this interest in teaching about diet. The Dietary Approaches to Stop Hyperten-sion (DASH) diet (see Chapters 1 and 14) or the MyPyramid plan
Text continued on p. 364.

Table13-1   Nutritional Impacts of Medications Commonly Prescribed for Persons with HIV Infection

Drug	Side Effect					
	Nausea/Vomiting	Diarrhea	Sore Mouth/Abdominal Pain	Dry Mouth/Throat	Unpleasant Taste	Anorexia
Antiretroviral (AIDS Chemotherapy) Agents						
Abacavir	X	X				X
Atazanavir	X	X				
Delavirdine	X	X		X	X	X
Didanosine		X				
Efavirenz	X	X	X			X
Emtricitabine	X	X				
Fosamprenavir	X					
Indinavir	X	X				
Lamivudine	X	X	X	X		X
Lopinavir	X	X				
Nelfinavir	X	X	X	X		
Nevirapine	X	X	X	X		
Ritonavir	X	X	X	X	X	
Saquinavir	X	X		X		
Stavudine	X	X		X		X
Tenofovir	X	X				

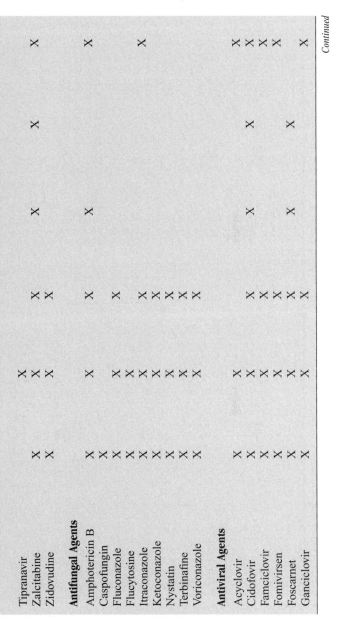

Agent						
Tipranavir	X	X				X
Zalcitabine	X	X	X			
Zidovudine	X	X	X	X		X
Antifungal Agents						
Amphotericin B	X	X	X	X		X
Caspofungin	X	X				
Fluconazole	X	X	X			
Flucytosine	X	X	X			
Itraconazole	X	X	X			X
Ketoconazole	X	X	X			
Nystatin	X	X	X			
Terbinafine	X	X	X			
Voriconazole	X	X	X			
Antiviral Agents						
Acyclovir	X	X	X			X
Cidofovir	X	X	X	X	X	X
Famciclovir	X	X	X			X
Fomivirsen	X	X	X			X
Foscarnet	X	X	X	X	X	
Ganciclovir	X	X	X			X

Continued

Table 13-1   Nutritional Impacts of Medications Commonly Prescribed for Persons with HIV Infection—cont'd

Drug	Side Effect					
	Nausea/Vomiting	Diarrhea	Sore Mouth/ Abdominal Pain	Dry Mouth/ Throat	Unpleasant Taste	Anorexia
Antiviral Agents						
Interferon alfa-2a	X	X	X			X
Interferon alfa-2b	X	X	X			X
Valacyclovir	X	X				
Valganciclovir	X	X	X			
Vidarabine	X	X	X			
Antiprotozoal Agents						
Atovaquone	X	X	X			X
Metronidazole	X	X	X	X	X	
Pentamidine						
IV or IM	X					
Inhalable	X		X	X	X	X

AIDS, Acquired immunodeficiency syndrome; *IM,* intramuscular; *IV,* intravenous.

Box 13-1   Nutrition Assessment of the HIV-Infected Individual

---

Protein-Energy Malnutrition (PEM) or Protein-Calorie Malnutrition (PCM)

History

Nutrient losses caused by diarrhea, malabsorption (from AIDS enteropathy, GI infections, medications), vomiting; increased needs related to infection and fever; poor intake related to anorexia (caused by respiratory or other infections, depression, medications), oral and esophageal pain (e.g., *Candida* or herpes esophagitis, endotracheal Kaposi sarcoma), dyspnea, dysphagia, distorted sense of taste caused by medication use or zinc deficiency, dementia, or CNS infections

Physical examination

Recent weight loss; weight <90% of desirable or BMI <18.5, or decline in percentiles for height or weight on growth chart for children; wasting of muscle and subcutaneous tissue; triceps skinfold <5th percentile

Laboratory analysis

↓ Serum albumin, transferrin, or prealbumin; negative nitrogen balance; ↓ creatinine-height index

Mineral Deficiencies

Iron

History

Poor intake (same causes as PEM); increased losses or impaired utilization related to medications such as pentamidine, amphotericin B, foscarnet; altered metabolism related to inflammation and chronic disease

Physical examination

Pallor, spoon-shaped nails, fatigue, tachycardia

Laboratory analysis

↓ Hct, Hgb, MCV, serum ferritin

Continued

Box 13-1   Nutrition Assessment of the HIV-Infected Individual—cont'd

Zinc

History

Poor intake (same causes as PEM); impaired absorption related to diarrhea

Physical examination

Poor sense of taste, distorted taste, delayed wound healing, alopecia, dermatitis, diarrhea

Laboratory analysis

↓ Serum zinc

Magnesium

History

Poor intake (same causes as PEM); impaired absorption related to diarrhea

Physical examination

Cardiac dysrhythmia, muscular weakness

Laboratory analysis

↓ Serum magnesium

Vitamin Deficiencies

A

History

Diarrhea and/or malabsorption; poor intake related to anorexia, nausea, vomiting

Physical examination

Drying of skin and cornea; papular eruption around hair follicles

Laboratory analysis

↓ Serum retinol, ↓ retinol binding protein (indicating PEM, with inadequate protein to manufacture vitamin A transport protein)

Box 13-1   Nutrition Assessment of the HIV-Infected Individual—cont'd

Vitamin D

History

Diarrhea and/or malabsorption; poor intake related to milk avoidance (lactose intolerance); little sun exposure

Laboratory analysis

↓ Bone mineral density

B₁₂

History

Poor intake because of poverty, difficulty chewing protein foods, vegetarian diet, anorexia; impaired absorption; diarrhea

Physical examination

Pallor, glossitis, fatigue, paresthesias

Laboratory analysis

↓ Hct, ↑ MCV, ↓ serum vitamin B_{12} and holotranscobalamin II (B_{12} and its transport protein)

Folate

History

Poor intake of fruits and vegetables related to mouth soreness, unconventional diet, poverty, anorexia; impaired absorption related to trimethoprim-sulfamethoxazole or pentamidine use

Physical examination

Pallor, glossitis, fatigue

Laboratory analysis

↓ Hct; ↑ MCV; ↓ serum or RBC folate

Dyslipidemia

History

Highly active antiretroviral therapy, especially PI therapy

Physical examination

Fat loss in the extremities with truncal fat accumulation

Continued

Box 13-1   Nutrition Assessment of the HIV-Infected
Individual—cont'd

Laboratory analysis
↑ Triglycerides, ↓ HDL cholesterol

Glucose Intolerance

History
Highly active antiretroviral therapy, especially PI therapy

Physical examination
Fat loss in the extremities with truncal fat accumulation

Laboratory analysis
↑ Fasting and postprandial plasma or blood glucose, ↑ Hb A_{1c}

AIDS, Acquired immunodeficiency syndrome; *BMI,* body mass index; *CNS,* central nervous system; *GI,* gastrointestinal; *Hb A_{1c},* hemoglobin A_{1c}; *Hct,* hematocrit; *HDL,* high-density lipoprotein; *Hgb,* hemoglobin; *HIV,* human immunodeficiency virus; *MCV,* mean corpuscular volume; *PI,* protease inhibitor; *RBC,* red blood cell.

(www.MyPyramid.gov) provides a healthful eating pattern that can be used as a teaching tool. In addition, a compilation of selected sources of teaching materials and information related to HIV infection is available (American Dietetic Association, Dietitians of Canada, 2004).

Weight loss and undernutrition. If oral intake is possible, nutrition counseling with frequent follow-up, use of supplements as appropriate, and enteral nutrition support can be attempted (in that order); total parenteral nutrition (TPN) is indicated only if oral or enteral feeding is impossible or inadequate (Ockenga et al., 2006). Energy needs can be estimated (see Box 2-4) if indirect calorimetry is not available to measure them. In stable phases of the disease, a protein intake of approximately 1.2 g/kg/day appears adequate, although 1.5 g/kg/day may be needed during acute infection (Ockenga et al., 2006). Issues to consider include the following:

■ Small, frequent meals are usually best tolerated if dyspnea is present, and foods of high energy density (e.g., cheese, meats, muffins, vegetables with sauces) are preferable to foods with low energy density (e.g., raw green leafy vegetables, no- or low-calorie beverages). If oxygen is needed, use of a nasal cannula during meals often improves eating ability.

- A diet that provides sufficient micronutrients to meet the Recommended Dietary Allowance (RDA) (see Appendix A on Evolve) should be encouraged. If dietary intake is likely to be inadequate, a daily multivitamin and mineral supplement that supplies 100% of the RDA may be beneficial. No evidence exists that higher levels of supplementation improve outcome in adults. Children in limited-resource settings appear to benefit from vitamin A supplementation (Irlam et al., 2005).
- Antiemetic medications (if ordered) should be scheduled to be taken before mealtimes.
- Individuals with dementia or neurologic dysfunction may need to be reminded and encouraged to eat. Occupational therapists can assist in evaluating patients with motor problems and selecting special eating utensils that can improve their ability to feed themselves. Those who cannot feed themselves should be fed in a calm, unhurried manner, with family members or friends being involved whenever possible.
- Lactose intolerance is common in individuals with HIV infection and can cause diarrhea, cramping, and bloating. Yogurt and hard cheeses are usually better tolerated than liquid milk in lactose intolerance. Milk treated with lactase enzyme is available commercially, or lactase capsules can be taken along with milk. Lactose-free products should be chosen if oral supplements or enteral tube feedings are used.
- Modular ingredients, including protein (e.g., Beneprotein [Nestle], ProPass [Hormel Health Labs]), carbohydrate (e.g., Polycose [Abbott]), fat (e.g., Microlipid or medium-chain triglyceride [MCT] oil [both from Nestle]), or combination modules (e.g., Benecalorie [Nestle], HiProCal [Hormel Health Labs]) may be added to foods and beverages to increase the protein and energy content. If the patient has malabsorption, MCT oil may be better absorbed than long-chain triglycerides (see Chapter 8 for a discussion of fat absorption).
- If oral supplements are needed to improve intake, various drinks, shakes, and fortified puddings, ice creams, or other foods are available. If the patient has difficulty consuming large volumes of supplements, some drinks and shakes are concentrated to provide approximately 2 kcal/ml (e.g., Resource Plus [Nestle],

Mighty Shakes Plus [Hormel Health Labs]). Supplements containing MCTs are likely to be better absorbed if malabsorption is present. Carnation Instant Breakfast and similar products made with milk can be used if lactose tolerance is not a problem. Lactose-free products such as Ensure Plus (Abbott) are available for individuals with lactose intolerance.

- Dronabinol, a marijuana derivative, and megestrol acetate, a progesterone-like drug, are approved for treatment of anorexia. These agents have been successful in promoting weight gain in some HIV-infected individuals, but much of the weight gained by adults using these drugs has been fat rather than lean body tissue (Grinspoon and Mulligan, 2003). If appetite stimulants are prescribed, the patient should take them about 30 minutes before meals, usually twice daily. Other drug treatments have been used to maintain or increase lean body mass in patients with HIV infection. Human growth hormone (hGH) increased lean body mass in patients with HIV infection, but the drug is very expensive and can cause glucose intolerance and other adverse effects (Grinspoon and Mulligan, 2003). Testosterone and synthetic anabolic steroids (e.g., oxandrolone, nandrolone) also improve muscle mass, but they are associated with liver dysfunction and can reduce high-density lipoprotein (HDL) cholesterol, which could contribute to cardiovascular disease. In females these drugs can lead to irreversible virilization (Brunton, 2007).

In some states, multivitamin-multiminerals, other nutrition supplements, and/or appetite stimulants are available under the AIDS Drug Assistance Program (ADAP); consult http://www.kff.org/hivaids/ADAP.cfm for a state-by-state listing of the ADAP formularies.

Micronutrient deficiencies. Micronutrient intakes have been found to be inadequate in many individuals with HIV (Jones et al., 2006). Anemia may occur because of poor intake, malabsorption, or altered metabolism of iron, folate, vitamin B_{12}, protein, or other nutrients. Nutritional status should be assessed if anemia is present. However, anemia of chronic disease (see Chapter 2) or anemia resulting from drug interactions is even more likely than anemias from nutritional deficits (American Dietetic Association, Dietitians of Canada, 2004). Some drugs, such as indinavir, can cause hemolytic anemia and others, such as Trizivir (composed of abacavir, lamivudine, and zidovudine), bring about anemia because of bone marrow suppression (Brunton, 2007). These anemias are not nutrition related.

Specialized nutrition support. Various oral nutritional supplements are available for patients with difficulty consuming an adequate diet from regular food (see Chapter 8). HAART involves numerous doses of medication daily. Taking oral medications with an oral nutritional supplement (unless the medication should be taken without food; see "Drug-Nutrient Interactions" below) offers several opportunities daily to obtain extra nutrients.

For patients who cannot consume or absorb enough nutrients administered orally, enteral or parenteral (TPN) feedings may be necessary. The enteral route is preferred whenever possible because it is less likely to be associated with sepsis, is more economical, and is possibly more effective in maintaining normal GI mucosa and immune function, an important barrier to infection. TPN may be necessary if the GI tract is nonfunctional or the energy requirements are so high that they cannot be met entirely by the enteral route. Careful attention to infection control measures is important during both enteral and parenteral feedings (as is the case in all patients, not just those with HIV infection).

Individuals with malabsorption usually tolerate enteral tube feedings better if they are given slowly rather than as bolus feedings. If malabsorption is present, formulas in which a substantial portion of the fat is in the form of MCTs are likely to be better absorbed than formulas that are rich in long-chain triglycerides. Where oral or esophageal infections are present, the patient may be unable to tolerate a nasogastric, nasoduodenal, or nasojejunal tube. Gastrostomy or jejunostomy feedings may be more appropriate. Chapters 8 and 9 provide additional information about nutrition support.

Complications of the infection and therapy. Many of the disease- and drug-related symptoms (anorexia, nausea and vomiting, stomatitis and esophagitis, dysphagia, neutropenia, diarrhea) are similar to those in the person with cancer. Interventions for these problems are summarized in Box 12-2.

Drug-nutrient interactions. In addition to the general side effects of the antiretroviral drugs, some of the drugs are associated with specific drug-nutrient interactions (Brunton, 2007). The presence or absence of food in the stomach at the time the medication is taken is especially important in determining absorption. Drugs that require special instructions include the following:

- *Atazanivir*: Take with a low-calorie, low-fat meal or snack to improve absorption.
- *Delavirdine*: Take with an acidic beverage, such as orange or cranberry juice, if achlorhydria (inadequate gastric acid production) is present.
- *Didanosine*: Do not take with food, which can reduce absorption as much as 50%. Take at least 1 hour before or 2 hours after a meal. Didanosine powder supplies 1360 mg sodium per single-dose packet. The capsule form is preferred for patients needing a sodium-restricted diet.
- *Efavirenz*: Take on an empty stomach, preferably at bedtime.
- *Fosamprenavir*: Adults should take liquid fosamprenavir on an empty stomach; pediatric patients should take it with food. Tablets can be taken with or without food.
- *Indinavir*: Take with water on an empty stomach. Do not take with grapefruit or grapefruit juice. Indinavir increases the risk of kidney stones. Adults taking this drug should consume a minimum of 1500 ml fluid daily to reduce the risk.
- *Lopinavir/ritonavir*: Take with food.
- *Nelfinavir*: Take within 1 hour before or after a meal. The meal needs to be more substantial than just fruit or fruit juice. Taking nelfinavir with acidic juices may leave a very bitter aftertaste.
- *Saquinavir*: Take within 2 hours after a full meal.
- *Tipranavir*: Take with fat-containing food to improve absorption.
- *Zalcitabine*: Do not take with food. Take at least 1 hour before or 2 hours after a meal.

Lipodystrophy. With more successful combination therapy, many individuals with HIV infection experience weight gain during therapy. Unfortunately this weight may not reflect an increase in lean body mass but instead may represent an increase in fat. PIs have been associated with **lipodystrophy syndrome** (redistribution of body fat, particularly accumulation of fat in the truncal region, accompanied by wasting of fat in the extremities). This creates body image disturbances for some patients and may cause them to discontinue the medication. Lipodystrophy is associated with elevated triglyceride levels, insulin resistance, and diabetes. Hyperglycemia and diabetes are especially common with use of abacavir and delavirdine; hypertriglyceridemia is most frequently found during use of abacavir, delavirdine, and ritonavir. Patients taking PIs must be regularly screened for lipid abnormalities and hyperglycemia. In addition, maraviroc is associated with increases in total and low-density lipoprotein (LDL) cholesterol (Brunton, 2007). Diet and lifestyle recommendations that may improve serum lipid and glucose levels include the following (Hadigan, 2003; American Dietetic Association, Dietitians of Canada, 2004):

- Be moderately physically active, as tolerated, daily or almost every day. Aerobic exercise improves cardiovascular fitness, and strength training helps to maintain or improve muscle mass.
- Determine energy needs (e.g., indirect calorimetry or estimate with calculations in Table 2-6). Monitor weight frequently, and adjust energy intake as needed to maintain or achieve a desirable body mass index (BMI; see inside back cover).
- Limit high-fat and high-energy foods that are low in nutritional value (e.g., snack foods, pastries, doughnuts, cakes). Limit saturated fat to 10% of total energy intake, and avoid *trans* fats as much as possible. A diet high in whole grains, fruits, and vegetables, such as the Dietary Approaches to Stop Hypertension (DASH) diet described in Chapter 14, is consistent with the nutrition goals.
- Divide dietary carbohydrate into three or more meals or snacks, and spread it throughout the day rather than consuming it in one or two large meals.

  If hypertriglyceridemia is present, do the following:
- Limit intake of sugars, sweets, and other simple carbohydrates. If additional energy is needed, a modest increase in intake of monounsaturated fat (e.g., olive, canola, and high oleic forms of sunflower and safflower oils; almonds; hazelnuts; avocados) can be made.
- Avoid alcohol or drink infrequently and in small amounts (never more than 1 drink daily for women or 2 drinks for men).

Bone mineral density. Decreased bone mineral density (BMD) is common among individuals with HIV infection. The cause or causes are undetermined but may include chronic inflammatory changes promoting bone resorption; secondary effects of the infection, including weight loss, hypogonadism, and impaired vitamin D metabolism; and side effects of antiretroviral medications, especially the PIs (Yin et al., 2005). Treatment with the bisphosphonate alendronate, along with vitamin D and calcium, improved BMD more than calcium and vitamin D supplementation alone but did not reduce fracture risk in a small group of subjects studied for 1 year (Lin and Rieder, 2007). Adequate calcium and vitamin D intakes are needed if bisphosphonates are used. If lactose intolerance is apparent, the patient may be able to consume yogurt, cheese, or milk treated with lactase enzyme. If intakes appear inadequate, supplements of calcium and vitamin D may be needed.

Complementary and alternative medical therapies. Use of **complementary** and **alternative medical (CAM) therapies** is very prevalent among HIV-positive individuals. In one large-scale survey, 50% of individuals with HIV were using one or more forms of CAM, and 26% of patients using these therapies had not told their health care providers about their CAM use (Hsiao et al., 2003). Nearly 30% of CAM usage involved herbal therapies or megadoses of vitamins. These are of concern because of possible toxicity and also because of potential interactions with conventional retroviral therapy (e.g., St. John's wort, an herbal treatment for depression, decreases blood levels of indinavir, and two African herbal therapies inhibit enzymes involved in retroviral drug metabolism [Liu et al., 2005]).

A review of controlled trials of herbal therapies in HIV infection was carried out; the therapies included four Chinese herbal preparations: IGM-1, "35 herb," SH, and Qiankunning; curcumin from tumeric; SP-303 extract (sangre de drago [blood of the dragon]) from the *Croton lechleri*; SPV30 *Buxus sempervirens* (boxwood) extract; and capsaicin cream derived from chili peppers. The authors concluded that evidence is insufficient to recommend these herbal therapies, although promising results with some products deserve further study (Liu et al., 2005).

Vitamin and mineral supplementation should be carefully assessed, because the effect in HIV-infected people is not always easy to predict. Vitamin A is a case in point. Multivitamin supplements, but not vitamin A alone, reduced the risk of transmission of HIV from mothers to their infants in a population with little access to antiretroviral therapy. In the same study, vitamin A supplementation actually increased the risk of transmitting HIV through breastfeeding (Tang et al., 2005). In a series of patients receiving HAART, the lowest viral loads among women were found in the quartile with the lowest serum vitamin A concentrations, and men tended to follow the same pattern (Jones et al., 2006). Lower viral load indicates that their disease was progressing more slowly toward AIDS than in the patients with higher viral load. Thus there is little evidence suggesting that vitamin A supplements, given alone, benefit adults with HIV or the breastfed infants of HIV-postive mothers, and the supplements might even be harmful for some individuals. In any event, chronic vitamin A intakes above 30,000 mcg/day should be avoided because of possible toxicity (Institute of Medicine, 2000).

Health care providers need to question each patient thoroughly about the use of CAM therapies and familiarize themselves with the types of therapies being used in order to evaluate them and give informed advice. Reliable information about CAM can be found at www.naturalstandard.com and www.nccam.nih.gov. Many CAM treatments have not been examined rigorously in large-scale randomized trials, and therefore their potential risks and benefits are not fully known. Most CAM therapies have not been carefully tested in pregnant and lactating women or in children, and they cannot be recommended in those groups until known to be safe.

Safe handling practices for food. Infection with food-borne organisms is more common in individuals with HIV than in the general population, although the use of HAART has decreased the likelihood of contracting food-borne illnesses (Hoffman et al., 2005). If infection does occur, it is more likely to lead to sepsis and other severe complications in HIV-infected patients than in healthy individuals. People with HIV and their families or caregivers, if appropriate, need instruction in choosing, preparing, and storing foods carefully. Appendix J on Evolve summarizes important food safety guidelines. In addition, the U.S. FDA offers specific guidelines for food safety in AIDS and other immune deficiency states at http://www.foodsafety.gov/~fsg/immuned.html.

Conclusion

HIV treatment is a complicated process requiring numerous therapeutic agents taken one or more times daily. Optimal antiviral therapy may conflict with the nutrition care plan. For example, the dyspneic individual may be able to eat more if he or she consumes small amounts frequently, but many of the antiretroviral agents are better absorbed if taken on an empty stomach. Individualization of the therapeutic regimen is vital to maximize quality of life and response to therapy.

REFERENCES

American Dietetic Association, Dietitians of Canada: Position statement: nutrition intervention in the care of persons with human immunodeficiency virus infection, *J Am Diet Assoc* 104:1425, 2004.

Brunton LL, editor: *Goodman and Gilman's pharmacologic basis of therapeutics* (on-line edition), ed 11, www.accessmedicine.com, 2007, McGraw-Hill.

Grinspoon S, Mulligan K: Weight loss and wasting in patients infected with human immunodeficiency virus, *Clin Infect Dis* 36(suppl 2):69, 2003.

Hadigan C: Dietary habits and their association with metabolic abnormalities in human immunodeficiency virus-related lipodystrophy, *Clin Infect Dis* 37(suppl 2):101, 2003.

Hendricks KM et al: Dietary intake in HIV-positive persons with and without malabsorption, *Nutr Clin Care* 8(1):37, 2005.

Hoffman EW et al: Application of a five-step message development model for food safety education materials targeting people with HIV/AIDS, *J Am Diet Assoc* 105(10):1597, 2005.

Hsiao AF et al: Complementary and alternative medicine use and substitution for conventional therapy by HIV-infected patients, *J Acquir Immune Defic Syndr* 33(2):157, 2003.

Institute of Medicine: *Dietary reference intakes for vitamin A, vitamin K, arsenic, boron, chromium, copper, iodine, iron, manganese, molybdenum, nickel, silicon, vanadium, and zinc*, Washington, DC, 2000, National Academies Press.

Irlam JH et al: Micronutrient supplementation in children and adults with HIV infection, *Cochrane Database Syst Rev* 4:CD003650, 2005.

Jones CY et al: Micronutrient levels and HIV disease status in HIV-infected patients on highly active antiretroviral therapy in the nutrition for healthy living cohort, *J Acquir Immune Defic Syndr* 43(4):475, 2006.

Lin D, Rieder MJ: Interventions for the treatment of decreased bone mineral density associated with HIV infection, *Cochrane Database Syst Rev* 2:CD005645, 2007.

Liu JP, Manheimer E, Yang M: Herbal medicines for treating HIV infection and aids, *Cochrane Database Syst Rev* 3:CD003937, 2005.

Ockenga J et al: ESPEN guidelines on enteral nutrition: wasting in HIV and other chronic infectious diseases, *Clin Nutr* 25(2):319, 2006.

Owens SR, Greenson JK: The pathology of malabsorption: current concepts, *Histopathology* 50(1):64, 2007.

Tang AM et al: Micronutrients: current issues for HIV care providers, *AIDS* 19(9):847, 2005.

Yin M et al: Bone mass and mineral metabolism in HIV+ postmenopausal women, *Osteoporos Int* 16(11):1345, 2005.

SELECTED BIBLIOGRAPHY

Jacobson DL et al: Incidence of metabolic syndrome in a cohort of HIV-infected adults and prevalence relative to the US population (National Health and Nutrition Examination Survey), *J Acquir Immune Defic Syndr* 43(4):458, 2006.

Lynch GS, Schertzer JD, Ryall JG: Therapeutic approaches for muscle wasting disorders, *Pharmacol Ther* 113(3):461, 2007.

Mills E, Wu P, Ernst E: Complementary therapies for the treatment of HIV: in search of the evidence, *Int J STD AIDS* 16(6):395, 2005.

CARDIOVASCULAR DISEASE

Cardiovascular disease (CVD), the leading cause of death in the United States, encompasses a variety of conditions, including coronary heart disease, stroke, and heart failure.

Primary Prevention of Cardiovascular Disease

Diet and lifestyle factors are extremely important in the prevention of cardiovascular diseases, and because of this, measures for primary prevention of CVD are emphasized in the *Dietary Guidelines for Americans* (http://www.health.gov/dietaryguidelines/dga2005). Specific guidelines consistent with and very similar to the *Dietary Guidelines* have been developed for diet and lifestyle measures in prevention of CVD in adults and children older than the age of 2 years (Box 14-1). Weight control, a diet low in cholesterol and saturated fat, moderation in the use of alcohol and intake of sodium, regular physical activity, and smoking cessation are key elements of risk reduction. A diet containing no more than 2.3 g (100 mmol) sodium daily is an achievable goal at present (Lichtenstein et al., 2006), although a sodium intake of 1.5 g (65 mmol) daily is likely to be even more effective in reducing the risk of hypertension (Appel et al., 2006). Moderate alcohol intake refers to no more than 1 drink per day for most adult women and 2 drinks for adult men. One drink is 5 oz (150 ml) of wine, 12 oz (360 ml) of beer, or 1.5 oz (45 ml) of 80-proof alcohol. Pregnant women should not drink alcohol.

The Dietary Approaches to Stop Hypertension (DASH) diet (Table 14-1) is one plan that is recommended for prevention of CVD (Lichtenstein et al., 2006), particularly the prevention of hypertension and ischemic stroke (Appel et al., 2006; Goldstein et al., 2006). It is a carbohydrate- and fiber-rich diet that emphasizes fruits, vegetables, and low-fat dairy products; includes whole grains, poultry, fish, and nuts; and is reduced in fat, saturated fat,

---

Box 14-1   AHA Diet and Lifestyle Recommendations
for Cardiovascular Disease Risk Reduction

■ Balance calorie intake and physical activity to achieve or
  maintain a healthy body weight.
■ Consume a diet rich in vegetables and fruits.
■ Choose whole-grain, high-fiber foods.
■ Consume fish, especially oily fish, at least twice per week.
■ Limit your intake of saturated fat to <7% of energy, *trans* fat
  to <1% of energy, and cholesterol to <300 mg per day by
  doing the following:
  ■ Choosing lean meats and vegetable alternatives
  ■ Selecting fat-free (skim), 1%-fat, and low-fat dairy prod-
    ucts
  ■ Minimizing intake of partially hydrogenated fats
■ Minimize your intake of beverages and foods with added
  sugars.
■ Choose and prepare foods with little or no salt.
■ If you consume alcohol, do so in moderation.
■ When you eat food that is prepared outside the home, follow
  the AHA Diet and Lifestyle Recommendations.

Used with permission from Lichtenstein AH et al: Diet and lifestyle recommenda-
tions revision 2006: a scientific statement from the American Heart Association
Nutrition Committee, *Circulation* 114:82, 2006.
AHA, American Heart Association.

cholesterol, sweets, and sugar-containing beverages compared with
the usual American diet (Champagne, 2006; U.S. Department of
Health and Human Services, 2006). The DASH diet significantly
reduced blood pressure and total and low-density lipoprotein
(LDL) cholesterol in large multicenter trials (Champagne, 2006).
The DASH diet and modifications of it that were also effective in
reducing blood pressure (Miller et al., 2006) had a number of common characteristics. They were relatively high in dietary fiber, potassium, calcium, and magnesium, which appear to have blood
pressure–lowering effects (Myers and Champagne, 2007), and they
were low in cholesterol and saturated fats. This suggests that individuals aiming for a heart-healthy diet have flexibility in choosing
from a variety of diet patterns that share certain common characteristics (Miller et al., 2006).

Table 14-1   DASH Eating Plan

The DASH eating plan shown here is based on 2000 calories per day. The number of daily servings in a food group may vary from those listed, depending on energy needs.

Food Group	Daily Serving (Except Where Noted)	Serving Sizes	Examples and Notes	Significance to the DASH Diet Pattern
Grains*	6-8	1 slice bread 1 oz dry cereal† ½ C cooked rice, pasta, or cereal	Whole-wheat bread, English muffin, pita bread, bagel; cereals; grits; oatmeal	Major source of energy and fiber
Vegetables	4-5	1 C raw, leafy vegetables ½ C raw or cooked vegetables 6 oz vegetable juice	Tomatoes, potatoes, carrots, peas, squash, broccoli, turnip greens, collards, kale, spinach, artichokes, beans, sweet potatoes	Rich sources of potassium, magnesium, and fiber
Fruits	4-5	1 medium fruit ¼ C dried fruit ½ C fresh, frozen, or canned fruit 4 oz fruit juice	Apricots, bananas, dates, grapes, oranges, orange juice, tangerines, strawberries, mangoes, melons, peaches, pineapple, prunes, raisins	Important sources of potassium, magnesium, and fiber
Fat-free or low-fat dairy foods	2-3	8 oz milk 1 C yogurt 1½ oz cheese	Fat-free or 1% milk, fat-free or low-fat buttermilk; nonfat or low-fat yogurt; part-skim mozzarella cheese, nonfat cheese	Major sources of calcium and protein

Lean meats, poultry, and fish	6 or less	1 oz cooked meats, poultry, or fish 1 egg[‡]	Select only lean meats; trim away visible fats; broil, roast, or boil, instead of frying; remove skin from chicken	Rich sources of protein and magnesium
Nuts, seeds, and legumes	4-5/wk	1½ oz or ⅓ C nuts ½ oz or 2 tbsp seeds ½ C cooked legumes 2 tbsp peanut butter	Almonds, filberts, mixed nuts, peanuts, walnuts, sunflower seeds, kidney beans, lentils	Rich sources of energy, magnesium, potassium, protein, and fiber
Fats and oils[§]	2-3	1 tsp soft margarine 1 tbsp mayonnaise 2 tbsp salad dressing 1 tsp vegetable oil	Soft margarine, low-fat mayonnaise, light salad dressing, vegetable oil (e.g., olive, corn, canola, or safflower)	DASH has 27% of kcal as fat, including that in or added to foods
Sweets	5 or less/wk	1 tbsp sugar 1 tbsp jelly or jam ½ C sorbet, gelatin 8 oz lemonade	Maple syrup, sugar, jelly, jam; fruit-flavored gelatin, fruit punch, sorbet, ices, hard candy	Sweets should be low in fat

From U.S. Department of Health and Human Services: *Your guide to lowering your blood pressure with DASH: the DASH eating plan*, Washington, DC, 2006 (revised), National Institutes of Health (NIH), National Heart, Lung, and Blood Institute (NHLBI).

DASH, Dietary Approaches to Stop Hypertension.

*Whole grains are recommended for most grain servings as a good source of fiber and nutrients.

[†]Serving sizes vary between ½ and 1¼ C, depending on cereal type. Check the product's Nutrition Facts label.

[‡]Since eggs are high in cholesterol, limit egg yolk intake to no more than 4/wk; two egg whites have the same protein as 1 oz of meat.

[§]Fat content changes serving amount for fats and oils. For example, 1 tbsp of regular salad dressing equals 1 serving; 1 tbsp of a low-fat dressing equals ½ serving; 1 tbsp of a fat-free dressing equals 0 servings.

Treatment of Cardiovascular Disease

Hypertension

Hypertension—defined as systolic blood pressure greater than 140 mm Hg or diastolic pressure greater than 90 mm Hg—affects approximately 50 million individuals in the United States. Nearly 30% of adults in the United States have hypertension (Dickinson et al., 2007). Systolic blood pressure between 120 and 139 mm Hg or diastolic blood pressure between 80 and 89 mm Hg is regarded as prehypertension and indicates that the person is at risk for developing hypertension (USDHHS, 2003). Increases in blood volume, heart rate, and peripheral vascular resistance can lead to hypertension, but a large percentage of cases are essential hypertension—that is, no cause is known. Nevertheless, it is clear that there is a close association of hypertension with CVD. For each increment of 20 mm Hg in systolic blood pressure or 10 mm Hg in diastolic blood pressure, the risk of heart attack, heart failure, stroke, or kidney disease is doubled (Grundy et al., 2004).

The National High Blood Pressure Education Program (Grundy et al., 2004) states that specific lifestyle changes can reduce blood pressure; the program has provided the following estimates of the reduction in systolic blood pressure for each change:

- Weight reduction for individuals who are overweight or obese, 5 to 20 mm Hg decrease per 10 kg (22 lb) loss
- Adhering to the DASH eating plan, 8 to 14 mm Hg decrease
- Reducing sodium intake to no more than 100 mmol (2.3 g, equivalent to 6 g of sodium chloride) daily, 2 to 8 mm Hg decrease
- Engaging in regular aerobic activity at least 30 minutes on most days of the week, 4 to 9 mm Hg decrease
- Moderation of alcohol intake to no more than 2 drinks/day in most men and 1 drink/day in women or small men, 2 to 4 mm Hg decrease

For those people who are unable to reduce their blood pressure enough with lifestyle changes, an extensive list of pharmacologic agents is available. Drugs used in treatment of hypertension include diuretics, aldosterone receptor blockers, β-adrenergic blocking agents, calcium channel blockers, angiotensin-converting enzyme

(ACE) inhibitors, angiotensin II antagonists, and renin inhibitors. Commonly two or more drugs are used in treatment of hypertension, increasing the risk of drug-drug and drug-nutrient interactions (see Appendix G on Evolve).

Nutrition assessment and care

The goal is to reduce blood pressure to normal if possible, but even small changes are beneficial in reducing CVD risk. For example, a reduction of only 3 mm Hg in systolic blood pressure by a hypertensive person reduces the risk of stroke by 8% (Goldstein et al., 2006). A thorough nutrition assessment should be performed as described in Chapter 2. Box 14-2 highlights common or especially serious findings in hypertension.

Intervention and education
Lifestyle changes to reduce blood pressure. Overweight and insulin resistance are linked with hypertension in the metabolic syndrome, described in Chapter 5. The overweight hypertensive or prehypertensive individual should be encouraged to lose weight. Chapter 7 provides more information about weight loss measures.

The DASH eating plan (see Table 14-1) is suited both for prevention (discussed above) and treatment of hypertension. Exactly which component or components of the diet are responsible for its effect on blood pressure is not clear. Diets that are high in calcium, magnesium, and potassium have been found to be associated with a reduced risk of hypertension, but supplements of these nutrients alone have not been as effective (Myers and Champagne, 2007). Thus a diet plan, rather than just nutritional supplements, offers the most promise for blood pressure–lowering effects. Table 14-1 shows an eating plan providing 2000 kcal/day, but the diet can easily be adapted to fewer or greater numbers of kcal by altering the numbers of servings.

The DASH diet itself is not a low-sodium diet, although the fruits, vegetables, and whole grains suggested by the eating plan provide healthful, low-sodium food choices. The DASH eating plan has been found to be more effective in reducing blood pressure if combined with a moderate sodium restriction of 65 mmol, or 1.5 g of sodium (3.8 g salt) per day (Sacks et al., 2001). About 80% of the sodium in the U.S. diet comes from commercially prepared or processed foods (Dickinson et al., 2007), and thus a diet with ample amounts of unprocessed vegetables, fruits, and whole grains helps to

Box 14-2   Assessment in Cardiovascular Disease

Overweight/Obesity

History

Excessive energy intake; sedentary lifestyle

Physical examination

Weight >120% of desirable or BMI >25; triceps skinfold >95th percentile for age and gender

Underweight (Seen Primarily in Heart Failure)

History

Poor intake related to dyspnea or fatigue; impaired absorption related to inadequate bowel perfusion; increased energy needs if dyspneic or experiencing concomitant infection; loss of 6% or more of body weight over 6 months in the absence of edema

Physical examination

Weight <90% of desirable or BMI <18.5 (adults); BMI, height, or weight <5th percentile for age (children)

Elevated Serum Lipid Levels

History

Daily use of foods high in saturated fat and cholesterol; sedentary lifestyle; family history of hyperlipidemia; diabetes; obesity

Physical examination

Xanthomas, or yellowish plaques deposited on the skin

Laboratory analysis

↑ Total serum cholesterol; HDL <40 mg/dl; LDL >130 mg/dl

Elevated Blood Pressure

History

Daily use of high-sodium (processed) foods and salt at the table; psychosocial stress; family history of hypertension; obesity; excessive alcohol intake; diabetes

Fluid Status

Physical examination

Edema, pulmonary congestion

BMI, Body mass index; *HDL,* high-density lipoprotein; *LDL,* low-density lipoprotein.

control sodium intake. Box 14-3 lists high-sodium foods to be avoided by those trying to reduce their sodium intake, and Box 14-4 provides useful tips for those following a low-sodium diet. A sample daily intake, providing approximately 2.3 g sodium, and a version modified to provide only 1.5 g are shown in Table 14-2 as a guide to demonstrating to patients how to make the necessary modifications.

Most commercial salt substitutes contain potassium chloride rather than sodium chloride. The patient should consult with the physician about using them; generally their use is allowed if the

---

Box 14-3   Foods to Be Restricted on a Low-Sodium Diet (2 to 3 g Sodium/Day)*

Foods to Avoid

1. Salt at the table (use salt lightly in cooking; 1 tsp table salt, sea salt, or Kosher salt ≈2300 mg sodium)
2. Salt-preserved foods, such as salted or smoked meat (bacon, bacon fat, bologna, dried or chipped beef, frankfurters, ham, sausage, kosher meats, luncheon meats, salt pork, smoked tongue), salted or smoked fish (anchovies, caviar, salted and dried cod), sauerkraut, olives
3. Highly salted snack foods such as crackers*; potato, corn, and tortilla chips; pretzels; salted popcorn; salted nuts
4. Canned and dried soups,* chili con carne
5. Spices and condiments such as bouillon cubes or powder,* celery salt, garlic salt, miso, onion salt, monosodium glutamate, and meat tenderizers; pickles; condiments such as ketchup,* prepared mustard,* relishes,* soy sauce, Worcestershire sauce
6. Cheese,*† peanut butter*
7. Biscuits, self-rising flour, pies, muffins, and other quick breads containing regular baking powder* or baking soda*

Adapted from Williams SR: *Basic nutrition and diet therapy*, ed 11, St Louis, 2001, Mosby; USDA National Nutrient Database for Standard Reference, Release 20, updated September 26, 2007. Available at http://www.nal.usda.gov/fnic/foodcomp/. Accessed November 27, 2007.
For some items, home-prepared products with no added salt (e.g., pies and pie crust) may be substituted for commercial, high-sodium versions.
*Low- or no-sodium types are available commercially and may be used.
†Dry curd, nonfat cottage cheese is low sodium.

Box 14-4   Tips for Reducing Sodium in the Diet

- Use the Nutrition Facts label as a guide to choosing food with less sodium. The sodium content is shown per serving, so check the serving size. If you eat 2 servings, multiply the sodium content by 2. The following terms used on labels are a quick guide to sodium content:
  - Sodium free—less than 5 mg of sodium per serving
  - Very low sodium—35 mg or less per serving
  - Low sodium—140 mg or less per serving
  - Reduced sodium—at least 25% less than the sodium in usual food of this type
  - Unsalted, no salt added, or without added salt—made without any added salt but still contains sodium if the food is a natural source of sodium
- Buy fresh, plain frozen, or canned "with no salt added" vegetables.
- Use herbs, spices, lemon juice or peel, and salt-free seasoning blends in cooking and at the table.
- Cook rice, pasta, and hot cereals without salt. Cut back on instant or flavored rice, pasta, and cereal mixes, which usually have added salt.
- Choose "convenience" foods that are lower in sodium. Cut back on frozen dinners, pizza, packaged mixes, canned soups or broths, and salad dressings—these often have a lot of sodium.
- Rinse canned foods, such as tuna, to remove some sodium.
- When available, buy low- or reduced-sodium or no-salt-added versions of foods.
- Choose ready-to-eat breakfast cereals that are lower in sodium.

From National Heart, Lung, and Blood Institute: Your guide to lowering high blood pressure. Available at http://www.nhlbi.nih.gov/hbp/prevent/sodium/tips.htm; U.S. FDA: A little 'lite' reading. Available at http://www.fda.gov/fdac/graphics/foodlabelspecial/pg32.pdf. Both accessed November 27, 2007.

individual has no renal impairment. Some drugs, including antibiotics (especially the penicillins), sulfonamides, and barbiturates, are high in sodium. Their sodium content should be considered for the individual who is following a sodium-restricted diet. The pharmacist can provide additional information about the sodium content of drugs. A number of over-the-counter medications, including

Table 14-2 The DASH Plan and Ways to Reduce Sodium Intake

2300-mg Sodium Menu	Sodium (mg)	Substitution to Reduce Sodium to 1500 mg	Sodium (mg)
Breakfast			
1 C whole grain oat rings cereal	200	1 C frosted shredded wheat	4
1 Medium banana	1		
1 C skim milk	103		
1 Medium cinnamon raisin bagel	287		
1 Tbsp peanut butter	81	1 Tbsp peanut butter, unsalted	3
1 C orange juice	2		
Lunch			
Tuna salad plate:			
½ C tuna salad (canned tuna, no salt; low-fat mayonnaise, celery, green onion)	171		
1 Large leaf romaine lettuce	1		
7 Baked whole-wheat crackers (Triscuit type)	140	7 Baked whole-wheat crackers, low sodium	75

Continued

Table 14-2   The DASH Plan and Ways to Reduce Sodium Intake—cont'd

2300-mg Sodium Menu	Sodium (mg)	Substitution to Reduce Sodium to 1500 mg	Sodium (mg)
Lunch			
Cucumber salad			
1 C fresh cucumber slices	2		
½ C tomato wedges	5		
1 Tbsp vinaigrette dressing	133	1 Tbsp vinaigrette dressing, homemade without salt	1
½ C cottage cheese, low-fat	459		
½ C canned peaches, juice pack	5		
1 Tbsp almonds, unsalted	0		
Dinner			
3 oz Turkey meatloaf, made with regular ketchup	205	Substitute low-sodium ketchup in recipe	74
1 Small baked potato	14		
1 Tbsp sour cream, fat free	21		
1 Tbsp natural cheddar cheese, reduced fat, grated	67	1 Tbsp natural cheddar cheese, reduced fat, low sodium	1
1 Tbsp chopped chives	0		

Food		
1 C collard greens, sauteed with:	85	
1 Tsp canola oil	0	
1 Small whole-wheat roll	148	
½ C fresh pineapple chunks	1	
6 Small melba toast crackers, unsalted		1
Snacks		
1 C fruit yogurt, fat free, no added sugar	173	
2 tbsp sunflower seeds, unsalted	0	
TOTALS	2304	1489

From U.S. Department of Health and Human Services: *Your guide to lowering your blood pressure with DASH: the DASH eating plan*, Washington, DC, 2006 (revised), National Institutes of Health (NIH), National Heart, Lung and Blood Institute (NHLBI).

DASH, Dietary Approaches to Stop Hypertension.

Total kcal approximately 2000; approximately 25% kcal from fat and 5% from saturated fat; 158 mg cholesterol.

antacids (except those containing magaldrate), aspirins, cough medicines, and laxatives, contain sodium.

Coronary Heart Disease

Coronary heart disease (CHD) occurs when plaques containing **lipoproteins**, cholesterol, tissue debris, and calcium form on the intima, or interior surface of blood vessels. The plaques roughen the intima, and platelets are attracted to the roughened areas, forming clots. When the plaques enlarge sufficiently to occlude the blood flow, tissues distal to the occlusion are deprived of oxygen and nutrients, creating an area of infarct. CHD is manifested when a myocardial infarction (MI) occurs or when myocardial ischemia is present, causing the painful disorder known as angina pectoris.

Serum cholesterol, one of the determinants of the likelihood of CHD, is carried by several lipoproteins classified by their density. In order of increasing density, the lipoproteins are **chylomicrons**, **very–low-density lipoproteins (VLDLs)**, **LDLs**, and **high-density lipoproteins (HDLs)**. LDLs carry the most cholesterol and are the most closely correlated with CHD. HDLs reduce the risk from CHD by transporting cholesterol from the tissues to the liver, where it is metabolized and excreted.

Treatment

Total cholesterol levels below 200 mg/dl are desirable, with levels between 200 and 239 mg/dl being borderline high and levels of 240 mg/dl or greater being high. However, the LDL cholesterol level is a more specific indicator of CHD risk than total cholesterol is, and treatment goals are based on LDL cholesterol levels and the presence or absence of other risk factors (Table 14-3). The initial approach recommended for elevated LDL cholesterol and CHD risk factors involves lifestyle changes (increased physical activity, weight reduction if necessary, and a diet low in saturated fat and cholesterol, moderate in total fat, and relatively high in fiber). The Adult Treatment Panel III (ATP III, 2002) recommended a system of lifestyle measures known as **therapeutic lifestyle changes (TLC)**. These changes are described in more detail below. If goals for LDL cholesterol are not achieved with the TLC, drug therapy may be necessary (ATP III, 2002). Drugs used include the HMG-CoA reductase inhibitors (statins) that inhibit cholesterol synthesis; the bile acid sequestrants cholestyramine and colestipol; nicotinic acid, which lowers total and LDL cholesterol, as well as triglycerides; fibric acid derivatives

Table 14-3   LDL Cholesterol Goals

Risk Factors	LDL Goal
CHD or CHD risk equivalents (10-year risk >20%)[*]	<100 mg/dl[†]
2+ risk factors (10-year risk ≤20%)[‡]	<130 mg/dl
0-1 risk factor[§]	<160 mg/dl

From Adult Treatment Panel (ATP) III: *Third report of the national cholesterol education program (NCEP) expert panel on detection, evaluation, and treatment of high blood cholesterol in adults (adult treatment panel III),* Washington, DC, 2002, National Institutes of Health, National Heart, Lung and Blood Institute. *CHD,* Coronary heart disease; *LDL,* low-density lipoprotein.

[*]Known CHD or CHD risk equivalent noncoronary forms of atherosclerotic disease (peripheral arterial disease, abdominal aortic aneurysm, and carotid artery disease [transient ischemic attacks or stroke of carotid origin or >50% obstruction of a carotid artery]), diabetes, and 2+ risk factors with 10-year risk for "hard" CHD (myocardial infarction or coronary death) >20%.

[†]For patients at very high risk, a goal of 70 mg/dl is an optional target (Grundy et al., 2004).

[‡]Risk factors include cigarette smoking, hypertension (blood pressure ≥140/90 mm Hg or use of an antihypertensive medication), low HDL cholesterol (<40 mg/dl for males or <50 mg/dl for females), family history of premature CHD (CHD in male first-degree relative before age 55 years; CHD in female first-degree relative before age 65 years), age (≥45 years in men and ≥55 years in women). Risk factors are scored to yield the risk of developing hard CHD. (Hard CHD includes myocardial infarction or death from cardiovascular disease.) An on-line calculator for estimating 10-year risk is available at www.nhlbi.nih.gov/guidelines/cholesterol.

[§]Most individuals with 0 or 1 risk factors have 10-year risk <10%, and calculating risk is unnecessary.

such as gemfibrozil and clofibrate, which reduce triglycerides and raise HDL cholesterol; and ezetimibe, which inhibits cholesterol absorption. The presence of the metabolic syndrome, defined as three or more of the following findings—abdominal obesity (waist circumference >40 inches in men or >35 inches in women), glucose intolerance (fasting glucose >110 mg/dl), blood pressure above 130/85 mm Hg, high triglycerides (>150 mg/dl), or low HDL (<40 mg/dl in men or <50 mg/dl in women)—increases the degree of risk (ATP III, 2002). More aggressive weight control measures and increases in physical activity are likely to be needed to combat the metabolic syndrome (ATP III, 2002). The insulin-sensitizing thiazolidinedione drugs, e.g., pioglitazone, have been used in treatment of metabolic syndrome for their triglyceride-lowering and HDL-raising effects.

Nutrition assessment and care

The primary goal of care is to achieve LDL cholesterol levels associated with low risk (<160 mg/dl for those with no risk factors or only one, <130 mg/dl for those with two or more risk factors, and <100 mg/dl for those with established CHD or a CHD equivalent) (ATP III, 2002).

Assessment is summarized in Box 14-2. The MEDFICTS (Meats, Eggs, Dairy, Frying foods, In baked goods, Convenience foods, Table fats, Snacks) assessment tool (Figure 14-1) provides a guide for assessing the current diet of an individual.

Intervention and education
Therapeutic lifestyle changes. The TLC are outlined in Table 14-4, and Box 14-5 describes in more detail the specific diet pattern, weight loss goals, and activity recommendations. Whereas the TLC plan is primarily designed for cholesterol lowering in individuals with established CVD or risk of CVD, the TLC diet and lifestyle habits are suited to the needs of most adults, whether or not they have established heart disease or a high risk of heart disease. Although the DASH diet and the TLC were developed separately and are shown separately here, the DASH diet can easily fit the TLC guidelines.

Adopting the TLC guidelines requires numerous changes for many patients. Motivational interviewing is one technique that can be used in helping patients to change their behaviors (ATP III, 2002). Motivational interviewing is a client-centered technique to help individuals recognize the discrepancies between their behavior and their goals. Setting step-wise goals (e.g., first to change from drinking regular 3.5% fat milk to 2% milk and then to change to skim milk) is a tool used in motivational interviewing.

To follow the guidelines, patients and their families can be encouraged to do the following (ATP III, 2002):

■ Emphasize consumption of vegetables; fruits; breads, cereals, rice, legumes, and pasta; skim milk and skim milk products; and poultry, fish, and lean meat to reduce saturated fat and cholesterol intake. Meats and dairy products are the primary sources of saturated fat and cholesterol in the diet. Combine meats with pasta, rice, or vegetables in a main dish, or use legumes in a meatless main dish, to reduce the amount of saturated fat and cholesterol.

Text continued on p. 393.

Sample Dietary Assessment Questionnaire
MEDFICTS

In each food category for both Group 1 and Group 2 foods check one box from the "Weekly Consumption" column (number of servings eaten per week) and then check one box from the "Serving Size" column. If you check Rarely/Never, do not check a serving size box. See p. 392 for score.

Food Category	Weekly Consumption		Serving Size			Score
	Rarely/ never	3 or less	4 or more	Small <5 oz/d 1 pt	Average 5 oz/d 2 pts	Large >5 oz/d 3 pts	

Meats

■ Recommended amount per day: ≤5 oz (equal in size to 2 decks of playing cards).
■ Base your estimate on the food you consume most often.
■ Beef and lamb selections are trimmed to 1/8" fat.

Group 1. 10 g or more total fat in 3 oz cooked portion
Beef – Ground beef, Ribs, Steak (T-bone, Flank, Porterhouse, Tenderloin). Chuck blade roast, Brisket, Meatloaf (w/ground beef). Corned beef
Processed meats – 1/4 lb burger or lg. sandwich, Bacon, Lunch meat Sausage/knockwurst, Hot dogs, Ham (bone-end). Ground turkey
Other meats, Poultry, Seafood – Pork chops (center loin), Pork roast (Blade, Boston, Sirloin). Pork spareribs, Ground pork, Lamb chops, Lamb (ribs), Organ meats*, Chicken w/skin, Eel, Mackerel, Pompano

Group 1 row: Weekly Consumption — 3 or less: **3 pts**; 4 or more: **7 pts**. Serving Size — Small: **1 pt**; Average: **2 pts**; Large: **3 pts**.

Group 2. Less than 10 g total fat in 3 oz cooked portion
Lean beef – Round steak (Eye of round, Top round), Sirloin†, Tip and bottom round*, Chuck arm pot roast*, Top loin†
Low-fat processed meats – Low-fat lunch meat, Canadian bacon, "Lean" fast food sandwich, Boneless ham
Other meats, Poultry, Seafood – Chicken, Turkey (w/o skin)§, most Seafood*, Lamb leg shank, Pork tenderloin, Sirloin top loin, Veal cutlets, Sirloin, Shoulder, Ground veal, Venison, Veal chops and ribs†, Lamb (whole leg, loin, fore-shank, sirloin)†

Group 2 row: Serving Size — Large: **6 pts**‡

Continued

Figure 14-1. For legend, see p. 393.

Sample Dietary Assessment Questionnaire
MEDFICTS

In each food category for both Group 1 and Group 2 foods check one box from the "Weekly Consumption" column (number of servings eaten per week) and then check one box from the "Serving Size" column. If you check Rarely/Never, do not check a serving size box. See p. 392 for score.

Eggs – Weekly consumption is the number of times you eat eggs each week.

	Weekly Consumption			Serving Size			Score
	Rarely/ never	3 or less	4 or more	Small <5 oz/d 1 pt	Average 5 oz/d 2 pts	Large >5 oz/d 3 pts	
				Check the number of eggs eaten each time			
Group 1. Whole eggs, Yolks	☐	☐ 3 pts	☐ 7 pts ×	☐ ≤1 1 pt	☐ 2 2 pts	☐ ≥3 3 pts	____
Group 2. Egg whites, Egg substitutes (1/2 cup)	☐						____

Dairy

Milk – Average serving 1 cup
| Group 1. Whole milk, 2% milk, 2% buttermilk, Yogurt (whole milk) | ☐ | ☐ 3 pts | ☐ 7 pts × | ☐ 1 pt | ☐ 2 pts | ☐ 3 pts | ____ |
| Group 2. Fat-free milk, 1% milk, Fat-free buttermilk, Yogurt (Fat-free, 1% low fat) | ☐ | ☐ | ☐ | | | | ____ |

Cheese – Average serving 1 oz
| Group 1. Cream cheese, Cheddar, Monterey Jack, Colby, Swiss, American processed, Blue cheese, Regular cottage cheese (1/2 cup), and Ricotta (1/4 cup) | ☐ | ☐ 3 pts | ☐ 7 pts | ☐ 1 pts | ☐ 2 pts | ☐ 3 pts | ____ |
| Group 2. Low-fat and fat-free cheeses, Fat-free milk mozzarella, String cheese, Low-fat, Fat-free milk and Fat-free cottage cheese (1/2 cup) and Ricotta (1/4 cup) | ☐ | ☐ | ☐ | | | | ____ |

Frozen Desserts – Average serving 1/2 cup
| Group 1. Ice cream, Milk shakes | ☐ | ☐ 3 pts | ☐ 7 pts | ☐ 1 pts | ☐ 2 pts | ☐ 3 pts | ____ |
| Group 2. Low-fat ice cream, Frozen yogurt | ☐ | ☐ | ☐ | | | | ____ |

Food Category	Weekly Consumption			Serving Size			Score
	Rarely/never	3 or less	4 or more	Small <5 oz/d 1 pt	Average 5 oz/d 2 pts	Large >5 oz/d 3 pts	
Frying Foods – Average servings: see below. This section refers to method of preparation for vegetables and meat.							
Group 1. French fries, Fried vegetables (1/2 cup), Fried chicken, fish, meat (3 oz)	☐	☐ 3 pts	☐ 7 pts	x ☐ 1 pt	☐ 2 pts	☐ 3 pts	—
Group 2. Vegetables, not deep fried (1/2 cup), Meat, poultry, or fish—prepared by baking, broiling, grilling, poaching, roasting, stewing (3 oz)	☐	☐	☐	☐	☐	☐	—
In Baked Goods – 1 Average serving							
Group 1. Doughnuts, Biscuits, Butter rolls, Muffins, Croissants, Sweet rolls, Danish, Cakes, Pies, Coffee cakes, Cookies	☐	☐ 3 pts	☐ 7 pts	x ☐ 1 pt	☐ 2 pts	☐ 3 pts	—
Group 2. Fruit bars, Low-fat cookies/cakes/pastries, Angel food cake, Homemade baked goods with vegetable oils, breads, bagels	☐	☐	☐	☐	☐	☐	—
Convenience Foods							
Group 1. Canned, Packaged, or Frozen dinners: e.g., Pizza (1 slice), Macaroni and cheese (1 cup), Pot pie (1), Cream soups (1 cup), Potato, rice and pasta dishes with cream/cheese sauces (1/2 cup)	☐	☐ 3 pts	☐ 7 pts	x ☐ 1 pt	☐ 2 pts	☐ 3 pts	—
Group 2. Diet/Reduced calorie or reduced fat dinners (1), Potato, rice and pasta dishes without cream/cheese sauces (1/2 cup)	☐	☐	☐	☐	☐	☐	—
Table Fats – Average serving: 1 Tbsp							
Group 1. Butter, Stick margarine, Regular salad dressing, Mayonnaise, Sour cream (2 Tbsp)	☐	☐ 3 pts	☐ 7 pts	x ☐ 1 pts	☐ 2 pts	☐ 3 pts	—
Group 2. Diet and tub margarine, Low-fat and fat-free salad dressing, Low-fat and fat-free mayonnaise	☐	☐	☐	☐	☐	☐	—

For legend, see p. 393.

Continued

Figure 14-1.

Sample Dietary Assessment Questionnaire
MEDFICTS

In each food category for both Group 1 and Group 2 foods check one box from the "Weekly Consumption" column (number of servings eaten per week) and then check one box from the "Serving Size" column. If you check Rarely/Never, do not check a serving size box.

	Weekly Consumption		Serving Size			Score
	Rarely/never	3 or less	4 or more	Small <5 oz/d 1 pt	Average 5 oz/d 2 pts	Large >5 oz/d 3 pts	

Snacks

Group 1. Chips (potato, corn, taco), Cheese puffs, Snack mix, Nuts (1 oz), Regular crackers (½ oz), Candy (milk chocolate, caramel, coconut) (about 1½ oz), Regular popcorn (3 cups)

| ☐ | ☐ 3 pts | ☐ 7 pts | ☐ 1 pt × | ☐ 2 pts | ☐ 3 pts | ___ |

Group 2. Pretzels, Fat-free chips (1 oz), Low-fat crackers (½ oz), Fruit, Fruit rolls, Licorice, Hard candy (1 med piece), Bread sticks (1–2 pcs), Air-popped or low-fat popcorn (3 cups)

| ☐ | ☐ | ☐ | ☐ | ☐ | ☐ | ___ |

Final Score ___

To Score: For each food category, multiply points in weekly consumption box by points in serving size box and record total in score column. If Group 2 foods checked, no points are scored (except for Group 2 meats, large serving = 6 pts).

Example:

| ☐ 3 pts | ☑ 7 pts × | ☐ 1 pt | ☐ 2 pts | ☑ 3 pts | 21 pts |

Add score to get final score.

Key:
≥70   Need to make some dietary changes
40–70 Heart-Healthy Diet
<40   TLC Diet

Figure 14-1
Sample dietary assessment questionnaire (MEDFICTS).
*Organ meats, shrimp, abalone, and squid are low in fat but high in cholesterol.
†Only lean cuts with all visible fat trimmed. If not trimmed of all visible fat, score as if in Group 1.
‡Score 6 points if this box is checked.
§All parts not listed in Group 1 have <10 g total fat.
(From Adult Treatment Panel [ATP] III: *Third report of the national cholesterol education program [NCEP] expert panel on detection, evaluation, and treatment of high blood cholesterol in adults [adult treatment panel III]*, Washington, DC, 2002, National Institutes of Health, National Heart, Lung and Blood Institute.)

- Choose low-fat meats, e.g., 98% fat-free cold cuts, rather than fatty meats, such as bologna, bacon, or sausages.
- Use lower-fat cooking and food preparation methods: broiling, baking, grilling, steaming, poaching without added fat, trimming fat from meat, draining fat after cooking, and removing skin from poultry.
- Use the Nutrition Facts label as a guide in making food choices.
- Choose nonfat or 1% milk and milk products, e.g., fat-free yogurt, reduced-fat cheese, low-fat or fat-free ice cream and frozen yogurt.
- Learn to identify "hidden" sources of saturated fat, such as baked goods, cheese, salad dressings, and many snack items.
- Keep snacks that are low in saturated fat and cholesterol available. Some examples are fresh or individually packed canned fruit; carrots, celery, cucumber slices, cauliflower, or other fresh vegetables to eat raw; ginger snaps; low-fat graham crackers; fat-free yogurt or cottage cheese.

The TLC diet is moderate in protein and fat (see Table 14-4), with unsaturated fatty acids encouraged. Partially **hydrogenated fats** (found especially in stick margarines, shortening, and fried and baked goods made with those products) contain *trans* forms of fatty acids, rather than the *cis* forms more common in nature

Table 14-4   Components of the TLC Diet

Component	Recommendation
Total fat intake	20%-35% of total calories*
Monounsaturated fat	Up to 20% of total calories
Polyunsaturated fat	Up to 10% of total calories
Saturated fat	<7% of total calories
Trans fat	Keep intake low
Cholesterol	<200 mg/day
Carbohydrate†	50%-60% of total calories*
Dietary fiber	20-30 g/day
Protein	Approximately 15% of total calories
Total calories (energy)	Adjust total caloric intake to maintain desirable body weight/prevent weight gain
Physical activity	Include enough moderate exercise to expend at least 200 kcal/day
Therapeutic Options for LDL Lowering	
Plant stanols/sterols	2 g/day
Increased viscous (soluble) fiber	At least 5-10 g/day

From Adult Treatment Panel (ATP) III: *Third report of the national cholesterol education program (NCEP) expert panel on detection, evaluation, and treatment of high blood cholesterol in adults (adult treatment panel III)*,Washington, DC, 2002, National Institutes of Health, National Heart, Lung and Blood Institute.
LDL, Low-density lipoprotein; *TLC,* therapeutic lifestyle changes.
*Total fat can be increased to 35% of total calories and carbohydrate can be reduced to 50% of calories for persons with the metabolic syndrome. Any increase in fat intake should be in the form of either polyunsaturated or monounsaturated fat.
†Carbohydrate should come mostly from foods rich in complex carbohydrates, including grains (especially whole grains), fruits, and vegetables.

(see Figure 1-4). Both saturated and *trans* fats raise LDL cholesterol (Lichtenstein et al., 2006). Liquid vegetable oil, soft (tub) margarine, and *trans*-fatty acid–free margarine are preferable to stick margarine and shortening and to butter, a source of saturated fat. Including plant *stanols* and *sterols* in the diet is an option that can help to reduce LDL cholesterol. Stanols and sterols are available in gelcaps and are also added to an increasing number of food products, including some margarines, orange juice, yogurt, snack and granola bars, rice beverages, and whole-grain bread.

Box 14-5   Guide to Therapeutic Lifestyle Changes (TLC): Healthy Lifestyle Recommendations for a Healthy Heart

Food Items to Choose More Often

Breads and Cereals

≥6 servings per day, adjusted to kcal needs

Breads, cereals, especially whole grains; pasta; rice; potatoes; dry beans and peas; low-fat crackers and cookies

Vegetables

3 to 5 servings per day fresh, frozen, or canned without added fat, sauce, or salt

Fruits

2-4 servings per day fresh, frozen, canned, dried

Dairy Products

2 or 3 servings per day fat-free, ½%, 1% milk, buttermilk, yogurt, cottage cheese; fat-free and low-fat cheese

Eggs

≤2 egg yolks per week

Egg whites or egg substitute

Meat, Poultry, Fish

≤5 oz per day

Lean cuts: loin, leg, round, extralean hamburger; cold cuts made with lean meat or soy protein; skinless poultry; fish

Fats and Oils

Amount adjusted to kcal level: unsaturated oils; soft or liquid margarines and vegetable oil spreads; salad dressings, seeds, and nuts

TLC Diet Options

Stanol/sterol–containing margarines; soluble-fiber food sources: barley, oats, psyllium, apples, bananas, berries, citrus fruits, nectarines, peaches, pears, plums, prunes, broccoli, Brussels sprouts, carrots, dry beans, soy products (tofu, miso)

Continued

Box 14-5   Guide to Therapeutic Lifestyle Changes (TLC): Healthy Lifestyle Recommendations for a Healthy Heart—cont'd

Food Items to Choose Less Often

Breads and Cereals

Many bakery products, including doughnuts, biscuits, butter rolls, muffins, croissants, sweet rolls, Danish, cakes, pies, coffeecakes, cookies

Many grain-based snacks, including chips, cheese puffs, regular crackers, buttered popcorn

Vegetables

Vegetables fried or prepared with butter, cheese, or cream sauce

Fruits

Fruits fried or served with butter or cream

Dairy Products

Whole milk, 2% milk, whole-milk yogurt, ice cream, cream, cheese

Eggs

Egg yolk, whole eggs

Meat, Poultry, Fish

Higher-fat meat cuts: ribs, T-bone steak, regular hamburger, bacon, sausage; cold cuts: salami, bologna, hot dogs; organ meats: liver, brains, sweetbreads; poultry with skin; fried meat; fried poultry; fried fish

Fats and Oils

Butter, shortening, stick margarine, chocolate, coconut

Recommendations for Weight Reduction

Weigh Regularly.

Record weight, body mass index (BMI), and waist circumference.

Lose Weight Gradually.

Goal: lose 10% of body weight in 6 months; lose ½ to 1 lb/wk.

Develop Healthy Eating Patterns.

Choose healthy foods (see "Food Items to Choose More Often").

Reduce intake of less healthy foods (see "Food Items to Choose Less Often").

Limit number of eating occasions.

Avoid second helpings.

Identify and reduce hidden fat by reading food labels to choose products lower in saturated fat and kcal, and ask about ingredients in ready-to-eat foods prepared away from home.

Identify and reduce sources of excess carbohydrates, such as fat-free and regular crackers; cookies and other desserts; snacks; and sugar-containing beverages.

Recommendations for Increased Physical Activity

Make Physical Activity Part of Daily Routine.

Reduce sedentary time.

Walk or wheel more; drive less. Take the stairs instead of an elevator. Get off the bus a few stops early, and walk the remaining distance. Mow the lawn with a push mower. Rake leaves. Garden. Push a stroller. Clean the house. Do exercises or pedal a stationary bike while watching television. Play actively with children. Take a brisk 10-minute walk or wheel before work, during your work break, and after dinner.

Make Physical Activity Part of Exercise or Recreational Activities.

Walk, wheel, or jog. Bicycle or use an arm pedal bicycle. Swim or do water aerobics. Play basketball. Join a sport team. Play wheelchair sports. Golf (pull cart or carry clubs). Canoe. Cross-country ski. Dance. Take part in an exercise program at work, home, school, or gym.

From Adult Treatment Panel (ATP) III: *Third report of the national cholesterol education program (NCEP) expert panel on detection, evaluation, and treatment of high blood cholesterol in adults (adult treatment panel III)*, Washington, DC, 2002, National Institutes of Health, National Heart, Lung, and Blood Institute. *TLC,* Therapeutic lifestyle changes.

The American Heart Association recommends at least 2 servings (8 oz, or 240 g) of oily fish, such as salmon, weekly. Oily fish are a source of the omega-3 (*n*-3) fatty acids eicosapentaenoic acid (EPA) and docosahexaenoic acid (DHA) (Table 14-5), which help to reduce serum triglycerides. By eating fish, the patient may also displace some of the sources of saturated fat, such as red meats, in the diet (Lichtenstein et al., 2006). Some fish are contaminated with methylmercury, and for this reason pregnant women, women who may become pregnant, nursing mothers, and young children should not eat the fish with the highest potential for contamination, including tilefish, shark, swordfish, and king mackerel. Local advisories are the best guide as to whether fish caught in local lakes, rivers, and coastal areas are safe to eat (U.S. Food and Drug Administration, 2004). Most commercially prepared fried fish (in restaurants and frozen convenience items) is low in omega-3 fatty acids. Certain vegetable oils (e.g., canola,

Table 14-5   Omega-3 (n-3) Fatty Acids in Fish

Type of Fish	Omega-3 (EPA and DHA), in g[*]
Salmon, Atlantic	2.1
Herring, Atlantic	2.1
Salmon, pink, canned	1.7
Tuna, bluefin	1.3
Mackerel, Atlantic	1.3
Trout, rainbow	1.1
Sardines, oil-canned	1.0
Tuna, water-canned, white	0.9
Bass, freshwater	0.8
Halibut	0.6
Sole/flounder	0.5
Crab, Alaskan king	0.4
Shrimp	0.3
Catfish, farmed	0.2
Tuna, water-canned, light	0.2

Data are derived from the *USDA National Nutrient Database for Standard Reference*, Release 20, updated September 26, 2007. Available at http://www.nal.usda.gov/fnic/foodcomp/search/. Accessed November 27, 2007.
[*]Values are for 100-g (≈3-oz) servings of broiled, steamed, or baked fish, except where canned is specified.

walnut, flaxseed [linseed], soybean) are also sources of omega-3 fatty acids. However, the omega-3 fatty acids they contain are not EPA and DHA, and it is not known if the benefits from these oils are the same as those from fish.

Soluble, or viscous, fiber has a cholesterol-lowering effect (Lichtenstein et al., 2006). Good sources of soluble fiber are listed in Box 14-6. The so-called Mediterranean diet, modeled after the traditional diet of Mediterranean countries, has been found in one large prospective study to reduce recurrence of MI in patients who had had one MI. The diet is effective in reducing LDL cholesterol levels and inflammatory markers. The traditional Mediterranean diet emphasizes fruits, vegetables, breads and

---

Box 14-6   **Good Dietary Sources of Viscous (Soluble) Fiber**

3 or More g/Serving*
Psyllium seeds, ground, 1 tbsp
Lima or kidney beans, ½ cup
Brussels sprouts, ½ cup

1.5 to 2 g/Serving*
Citrus fruit (orange, grapefruit), 1 medium
Pear, 1 medium
Black, navy, or pinto beans, ½ cup
Northern beans, ½ cup
Plums, dried, ¼ cup

1 g/Serving
Barley, oatmeal, or oat bran, cooked, ½ cup
Apple, banana, or plum, 1 medium
Blackberries, ½ cup
Nectarine or peach, 1 medium
Lentils, chickpeas, or black-eyed peas, ½ cup
Broccoli, ½ cup
Carrots, ½ cup

Adapted from National Heart, Lung, and Blood Institute: *How you can lower your cholesterol level.* Available at http://www.nhlbi.nih.gov/chd/Tipsheets/solfiber.htm. Accessed November 24, 2007.
*Within these categories, foods with the highest viscous fiber content are listed first.

other unrefined grains, potatoes, beans, nuts, and seeds. Olive oil, which is rich in monounsaturated fat, is an important component. Dairy products, fish, and poultry are included in low to moderate amounts, eggs are consumed 0 to 4 times weekly, and there is little red meat (4 or 5 servings/mo). Wine is consumed moderately (1 or 2 glasses/day). Overall, fiber intake is higher than that in the traditional American diet, and saturated fat and cholesterol intakes are lower (Panagiotakos et al., 2006; Willett, 2006). This diet is similar to the TLC diet and the dietary guidelines of the American Heart Association.

In a 1-year trial in hypercholesterolemic individuals, a diet low in saturated fat and high in soluble fiber, plant sterols, soy and other plant proteins, and almonds reduced LDL cholesterol as much as statin treatment in a substantial number of the subjects, with none of the side effects that might be experienced with drug therapy (Jenkins et al., 2006). This underscores the potential for risk factor reduction with appropriate diet and lifestyle practices. Changes do not have to result in a restrictive or unpalatable diet; the sample diet in Table 14-2 meets the TLC guidelines yet includes tasty, attractive meals that can be prepared with ingredients that are readily available.

Eating away from home is likely to pose challenges for the person trying to follow the TLC diet. Some suggestions to make the experience easier include the following:

- Ask service personnel in restaurants about preparation methods and fat content of foods if this information is not clear from the menu.
- Avoid fried foods and large portions of red meats. Salads (with as few high-fat ingredients such as cheese or bacon bits as possible) or grilled items are preferable.
- Order foods without sauces, butter, and sour cream.
- Ask that salad dressings be served on the side, and use limited amounts, or request low-fat dressings.
- Choose small amounts of sunflower seeds and olives over high-saturated fat toppings, such as bacon and cheese.
- Avoid eating everything if portions are large. Share with a companion, or plan to take some food home for another meal.
- Move away from buffet tables or other areas where food is available at parties.

Hypertriglyceridemia. Hypertriglyceridemia, or elevated serum triglycerides, is an independent risk factor for CHD. In addition to weight loss and increased activity, the following measures are recommended to reduce triglyceride concentrations (ATP III, 2002; Lichtenstein et al., 2006):

- Avoid alcohol intake. If this is not acceptable to the patient, intake should be limited as much as possible. In no case should intake be more than 1 drink daily for women and 2 for men.
- Consult with the physician; a supplement of EPA+DHA (2 to 4 g daily) is recommended. Belching and a fishy taste in the mouth are the major side effects of the supplement.
- Avoid simple sugars; most dietary carbohydrates should be complex (starches and fiber).
- Avoid very–low-fat diets; in particular, keep carbohydrate intake less than 60% of energy intake.

Chronic Heart Failure

Chronic heart failure (CHF) is "a complex clinical syndrome that can result from any cardiac disorder that impairs the ability of the ventricle to fill with or eject blood" (Hunt, 2005). The characteristic symptoms of CHF are dyspnea, fatigue, and fluid retention. Patients with the disorder may or may not have pulmonary or peripheral edema. CHF is most common among individuals with diabetes, hypertension, atherosclerotic heart disease, presence of the metabolic syndrome, and obesity. Levels of inflammatory cytokines are elevated in CHF, and this likely contributes to cardiac cachexia (physical wasting and weakness) that occurs in some patients (Krack et al., 2005). Poor perfusion of the gastrointestinal tract, which might allow bacteria to translocate from the gut lumen into the body and also impair intestinal absorption, is an additional factor that may contribute to cachexia (Krack et al., 2005). Patients with CHF have elevated levels of hormones including catecholamines, cortisol, and aldosterone, which could also contribute to tissue catabolism (Anker et al., 2006). Anorexia, dyspnea, and weakness or fatigue also play a role in poor nutrient intake and wasting. Overweight patients actually seem to have a survival advantage in CHF, but this observation does not justify recommending that individuals with CHF become overweight (Curtis et al., 2005).

Treatment

Most medications used for treating hypertension are applicable to the treatment of CHF. ACE inhibitors and other vasodilatory agents and diuretics (used to reduce total body water) are used in the treatment of CHF. Inotropic agents such as digitalis are often given to improve cardiac contractility.

Nutrition assessment and care

A thorough nutrition assessment should be performed as described in Chapter 2. Box 14-2 highlights common or especially serious findings in CHF. A loss of 6% of body weight over 6 months, in the absence of edema, is an indicator of cardiac cachexia (Anker et al., 2006).

Intervention and education

Prevention and treatment. Prevention and treatment of CHF require lifestyle changes to correct or control the contributing conditions, including hypertension, hyperlipidemia, diabetes (see Chapter 17), the metabolic syndrome (see Chapter 5), and obesity (see Chapter 7). Patients with reduced left ventricular ejection fraction and fluid retention benefit from a low-sodium diet, along with diuretics (Hunt, 2005).

For those patients with undernutrition or cachexia, try dividing daily food intake into five or six small meals and snacks. Small meals are often better tolerated by the dyspneic individual than three large meals per day. Box 12-3 provides tips for increasing food intake if dyspnea or other symptoms interfere with eating. Modular ingredients (see Chapter 8) can be used to increase the energy density of foods and beverages or of infant formulas, if applicable, to allow provision of adequate energy within the fluid volume tolerated. If oral feedings are not sufficient, enteral tube feedings can be used, with care to prevent fluid overload (Anker et al., 2006).

Conclusion

Primary prevention is central to reducing the risk of CVD. Limiting intake of saturated and *trans* fats and cholesterol, achieving and maintaining a healthy weight, choosing a diet moderate in sodium, drinking alcohol moderately if at all, and being physically active on a regular basis are measures appropriate for almost all individuals over 2 years of age.

REFERENCES

Adult Treatment Panel (ATP) III: *Third report of the national cholesterol education program (NCEP) expert panel on detection, evaluation, and treatment of high blood cholesterol in adults (adult treatment panel III),* Washington, DC, 2002, National Institutes of Health, National Heart, Lung and Blood Institute.

Anker SD et al: ESPEN guidelines on enteral nutrition: cardiology and pulmonology, *Clin Nutr* 25(2):311, 2006.

Appel LJ et al: Dietary approaches to prevent and treat hypertension: a scientific statement from the American Heart Association, *Hypertension* 47(2):296, 2006.

Champagne CM: Dietary interventions on blood pressure: the Dietary Approaches to Stop Hypertension (DASH) trials, *Nutr Rev* 64(2 pt 2): S53, 2006.

Curtis JP et al: The obesity paradox: body mass index and outcomes in patients with heart failure, *Arch Intern Med* 165(1):55, 2005.

Dickinson BD et al: Reducing the population burden of cardiovascular disease by reducing sodium intake: a report of the Council on Science and Public Health, *Arch Intern Med* 167(14):1460, 2007.

Goldstein LB et al: Primary prevention of ischemic stroke: a guideline from the American Heart Association/American Stroke Association Stroke Council, *Circulation* 113(24):e873, 2006.

Grundy SM et al: Implications of recent clinical trials for the National Cholesterol Education Program Adult Treatment Panel III Guidelines, *J Am Coll Cardiol* 44(3):720, 2004.

Hunt SA: ACC/AHA 2005 guideline update for the diagnosis and management of chronic heart failure in the adult: a report of the American College of Cardiology/American Heart Association Task Force on Practice Guidelines (Writing Committee to Update the 2001 Guidelines for the Evaluation and Management of Heart Failure), *J Am Coll Cardiol* 46(6):e1, 2005.

Jenkins DJ et al: Assessment of the longer-term effects of a dietary portfolio of cholesterol-lowering foods in hypercholesterolemia, *Am J Clin Nutr* 83(3):582, 2006.

Krack A et al: The importance of the gastrointestinal system in the pathogenesis of heart failure, *Eur Heart J* 26(22):2368, 2005.

Lichtenstein AH et al: Diet and lifestyle recommendations revision 2006: a scientific statement from the American Heart Association Nutrition Committee, *Circulation* 114(1):82, 2006.

Miller ER 3rd, Erlinger TP, Appel LJ: The effects of macronutrients on blood pressure and lipids: an overview of the DASH and OmniHeart trials, *Curr Atheroscler Rep* 8(6):460, 2006.

Myers VH, Champagne CM: Nutritional effects on blood pressure, *Curr Opin Lipidol* 18(1):20, 2007.

Panagiotakos DB et al: The relationship between adherence to the Mediterranean diet and the severity and short-term prognosis of acute coronary syndromes (ACS): The Greek Study of ACS (The GREECS), *Nutrition* 22(7-8):722, 2006.

Sacks FM et al: Effects on blood pressure of reduced dietary sodium and the Dietary Approaches to Stop Hypertension (DASH) diet. DASH-Sodium Collaborative Research Group, *N Engl J Med* 344(1):3, 2001.

U.S. Department of Health and Human Services (USDHHS): *The seventh report of the joint national committee on prevention, detection, evaluation, and treatment of high blood pressure (JNC 7)*, Washington, DC, 2003, The Department.

U.S. Department of Health and Human Services: *Your guide to lowering your blood pressure with DASH: the DASH eating plan*, Washington, DC, 2006 (revised), National Institutes of Health (NIH), National Heart, Lung, and Blood Institute (NHLBI).

U.S. Food and Drug Administration: What you need to know about mercury in fish and shellfish, 2004. Available at http://www.cfsan.fda. gov/~dms/admehg3.html. Accessed November 24, 2007.

Willett WC: The Mediterranean diet: science and practice, *Public Health Nutr* 9(1A):105, 2006.

PULMONARY DISEASE

Nutrition and acute or chronic respiratory diseases interact in a variety of ways. Increased work of breathing increases energy needs, whereas dyspnea interferes with nutrient intake. These factors contribute to weight loss and inadequate nutritional status. In addition, chronic obstructive pulmonary disease (COPD) and **cystic fibrosis (CF)** are associated with chronic inflammation that can contribute to cachexia, or wasting of fat-free mass (FFM, or lean body mass) and weakness (Sinaasappel et al., 2002; Gan et al., 2004).

Chronic Obstructive Pulmonary Disease

COPD is a group of diseases, including chronic bronchitis, emphysema, and small airways disease, characterized by chronic and progressive airflow obstruction. By far the most common cause is smoking. COPD is the fourth leading cause of death among adults in the United States. The symptoms of COPD can include chronic cough, sputum production, wheezing, dyspnea, and poor exercise tolerance (Kasper et al., 2005; Qaseem et al., 2007). Forced expiratory volume at 1 second (FEV_1), obtained by spirometry, is used as an index of the severity of airflow obstruction.

Never smoking or stopping smoking is the best preventive measure for COPD. Diets rich in fruits, vegetables, and fish are associated with the lowest risk of COPD, whereas diets high in refined grains, cured and red meats, desserts, and French fries may increase the risk (Varraso et al., 2007a, 2007b).

Treatment

Smoking cessation is the most important measure to treat COPD (Kasper et al., 2005). Inhaled bronchodilators, such as long-acting anticholinergic agents (e.g., tiotropium), β-agonists (e.g., salmeterol), or glucocorticoids (e.g., fluticasone), are recommended for maintenance therapy for symptomatic patients with FEV_1 less than

60% of predicted (Qaseem et al., 2007). For patients with severe hypercapnia, noninvasive positive pressure ventilation can improve exercise tolerance and functional status, and oxygen therapy is recommended for patients with resting hypoxemia (Nici et al., 2006; Qaseem et al., 2007).

Nutrition Assessment and Care

Malnutrition is common among individuals with COPD, especially those with emphysema. As many as 30% of outpatients with COPD have lost weight, are underweight, and/or show signs of muscle or fat wasting (Nici et al., 2006; Budweiser et al., 2008). Resting energy expenditure is increased approximately 25% in people with moderate to severe COPD (Nici et al., 2006). Underweight or a history of recent weight loss (>10% of body weight in 6 months or >5% in 1 month) is an indication of poor prognosis in COPD, and weight gain in COPD patients with a body mass index (BMI) below 25 kg/m^2 reduces mortality (Nici et al., 2006). FFM has been found to be an even better predictor of morbidity and mortality than BMI (Vestbo et al., 2006; Budweiser et al., 2008).

COPD is suggested to involve an imbalance between oxidants and antioxidants. The plasma concentrations of the retinoids lutein/zeaxanthin, lycopene, β-cryptoxanthin, retinol, and β-carotene have been noted to be directly related to lung function in COPD (Ochs-Balcom et al., 2006), suggesting that adequate antioxidant status might improve outcome. However, supplementation of patients with COPD with retinoids and other antioxidants has not brought about clear-cut improvements in clinical status (Kelly, 2005; Roth et al., 2006). A diet with ample amounts of antioxidant nutrients, such as vitamins C, E, A, and other retinoids (e.g., rich in fruits, vegetables, and whole grains), might have benefits that a single supplement does not.

A thorough nutrition assessment should be performed as described in Chapter 2. Box 15-1 highlights common or especially serious findings in patients with COPD.

Intervention and education
Preventing or correcting underweight/undernutrition. Intervention and patient and family education can include the following:

■ Increase energy intake through use of energy-dense foods or supplements; Box 12-3 provides a list of suggestions. Individuals

Text continued on p. 411.

Box 15-1   Assessment in Pulmonary Disease

Protein-Energy Malnutrition (PEM) or Protein-Calorie Malnutrition (PCM)

History

COPD or *CF*: inadequate intake of protein and energy related to pressure of a full stomach on the diaphragm, unpleasant taste in the mouth from chronic sputum production, gastric irritation from bronchodilator therapy, smoking; increased needs related to increased work of breathing, frequent infections; short bowel syndrome after meconium ileus in CF

Acute respiratory failure: inadequate intake of protein and energy related to upper airway intubation, altered state of consciousness, dyspnea; increase in protein and energy requirements related to increased work of breathing or acute pulmonary infections

Physical examination

Evidence of weight loss (muscle wasting, lack of fat); weight for height <90% of desirable or BMI <18.5 (adults) or <25th percentile for age and gender (children); triceps skinfold <5th percentile

Laboratory analysis

↓ Serum albumin, transferrin, or prealbumin; ↓ creatinine-height index (all uncommon in COPD)

Overweight

History

COPD: decreased energy needs related to decreased basal metabolic rate with aging, decreased activity to compensate for impaired respiratory function, weight gain after smoking cessation

Physical examination

Weight for height >120% of desirable or BMI >25; triceps skinfold >95th percentile

Continued

Box 15-1   Assessment in Pulmonary Disease—cont'd

Vitamin A Deficiency

History

Diet inadequate in vitamin A or retinoids; oxidative stress; *CF:* steatorrhea with loss of fat-soluble vitamins in stools, short bowel syndrome

Physical examination

Follicular hyperkeratosis; poor light-dark visual adaptation; dryness of the skin or cornea

Laboratory analysis

↓ Serum retinol

Vitamin D Deficiency

History

Little sun exposure (northern latitudes, clothing covering most of skin, use of high-SPF sunscreens*); diet inadequate in foods fortified with vitamin D, such as milk and ready-to-eat cereals; *CF:* steatorrhea

Laboratory analysis

↓ Serum 25-OH-D; bone mineral density

Vitamin E Deficiency

History

Oxidative stress; *CF:* steatorrhea

Physical examination

Musculoskeletal pain

Laboratory analysis

Hemolytic anemia, ↓ serum α-tocopherol

Vitamin K Deficiency

History

Chronic or repeated antibiotic treatment that decreases normal intestinal flora; *CF:* steatorrhea

Box 15-1   Assessment in Pulmonary Disease—cont'd

Physical examination

Easy bruisability, petechiae

Laboratory analysis

Prolonged prothrombin time; more sensitive: ↓ PIVKA-II (not widely available)

Mineral Deficiencies

Calcium Deficiency

History

CF: steatorrhea with loss in stool, vitamin D deficiency, short bowel syndrome after meconium ileus

Physical examination

Weakness, fatigue, muscle cramping and spasm, abdominal pain, paresthesias

Laboratory analysis

↓ Serum calcium; chronic: ↓ bone mineral density

Magnesium Deficiency

History

Inadequate food intake, undernutrition; *CF:* steatorrhea, short bowel syndrome

Physical examination

Diminished ventilation, difficulty weaning from the ventilator (decreased respiratory muscle strength)

Laboratory analysis

↓ Serum magnesium

Zinc Deficiency

History

Inadequate intake, especially meats and whole grains; *CF:* steatorrhea

Continued

Box 15-1   Assessment in Pulmonary Disease—cont'd

Physical examination

Loss of taste acuity, diarrhea, dermatitis

Laboratory analysis

↓ Serum zinc (not a sensitive measurement)

Elevated Respiratory Quotient (RQ)

History

Overfeeding

Physical examination

Tachypnea (>20 breaths/min in a non–mechanically ventilated adult); shortness of breath

Laboratory analysis

RQ ≥1; ↑ partial pressure of CO_2 (P_{CO_2})

Fluid Excess

History

Administration of more than 35-50 ml fluid/kg/day in an adult, including fluids in IVs, medications, tube feedings, TPN, and oral intake; ventilator dependency or recent surgery, which can cause increased release of antidiuretic hormone (ADH)

Physical examination

Bounding pulse; sacral or peripheral edema; shortness of breath; pulmonary rales; acute weight gain

Laboratory analysis

↓ Serum sodium; ↓ Hct

Essential Fatty Acid Deficiency

History

Very-high–carbohydrate formula feedings with inadequate essential fatty acids (uncommon); *CF*: steatorrhea

Physical examination

Dermatitis, failure to thrive

Box 15-1   Assessment in Pulmonary Disease—cont'd

Laboratory analysis

Plasma triene/tetraene (eicosatrienoic acid/arachidonic acid) ratio >0.2

Hyperglycemia

History

Use of glucocorticoid medications; *CF:* destruction of insulin-secreting beta cells of the pancreas

Physical examination

↑ Urination, thirst, and hunger; unexplained weight loss

Laboratory analysis

Fasting plasma glucose >100 mg/dl (impaired fasting glucose) or >126 mg/dl (diabetes); abnormal glucose tolerance test, with 2-hr postload plasma glucose >140 mg/dl (impaired glucose tolerance) or >200 mg/dl (diabetes); or casual blood glucose values >200 mg/dl with symptoms of diabetes

BMI, Body mass index; *CF,* cystic fibrosis; *COPD,* chronic obstructive pulmonary disease; *Hct,* hematocrit; *IVs,* intravenous lines; *PIVKA-II,* proteins induced by vitamin K absence or antagonism; *SPF,* sun protection factor; *TPN,* total parenteral nutrition.
*Should be encouraged.

with moderate to severe dyspnea may prefer liquid supplements (shakes, instant breakfast, or other commercial nutrient drinks; see Table 8-1). Approaches to specific problems are outlined as follows:

- *Early satiety or anorexia*: Eat small, frequent meals and snacks. Eat high–energy-density foods first (e.g., meats, grains) and then foods of low energy density (e.g., beverages, raw vegetables) at the end of the meal or between meals. Avoid high-fat meals, which may delay gastric emptying (Akrabawi et al., 1996). Limit liquids at mealtimes. Experiment to see if foods served cold cause fewer problems.
- *Bloating*: Eat small, frequent meals and avoid hurrying through meals, to reduce air swallowing. Avoid foods that have caused gas in the past; try reducing carbonated beverage intake.

- *Dyspnea*: Eat slowly; avoid overeating; eat small, frequent snacks and meals; avoid excessive fat intake, which may delay gastric emptying and increase pressure on the diaphragm.
- *Fatigue*: Rest before meals; eat larger meals in the morning or other times when less tired; have easy-to-prepare foods readily available for times when fatigued. Treatments and physical activity should be scheduled so that the individual has a chance to rest before meals.
- Ensure that patients have sufficient resources to secure an adequate diet. Many individuals with COPD are elderly or retired; they may have a limited income, or they may have an inadequate diet because of loneliness, apathy about food, or few food preparation skills (especially elderly men). Encouragement to eat at a group feeding site for the elderly (usually at senior citizen centers or in apartment houses for the elderly), or, if they are homebound, referral to a program for home-delivered meals can improve intake.
- Provide mouth care often or encourage the patient to perform mouth care, especially before meals, to clear the palate of the taste of sputum and improve the appetite.

Nutrition support. Oral nutrient supplements are the preferred form of nutrition support. To avoid worsening dyspnea and feelings of satiety, small amounts of energy-dense (1.5 to 2 kcal/ml) oral nutritional supplements can be taken frequently (see Table 8-1). If oral feedings are inadequate, enteral nutrition support in combination with exercise and anabolic agents (e.g., nandrolone) has the potential to improve the status of patients with COPD (Anker et al., 2006). In stable patients with COPD, there appears to be little need for special pulmonary formulas (with reduced carbohydrate and increased fat content); standard supplements are appropriate (Anker et al., 2006).

Bone mineral density. A decrease in bone mineral density (BMD), associated with osteoporosis and osteopenia, is common among individuals with COPD. This cannot be fully explained by chronic or repeated glucocorticoid use. The loss of BMD relates directly to the severity of the pulmonary symptoms (Jørgensen et al., 2007; Vrieze et al., 2007). Smoking, weight loss or low BMI, and chronic inflammation may be contributing factors. A diet adequate in calcium, vitamin D, vitamin K, and energy with supplements of calcium and vitamin D if necessary can help to reduce bone loss

(Ionescu and Schoon, 2003), but in a catabolic state, dietary measures are unlikely to be sufficient to maintain bone. Bisphos-phonates, such as alendronate and the newer ibandronate, are approved for treatment of osteoporosis.

Weight reduction (overweight or obese individuals). Obesity increases the work of breathing and may worsen the problems seen with COPD (Nici et al., 2006). Obese individuals often have low lung volumes and may experience hypoxia and hypercarbia because of this. Obstructive sleep apnea may also occur. Diet and lifestyle changes are appropriate for the obese individual with COPD (Nici et al., 2006). Counseling regarding reducing energy intake while maintaining a nutritious diet and increasing activity within physical limitations can help promote gradual weight loss. Walking, yoga, chair exercises, or water aerobics (if the individual is not oxygen dependent) may be tolerated. Start with short periods of low-intensity exercise if the person has been sedentary, and gradually increase the duration and intensity.

Acute Lung Injury/Acute Respiratory Distress Syndrome

Acute lung injury (ALI), with its most severe form, acute respiratory distress syndrome (ARDS), is one of the leading reasons for admission to intensive care units (ICUs). ALI/ARDS is not a disease but instead is a ventilatory disorder affecting a heterogeneous group of patients and characterized by new pulmonary infiltrates consistent with pulmonary edema and hypoxemia (PaO_2/FiO_2 ratio <40 kPa in ALI; PaO_2/FiO_2 ratio <26 kPa in ARDS) not caused by heart failure, chronic lung disease, or other identifiable causes (Leaver and Evans, 2007). It is most common in patients with sepsis and septic shock, severe pneumonia, and pulmonary aspiration of gastrointestinal (GI) contents (Leaver and Evans, 2007).

Treatment

Treatment of respiratory failure includes administration of oxygen or use of mechanical ventilation to maintain near-normal partial pressures of oxygen and CO_2 in the blood and use of antibiotics if infection is present. Inhaled nitric oxide and prostaglandins are controversial, as is extracorporeal oxygenation therapy (Kasper et al., 2005; Leaver and Evans, 2007).

Nutrition Assessment and Care

Patients with ARDS are extremely ill, with a mortality rate as high as 50% (Cheung et al., 2006; Leaver and Evans, 2007), and nutritional deficits often develop during treatment. In a group of 109 survivors of ARDS (median age 45 years), the mean weight loss during hospitalization was 18% of the previous weight. One year after hospital discharge, 71% had returned to their previous weight, but they still complained of weakness and loss of muscle mass (Herridge et al., 2003). Obese patients had longer lengths of stay and higher costs in the hospital (Cheung et al., 2006).

A thorough nutrition assessment should be performed as described in Chapter 2. Findings that are especially common or significant in ALI and ARDS are summarized in Box 15-1.

Intervention and education

Nutrition support. Critically ill patients should be given nutrition support early in their course, ideally within 24 to 48 hours (Heyland et al., 2007; Leaver and Evans, 2007). Enteral nutrition support is preferable, if there is no major malfunction of the GI tract. The following measures are recommended for optimizing enteral nutrition support (Heyland et al., 2007):

- Use prokinetic agents such as metoclopramide if gastric emptying is delayed.
- Position the patient in the supine recumbent position (head elevated 45 degrees if possible) to reduce the risk of aspiration of feedings.
- Avoid specialized formulas supplemented with arginine.
- Use "immune-enhancing" or antiinflammatory formulas supplemented with fish and/or borage oil (a source of γ-linolenic acid) and antioxidants.
- Avoid hyperglycemia (>180 mg/dl or >10 mM) by using insulin or reducing intravenous dextrose delivery. No studies of the effect of hyperglycemia in ARDS have been published, but hyperglycemia has adverse effects in other critically ill patients.

High-fat, low-carbohydrate formulas are made for patients with pulmonary disease, but evidence is insufficient to determine whether these are beneficial in patients with ARDS (Heyland et al., 2007). Fluid overload should be avoided (Kasper et al., 2005). Enteral formulas providing 1.5 to 2 kcal/ml rather than the standard 1 kcal/ml are available for patients needing fluid restrictions (see Table 8-1).

Patients able to eat are given a diet of nutrient-dense foods and supplements. Those who are unable to be fully fed by the GI tract may be given total parenteral nutrition (TPN). Supplementation with antioxidant nutrients such as vitamins C and E, retinoids, and especially selenium may be beneficial (Heyland et al., 2005; Kelly, 2005).

Overfeeding is particularly likely during nutrition support with enteral tube feedings or TPN because the feedings do not depend on the patient's voluntary food intake. Where indirect calorimetry is unavailable, physical examination and measurement of arterial blood gases can reveal some of the effects of overfeeding and high **respiratory quotient (RQ)**. Elevated PCO_2 (partial pressure of CO_2 in the blood), unexpected difficulty in weaning from the ventilator, tachypnea and shortness of breath (in non–ventilator-dependent patients), and hyperglycemia can be signs of overfeeding.

Cystic Fibrosis

CF results from a defect brought about by one of many possible mutations in the gene for a cell membrane protein, the cystic fibrosis transmembrane conductance regulator (CFTR), that regulates the passage of chloride out of cells. Approximately two thirds of the CF cases worldwide are related to a single mutation, deletion of phenylalanine at position 508 (Sinaasappel et al., 2002). Indirectly, the CFTR defect disrupts the sodium and water balance across cell membranes. Viscous mucus collects in the respiratory tract, which can obstruct the airways and provide a favorable environment for growth of microorganisms. Involvement of the pancreas (and, to a lesser extent, the common bile duct) results in malabsorption, with fat being the nutrient most affected. The defect in the CFTR results in increased losses of chloride in sweat and provides a key tool for diagnosis of CF.

Treatment

Prevention and correction of atelectasis and respiratory infections are an important part of care. Daily chest physiotherapy is useful in clearing the airways. Antibiotics are given as necessary to treat or prevent pneumonia; tobramycin is among the commonly used agents. Inhalation of human recombinant DNase (dornase alfa) assists in breaking up thick bronchial secretions. Lung transplantation is an option for some patients with end-stage pulmonary disease, although the 5-year survival is only 50% and organ donations have not equaled the number of candidates for transplantation (Yankaskas et al., 2004).

Eighty-five to ninety percent of individuals with CF have pancreatic insufficiency (PI) and require pancreatic enzyme replacement therapy (PERT) with meals and snacks (Borowitz et al., 2002). PI is associated with bulky, foul-smelling, greasy stools and complications such as distal intestinal obstruction syndrome. About 15% to 20% of infants with CF are born with meconium ileus, in which some portion of the intestine is blocked with thickened meconium. Simple cases can be cleared with hypertonic diatrizoate meglumine (Gastrografin) enemas, but complicated cases often require partial intestinal resection (Behrman et al., 2004). Nutritional implications depend on the site and amount of bowel resected.

The median age of survival is approximately 32 years (Yankaskas et al., 2004). As the life span has lengthened, new challenges have arisen. By the end of their second decade of life, 30% to 40% of patients are likely to have diabetes (cystic fibrosis–related diabetes [CFRD]), and an additional 25% to 30% may have **impaired glucose tolerance** (Sinaasappel et al., 2002; Yankaskas et al., 2004). CFRD is largely due to insulin deficiency because of pancreatic damage, but chronic and acute infections and inflammation, undernutrition, malabsorption, and liver dysfunction also contribute to the problem (Sinaasappel et al., 2002). Cirrhosis of the liver can occur as a result of biliary fibrosis (Yankaskas et al., 2004).

Nutrition Assessment and Care

A thorough nutrition assessment should be performed as described in Chapter 2. Findings that are especially common or significant in CF are summarized in Box 15-1.

Intervention and education

Promoting optimum growth and preventing or correcting malnutrition. Growth and development should be normal in individuals with CF (Borowitz et al., 2002). Adequate energy intake is needed to compensate for malabsorption, increased work of breathing, and increased needs imposed by infection. It has commonly been recommended that individuals with CF consume about 120% of the estimated average requirement for age and gender, but when energy expenditure is measured, it is rarely that high (Sinaasappel et al., 2002). A high-protein, moderate- to high-fat diet (30% to 40% of total energy) is recommended (Borowitz et al., 2002). Some individuals experience abdominal pain and severe steatorrhea with unrestricted fat intake. Adjustment of their pancreatic enzyme dosages usually improves their fat tolerance. Medium-chain triglyceride (MCT) oil may be used to increase caloric intake when steatorrhea is severe. Body image concerns become increasingly important as the child develops into an adolescent and adult and must be dealt with in an individualized and sensitive manner by heath care professionals. Sometimes concern over body image can be used as a way to promote an adequate, healthful diet (Borowitz et al., 2002).

If oral intake is inadequate to prevent or correct malnutrition, then enteral tube feedings can be used to supplement oral intake. Many times these are given nocturnally to avoid, as much as possible, interfering with daily activities and appetite. A polymeric (nonelemental or predigested) formula is normally used, with enzymes taken at the beginning and end of feeding (Sinaasappel et al., 2002). Nasal polyps are common in CF, and therefore nasogastric and nasointestinal tubes may be poorly tolerated. Gastrostomy feedings are an alternative.

Low BMD is present in both children and adults with CF. Nutritional deficits, delayed sexual maturation, and long-term corticosteroid use all play a role. To reduce bone loss, the patient should have laboratory testing for the adequacy of vitamins D and K and supplements given as needed, calcium intake should be at least as high as the Recommended Dietary Allowance (RDA) for age and gender, and weight-bearing exercise should be a part of the daily routine (Borowitz et al., 2002).

Micronutrient supplementation. There is a potential for the fat-soluble vitamins to be inadequately absorbed, and daily supplements are recommended by most centers. Multivitamins (e.g., AquADEKs and Source CF) are available in micelle or water-miscible formulations designed to improve absorption for individuals with steatorrhea. The consensus opinion regarding optimal doses for each pediatric age-group has been published (Borowitz et al., 2002). If a significant portion of the ileum was removed as a result of meconium ileus, the patient will need vitamin B_{12} supplementation delivered by parenteral injection or nasal gel or spray for the duration of life.

Zinc, magnesium, and calcium supplements may be necessary in individuals with steatorrhea. Food should be generously salted, especially in hot weather, to replace abnormal electrolyte losses in sweat.

Nutritional concerns in adolescent and adult CF patients. Diabetes becomes increasingly common as individuals with CF age. The goals of CFRD therapy are to maintain optimal nutritional status while controlling hyperglycemia, to reduce the risk of acute and chronic complications, and at the same time to avoid hypoglycemia (Yankaskas et al., 2004). The health care team can help the individual cope with the psychologic, emotional, and physical changes required by diabetes treatment and make the treatment regimen as flexible as possible. Diabetes care is discussed in more detail in Chapter 17.

Nutritional status should be optimized before pregnancy occurs, if possible. The pregnant woman's weight gain and nutritional status should be carefully assessed throughout pregnancy, with diet counseling and intervention carried out if nutrition appears inadequate. Women with CF appear to be especially likely to develop gestational diabetes (Yankaskas et al., 2004), and all should be screened for diabetes as outlined by the American Diabetes Association (www.diabetes.org). If CFRD is present before conception or gestational diabetes occurs during pregnancy, the guidelines for gestational diabetes in Chapter 17 are appropriate. Breastfeeding is not contraindicated as long as the woman can maintain an adequate nutritional status (Yankaskas et al., 2004).

Cirrhosis of the liver worsens malabsorption and makes deficiency of fat-soluble vitamins even more likely. Fat-soluble vitamin and overall nutritional status should be assessed regularly, with nutrient supplements as needed. Use of the bile acid ursodeoxycholic acid (UDCA) might delay progression of the disease (Yankaskas et al., 2004).

Lung transplantation usually takes place in individuals with end-stage disease, when severe nutritional deficits may be present. The immunosuppressive agents used after transplant are likely to worsen glucose tolerance in those patients with CFRD and cause additional cases of CFRD to become apparent, as well as to further reduce BMD. Hyperglycemia must be treated with insulin and medical nutrition therapy. BMD should be assessed with DEXA. A nutritious diet with supplements of vitamins D and K and calcium as needed can help to prevent bone loss, but pharmacologic treatment such as bisphosphonate therapy is likely to be needed (Borowitz et al., 2002).

Conclusion

Nutritional status, and particularly fat-free mass, is an important prognostic indicator in pulmonary diseases. In COPD and CF, optimal nutritional intake and regular exercise improve functional capability and quality of life (Borowitz et al., 2002; Yankaskas et al., 2004; Nici et al., 2006) and should be encouraged for all patients.

REFERENCES

Akrabawi SS et al: Gastric emptying, pulmonary function, gas exchange, and respiratory quotient after feeding a moderate versus high fat enteral formula meal in chronic obstructive pulmonary disease patients, *Nutrition* 12(4):260, 1996.

Anker SD et al: ESPEN guidelines on enteral nutrition: cardiology and pulmonology, *Clin Nutr* 25(2):311, 2006.

Behrman RE, Kliegman RM, Jenson HB, editors: *Nelson textbook of pediatrics,* ed 17, Philadelphia, 2004, Saunders.

Borowitz D, Baker RD, Stallings V: Consensus report on nutrition for pediatric patients with cystic fibrosis, *J Pediatr Gastroenterol Nutr* 35(3):246, 2002.

Budweiser S et al: Nutritional depletion and its relationship to respiratory impairment in patients with chronic respiratory failure due to COPD or restrictive thoracic diseases, *Eur J Clin Nutr*, 62(3):436, 2008.

Cheung AM et al: Two-year outcomes, health care use, and costs of survivors of acute respiratory distress syndrome, *Am J Respir Crit Care Med* 174(5):538, 2006.

Gan WQ et al: Association between chronic obstructive pulmonary disease and systemic inflammation: a systematic review and a meta-analysis, *Thorax* 59(7):574, 2004.

Herridge MS et al: One-year outcomes in survivors of the acute respiratory distress syndrome, *N Engl J Med* 348(8):683, 2003.

Heyland DK et al: Antioxidant nutrients: a systematic review of trace elements and vitamins in the critically ill patient, *Intensive Care Med* 31(3):327, 2005.

Heyland DK et al: Canadian clinical practice guidelines. Available at www.criticalcarenutrition.com. Accessed November 20, 2007.

Ionescu AA, Schoon E: Osteoporosis in chronic obstructive pulmonary disease, *Eur Respir J Suppl* 46:64, 2003.

Jørgensen NR et al: The prevalence of osteoporosis in patients with chronic obstructive pulmonary disease: a cross sectional study, *Respir Med* 101(1):177, 2007.

Kasper DL et al, editors: *Harrison's principles of internal medicine*, ed 16, Columbus, Ohio, 2005, McGraw-Hill.

Kelly FJ: Vitamins and respiratory disease: antioxidant micronutrients in pulmonary health and disease, *Proc Nutr Soc* 64(4):510, 2005.

Leaver SK, Evans TW: Acute respiratory distress syndrome, *BMJ* 335(7616):389, 2007.

Nici L et al: American Thoracic Society/European Respiratory Society statement on pulmonary rehabilitation, *Am J Respir Crit Care Med* 173(12):1390, 2006.

Ochs-Balcom HM et al: Antioxidants, oxidative stress, and pulmonary function in individuals diagnosed with asthma or COPD, *Eur J Clin Nutr* 60(8):991, 2006.

Qaseem A et al: Diagnosis and management of stable chronic obstructive pulmonary disease: a clinical practice guideline from the American College of Physicians, *Ann Intern Med* 147(9):633, 2007.

Roth MD et al: Feasibility of retinoids for the treatment of emphysema study, *Chest* 130(5):1334, 2006.

Sinaasappel M et al: Nutrition in patients with cystic fibrosis: a European consensus, *J Cyst Fibros* 1(2):51, 2002.

Varraso R et al: Prospective study of dietary patterns and chronic obstructive pulmonary disease among US men, *Thorax* 62(9):786, 2007a.

Varraso R et al: Prospective study of dietary patterns and chronic obstructive pulmonary disease among US women, *Am J Clin Nutr* 86(2):488, 2007b.

Vestbo J et al: Body mass, fat-free body mass, and prognosis in patients with chronic obstructive pulmonary disease from a random population sample: findings from the Copenhagen City Heart Study, *Am J Respir Crit Care Med* 173(1):79, 2006.

Vrieze A et al: Low bone mineral density in COPD patients related to worse lung function, low weight and decreased fat-free mass, *Osteoporos Int* 18(9):1197, 2007.

Yankaskas JR et al: Cystic fibrosis adult care: consensus conference report, *Chest* 125(1):1S, 2004.

RENAL DISEASE

The kidneys are responsible for maintaining the optimal chemical composition of body fluids, as well as for metabolic and endocrine actions. A variety of diseases can affect the kidneys; the ones included in this chapter are acute renal failure (ARF), chronic kidney disease (CKD), **nephrotic syndrome**, and calculi formation.

Acute Renal Failure and Chronic Kidney Disease

In ARF a sudden reduction in glomerular filtration rate (GFR) occurs, with impairment in excretion of wastes. Causes for this sudden reduction include inadequate renal perfusion, e.g., hemorrhage; acute tubular necrosis following trauma, surgery, or sepsis; nephrotoxic drugs or chemicals; acute glomerulonephritis; and obstruction, e.g., stricture of a ureter. The two phases are an oliguric phase with urinary output usually less than 400 ml/day (less than 0.5 to 1 ml/kg/hr in children) and then a diuretic phase when urine output increases. ARF may resolve, or it may instead progress to CKD. CKD is defined as having kidney damage for 3 months or more, with or without a fall in the GFR, or having a GFR of 60 ml/min/1.73 m^2 (body surface area) or less for 3 months or longer (National Kidney Foundation, 2000). The kidney is responsible for excretion of urea and creatinine derived from protein metabolism. With impaired renal function, circulating blood urea nitrogen (BUN) and creatinine levels rise, and retention of fluid, potassium, sodium, phosphorus, and other solutes normally excreted by the kidney occurs. CKD is divided into stages, based on the GFR (expressed per 1.73 m^2, the body surface area for an average adult), as follows: *stage 1*, or mild CKD, GFR 90 ml/min or higher; *stage 2*, GFR 60 to 89; *stage 3*, GFR 30 to 59; *stage 4*, GFR 15 to 29; and *stage 5*, GFR below 15 (or patient on dialysis) (NKF, 2002).

The leading cause of CKD in developed countries is diabetes, and hypertension is another common contributor to CKD (NKF, 2007b). Good control of both blood glucose and blood pressure reduces the risk of developing CKD or of progressing to a higher stage, once CKD has developed.

Nutrition-related problems are prevalent in renal disease. Decreased appetite is common among dialysis patients, possibly because they have chronic inflammation and elevated concentrations of inflammatory cytokines (Kalantar-Zadeh et al., 2004a). In addition, the kidney normally activates erythropoietin, which is required for red blood cell (RBC) formation, and vitamin D. Anemia, hypocalcemia, bone loss (osteodystrophy), and hyperphosphatemia are common. Retention of sodium and water contributes to hypertension, and potassium retention may lead to cardiac dysrhythmia. Impaired ability to excrete the organic acids produced in metabolic reactions and/or inadequate ability to conserve bicarbonate by the kidney results in metabolic acidosis. Cardiovascular disease is especially widespread among individuals with CKD . This may be related to the prevalence of diabetes among individuals with CKD and also to the existence of the inflammatory state, which appears to contribute to atherosclerotic heart disease (NKF, 2003b).

Treatment

Treatment involves removal or, if possible, correction of the cause of renal failure. The major complications during the oliguric phase include acidosis, hyperkalemia, infection, hyperphosphatemia, hypertension, and anemia. Alkalinizing agents (e.g., sodium bicarbonate or Shohl solution), cation-exchange resins to bind potassium, antibiotics, phosphate-binding drugs, antihypertensive agents, and diuretics are the most commonly used treatment measures.

Dialysis or hemofiltration is needed if these measures, combined with dietary restrictions, are insufficient to prevent or control hyperkalemia, fluid overload, symptomatic uremia (drowsiness, nausea, vomiting, tremors), or rapidly rising blood urea nitrogen (BUN) and creatinine levels. Different dialysis modalities include hemodialysis, chronic ambulatory peritoneal dialysis (CAPD), or automated peritoneal dialysis (APD). Transplantation is an option for some individuals with end-stage renal disease.

Nutrition Assessment and Care

The goals of medical nutrition therapy are to reduce the production of wastes that must be excreted by the kidney; avoid excessive fluid and electrolyte intake that will contribute to hypertension; prevent or correct nutritional deficits; prevent hyperkalemia; prevent or delay development of osteodystrophy; and control hyperlipidemia, which often occurs in these individuals.

A thorough nutrition assessment should be performed as described in Chapter 2. Box 16-1 highlights common or especially serious findings in renal disease. Because of the complexity of kidney disease and the impact that chronic illness can have on nutrition-related parameters, the NKF (NKF, 2000) recommends that a variety of measures, rather than only one or two, be used to evaluate protein-energy nutritional status in patients with CKD. The recommended schedule for maintenance dialysis patients is as follows: serum albumin (predialysis or "stabilized" [after hemodialysis or after drainage of peritoneal dialysate]), monthly; body weight (as a percentage of the usual postdialysis or postdrain body weight), monthly; body weight as a percentage of standard body weight, every 4 months; subjective global assessment (described in the following text), every 6 months; dietary interview and/or diary, every 6 months; protein equivalent of total nitrogen appearance (protein catabolic rate) normalized to body weight, monthly for hemodialysis and every 2 months for continuous peritoneal dialysis. Other measures that may be obtained as needed are prealbumin (predialysis or stabilized); skinfold thicknesses; dual energy x-ray absorptiometry; serum creatinine, urea nitrogen, and cholesterol (predialysis or stabilized; these parameters fall in malnourished renal patients); and creatinine-height index (as an indicator of muscle mass). The protein equivalent of total nitrogen appearance in a stable patient provides an estimate of protein intake and of tissue **catabolism** and is calculated (in g/kg/day) as follows: $6.25 \times$ (UNA + 1.81 + 0.31), where UNA (urea nitrogen appearance) is the total urea nitrogen output (measured in the urine and the dialysate fluid). For pediatric patients, the assessment should include measurement of height or length, as well as head circumference if 3 years old or less (NKF, 2000).

The subjective global assessment (SGA), which requires no laboratory testing or specialized equipment, is useful in many

Text continued on p. 428

Box 16-1   Assessment in Renal Disease

Protein-Energy Malnutrition (PEM) or Protein-Calorie Malnutrition (PCM)

History

Poor intake of protein-containing and energy-containing foods related to dietary restrictions or anorexia from uremia, abdominal fullness from peritoneal dialysate, zinc deficiency, or depression; losses of amino acids or serum proteins related to dialysis (hemodialysis losses ≈14 g/session, CAPD losses ≈5 to 15 g/day), steroid-induced tissue catabolism, and proteinuria; increased needs during infection

Physical examination

Muscle wasting; thinning of hair; dry weight <90% of desirable, BMI <18.5, or decline in growth percentile for height or weight (children); triceps skinfold <5th percentile; NOTE: loss of weight or decrease in subcutaneous fat may be masked by edema

Laboratory analysis

↓ Serum albumin, transferrin, or prealbumin*; nitrogen (N_2) losses in urine and dialysate greater than intake (negative N_2 balance)

Altered Lipid Metabolism

History

Nephrotic syndrome, excessive consumption of carbohydrates (CHO) related to dietary emphasis on CHO as an energy source or use of glucose as an osmotic agent in dialysis

Laboratory analysis

↑ Serum cholesterol, LDL and VLDL cholesterol, serum triglycerides

Fluid Excess

History

Oliguria or anuria

Box 16-1   Assessment in Renal Disease—cont'd

Physical examination

Edema; hypertension; acute weight gain (1% to 2% of body weight or more)

Laboratory analysis

↓ Hct

Potential for Mineral/Electrolyte Imbalance

Phosphorus (P) Excess

History

Oliguria or anuria

Laboratory analysis

↑ Serum P; Ca × P product (Ca in mg/dl × P in mg/dl) >55; renal calcification on radiographs

Calcium (Ca) Deficit

History

Metabolic acidosis; hyperphosphatemia

Physical examination

Renal osteodystrophy with bone pain and deformities; tetany

Laboratory analysis

↓ Serum Ca (NOTE: ≈45% of Ca is bound to albumin; if the person is hypoalbuminemic, then the Ca level will be misleading; it can be "corrected" by adding 0.8 mg/dl to the total Ca level for each 1 g/dl decrease in albumin below 4 g/dl.)

Zinc Deficit

History

↓ Intake related to dietary restrictions; loss during dialysis

Physical examination

Distorted taste, poor sense of taste; poor wound healing; alopecia; seborrheic dermatitis

Continued

Box 16-1   Assessment in Renal Disease—cont'd

Laboratory analysis

↓ Serum zinc

Iron Deficit

History

Decreased intake as a result of dietary restrictions, loss of RBC during hemodialysis

Physical examination

Fatigue; pallor

Laboratory analysis

↓ Hct and Hgb,[†] ↓ MCV, ↓ serum ferritin

Potassium (K+) Excess

History

Oliguria or anuria

Physical examination

Weakness, flaccid muscles

Laboratory analysis

↑ Serum K+; electrocardiogram: elevated T wave, depressed ST segment

Aluminum (Al) Excess

History

Use of Al-containing phosphate binders, especially if Al dosages >30 mg/kg/day; Al contamination in dialysis fluids or supplies

Physical examination

Ataxia, seizures, dementia; renal osteodystrophy with bone pain and deformities

Laboratory analysis

Plasma Al >100 mcg/L

Box 16-1   Assessment in Renal Disease—cont'd

Potential for Vitamin Imbalance

A Excess

History

Oliguria or anuria

Physical examination

Anorexia, fatigue; alopecia, dry skin; hepatomegaly; irritability (progressing to hydrocephalus and vomiting in infants and children)

Laboratory analysis

↑ Serum retinol

C Deficit

History

Losses in dialysis; ↓ intake caused by restriction of fruits and vegetables

Physical examination

Gingivitis; petechiae, ecchymoses

Laboratory analysis

↓ Serum or leukocyte ascorbic acid

B_6 Deficit

History

Failure of the diseased kidney to activate B_6; loss in dialysis

Physical examination

Dermatitis; ataxia, irritability, seizures

Laboratory analysis

↓ Plasma pyridoxal phosphate (PLP)

Folate

History

Loss of folate during dialysis; ↓ intake related to restriction of fruits, vegetables, whole grains, and meats

---

Continued

Box 16-1   Assessment in Renal Disease—cont'd

Physical examination

Glossitis (inflamed tongue); pallor

Laboratory analysis

↓ Hct, ↑ MCV; ↓ serum and RBC folate; ↑ serum homocysteine

D Deficit

History

Failure of the diseased kidney to activate vitamin D, poor intake
   related to restrictions of dairy products

Physical examination

Rickets (children), osteomalacia

Laboratory analysis

↓ $1,25\text{-OH}_2$ vitamin D

BMI, Body mass index; *CAPD,* continuous ambulatory peritoneal dialysis; *Hct,*
hematocrit; *Hgb,* hemoglobin; *LDL,* low-density lipoprotein; *MCV,* mean corpuscular
volume; *RBC,* red blood cell; *VLDL,* very-low–density lipoprotein.
[*]Serum proteins also fall in inflammation, which is common in renal failure.
[†]Decreased Hct and Hgb may occur because of decreased production of erythropoietic
factor by diseased kidney.

disease states and not just in kidney disease. However, the NKF
(NKF, 2000) recommends initial SGA screening, with regular
reassessment to detect changes. A sample format for the SGA is
shown in Figure 12-1. The primary parameters to be assessed in
the patient with kidney disease are weight loss within 6 months,
dietary intake and gastrointestinal symptoms, subcutaneous tissue, and muscle mass. Weight loss may be masked by edema, so
the health professional must be alert for this. Intentional weight
loss should not be rated as highly as unintentional loss (NKF,
2000). The Malnutrition-Inflammation Score (MIS) is an adaptation of the SGA that has been validated in both peritoneal and
hemodialysis patients (Afsar B et al., 2006; Kalantar-Zadeh et al.,
2004b). In addition to the information collected for the SGA, the
MIS includes the body mass index (BMI), serum albumin concentration, and total iron binding capacity.

Intervention and education. Modifications of fluid, electrolyte, mineral, and protein intakes are often needed because of the impairment of the kidney's ability to excrete fluid and wastes. Nutrition therapy is designed to reduce edema, hypertension, and uremia. Guidelines for daily nutrient allowances are given in Table 16-1, but individual needs vary, and continual monitoring and reassessment of the patient are the best guide. Malnutrition is associated with a poor prognosis in the patient with CKD, emphasizing the importance of aggressive nutrition intervention in these patients. Individuals with type 2 diabetes and CKD are apt to be overweight or obese, which should not be allowed to obscure evidence of undernutrition.

The renal diet is complex, and the registered dietitian should plan the diet and educate the patient and family. Individualization of the diet as much as possible (to incorporate favorite foods and respond to the demands of the individual's lifestyle) improves quality of life and compliance with the diet. Intensive nutrition counseling is needed, with follow-up at least every 1 to 2 months initially and updating of the plan of care at least every 3 to 4 months or more frequently if the patient's medical condition requires it.

Fluid needs. Fluid restriction is necessary when oliguria occurs. For the oliguric adult the daily fluid allowance is approximately 500 ml (to account for insensible losses) plus the volume lost from urine, diarrhea, vomitus, and any other sources during the previous 24 hours. For children the fluid allowance is equal to output plus a small amount to cover insensible losses. Hemodialysis allows fluid intake to be somewhat more liberal. Peritoneal dialysis is very effective at removing fluid, allowing an increased intake. Acute weight changes are the best guide to fluid deficits and excesses. Body weight should be measured daily, with the oral fluid intake adjusted so that gain is no more than 0.45 to 1 kg (1 to 2 lb) per day for adults on the days between dialyses.

Foods that are liquids at room temperature must be included in the fluid allowance. Water contents of some common foods are as follows: gelatins, 100% water; fruit ices, 90%; pudding or custard, 75%; sherbet, 67%; and ice cream, 50%. Raw fruits and vegetables need to be considered as well. For example, water makes up approximately 90% of the weight of watermelon, Asian pears, papayas, and cucumbers.

Table 16-1   Guidelines for Daily Nutrient Intakes in Renal Failure

Nutrient	Adults	Children
Energy	*Clinically stable* ≥60 years: 30-35 kcal/kg *Acutely ill* <60 yr: 35 kcal/kg <60 yr: ≥35 kcal/kg ≥60 years: ≥30-35 kcal/kg	DRI for age*
Protein	*Clinically stable* UD: 0.6-0.75 g/kg† HD: 1.2 g/kg PD: 1.2-1.3 g/kg *Acutely ill* HD: ≥1.2 g/kg PD: ≥1.3 g/kg	HD: DRI for age + 0.4 g/kg/day PD: DRI for age + amount equal to estimated losses in dialysis
Phosphorus	800-1000 mg (or 10-12 mg/kg) if serum phosphorus elevated (>4.6 mEq/L in stages 3 and 4, or >5.5 mEq/L in stage 5) *or* serum intact parathyroid hormone elevated above target range‡	800 mg if serum phosphorus >5.5 mEq/L (NOTE: infants may require higher serum phosphorus for bone mineralization.)

Calcium	800-1200 mg (do not exceed 2000 mg in food, supplements, and phosphate binders)	DRI for age (do not exceed 2500 mg in food, supplements, and phosphate binders) <20 kg: 2-3 g >20 kg: 3-4 g
Sodium	Individualize, 1-3 g	
Potassium	Individualize to maintain serum potassium ≤5 mEq/L	Individualize to maintain serum potassium ≤5 mEq/L

Data from American Dietetic Association: *Chronic kidney disease (non-dialysis) medical nutrition therapy protocol*, Chicago, 2002, The Association; National Kidney Foundation Disease Outcomes Quality Initiative (K/DOQI): Clinical practice guidelines for nutrition in chronic renal failure, *Am J Kidney Dis* 35(6 suppl 2):1, 2000; Kleinman RE, editor: *Pediatric nutrition handbook*, ed 5, Elk Grove Village, Ill, 2004, American Academy of Pediatrics.

NOTE: The numbers in this table represent an initial prescription and should be individualized as necessary based on the patient's response. Recommendations based on kg of body weight refer to dry weight.

HD, Hemodialysis; *PD*, peritoneal dialysis; *UD*, undialyzed.

*Dietary Reference Intake (see Appendix A on Evolve).

†0.6 is preferred; 0.75 for individuals who will not accept the more severe limitation or cannot maintain adequate energy intake with protein intake at 0.6 g/kg/day.

‡Target ranges for intact parathyroid hormone: stage 3, 35-70 pg/ml; stage 4, 70-110 pg/ml; stage 5, 150-300 pg/ml. In addition, restrict phosphorus if serum calcium × phosphorus product (Ca in mg/dl × P in mg/dl) is greater than 55.

Protein needs. Table 16-1 provides estimates of protein needs; intake should be adjusted as needed, depending on nutrition evaluation and measures of renal function. At least one half of dietary protein should be **high-biologic-value (HBV) protein**, rich in essential amino acids (those not synthesized in sufficient amounts by the body) in proportions favorable for synthesis and maintenance of human tissues. Good sources of HBV protein are eggs, meat, poultry, fish, and milk products. Approximately 7 g of HBV protein is contained in 1 oz of meat, fish, or poultry; 1 egg; or 210 ml (7 fluid oz) of milk.

Cereals, breads, pasta, and vegetables are sources of protein that is primarily of low biologic value (Table 16-2). Low-protein pasta and bread products—available through mail order, some pharmacies, and some larger supermarkets—are a source of complex carbohydrate for the person on a very-limited–protein diet (usually the undialyzed patient). An alternative approach to the standard low-protein diet is to use a very-low–protein diet (≈0.3 g/kg/day), supplemented with essential amino acids or a mixture of essential

Table 16-2   Examples of Foods Providing Protein with Primarily Low Biologic Value

Food	Serving Size	Protein (g)
Bagel, 4 in	1	9
Peanuts, oil roasted, unsalted	1 oz (30 g)	8
Rice, white, cooked	½ C	8
Beans and peas, dried, cooked (e.g., pinto, kidney, black beans; cowpeas, black-eye peas, chickpeas; refried beans)	½ C	6-8
Peas, green, cooked or canned	½ C	4
Potato, French fried, fast food	1 large	6
Pasta (macaroni, spaghetti) or egg noodles, plain, cooked	½ C	4
Oatmeal, regular, quick, or instant	½ C	3
Broccoli, Brussels sprouts, or edible-pod peas, cooked	½ C	3
Bread, white	1 slice	2

From U.S. Department of Agriculture: *National nutrient database for standard reference, SR20,* Washington, DC, updated September 2007, The Department. Available at http://www.nal.usda.gov/fnic/foodcomp/search/. Accessed November 18, 2007.

amino acids and ketoacid analogues (≈0.3 g/kg/day) (Fouque and Aparicio, 2007). A ketoacid analogue is the carbon backbone of an amino acid, with the nitrogen portion of the amino acid removed. The risk of malnutrition is increased among individuals consuming a highly restricted diet. It is especially important to consume adequate energy (see Table 16-1) to ensure that the amino acids in the diet are available for protein synthesis and not used for energy. Close monitoring of nutritional status is essential (ADA, 2002); the patient should not be allowed to become malnourished simply to delay the time when dialysis must be started.

Protein and amino acid losses during dialysis can result in protein malnutrition. One approach that appears to stimulate protein synthesis during peritoneal dialysis is to use a 1.1% amino acid mixture along with glucose as an osmotic agent in the dialysate (Tjiong et al., 2007).

Energy needs. Enough energy must be consumed to prevent catabolism because this process not only reduces the amount of functional tissue but also releases nitrogen, which must be excreted by the kidney. In most cases, fat provides about 25% to 30% of the energy intake and carbohydrate provides approximately 50% to 60%. Most carbohydrate should be complex (starches) to reduce the likelihood of hypertriglyceridemia.

In peritoneal dialysis, 1.5% to 4.25% glucose solutions (containing 15 to 42.5 g glucose/L) are commonly used as an osmotic agent to remove body fluid. About 60% of the glucose is absorbed by the body and must be considered in the energy allowance (NKF, 2000). Glucose monohydrate used in the dialysate provides 3.4 kcal/g. Thus the individual receives the following:

15 g/L × 60% × 3.4 kcal/g = 31 kcal/L of 1.5% dialysate

or

42.5 g/L × 60% × 3.4 kcal/g = 87 kcal/L of 4.25% dialysate

For most patients, carbohydrate absorption from the dialysate totals 100 to 200 g/day, or 340 to 680 kcal (NKF, 2000).

Electrolytes, minerals, and vitamins
Sodium and potassium. Sodium intake is restricted as necessary to reduce fluid retention, edema, and hypertension. Box 14-3 provides guidelines for sodium restriction, and Chapter 14 provides

further information for the person needing a sodium-restricted diet. The need for potassium restriction can be gauged from the serum potassium levels, which may not rise substantially until the GFR falls to 10 ml/hr. In teaching about potassium restriction, include the following points:

- Salt substitutes are not usually used in renal impairment because most are high in potassium.
- Low-sodium herbs and herb mixtures, lemon juice, and flavored oils and vinegars are good choices for seasoning foods.
- The richest potassium sources are fruits and vegetables, meats, and dairy products (Table 16-3). Choose canned, drained fruits or vegetables (processed without salt), rather than fresh or frozen. Decrease potassium in fresh vegetables and fruits by cutting them into small pieces, soaking or cooking them in a large amount of water, and then discarding the water.

Phosphorus/phosphate. Progression of renal insufficiency is delayed if phosphorus intake is limited; adults should consume no more than 800 to 1000 mg (or about 10 to 12 mg phosphorus per gram of protein consumed) daily if serum phosphorus is elevated (see Table 16-1). Sources rich in phosphorus include legumes, tofu, milk and other dairy products, meats, poultry, fish, eggs, whole grains, nuts (tree and peanuts), seeds, and peanut butter. In the past, aluminum hydroxide antacids were used as phosphate binders to reduce the absorption of phosphate, but their long-term use has resulted in aluminum toxicity, with ataxia, dementia, and worsening of renal osteodystrophy. Consequently, they are no longer used except for short-term treatment when other therapy is ineffective in reducing phosphorus levels (Goldman and Ausiello, 2008). Calcium carbonate or calcium acetate antacids are commonly used as phosphate binders, but there are risks in using large doses of calcium when phosphate levels are very high, especially the possibility that the combination of high levels of calcium and phosphorus will cause calcification of the soft tissues. Sevelamer hydrochloride is a phosphate binder that does not contain calcium, magnesium, or aluminum. It has the added advantage that it lowers levels of both total and low-density lipoprotein (LDL) cholesterol.

Calcium. Calcium is needed to prevent or delay the progression of renal osteodystrophy, resulting from chronic acidosis and impaired

Table 16-3   Examples of Foods High in Potassium

Food	Serving Size	Potassium (mg)
Potato, baked	1 medium	1081
Potatoes, French fried, fast food	1 large	930
Beet greens, cooked, drained	½ C	650
Banana, raw	1 C	537
Yogurt, fruit, low fat	8 oz	443
Spinach, cooked, drained	½ C	420
Sweet potato, canned	½ C	398
Sauce, pasta, marinara	½ C	395
Beans, dried, cooked (e.g., baked, pinto, kidney)	½ C	370
Milk, 1% milk fat	1 C	366
Fish, cooked, dry heat (e.g., salmon, haddock)	3 oz (90 g)	354
Beef, rib, lean meat only, roasted	3 oz (90 g)	318
Squash, winter varieties, cooked	½ C	247
Orange juice	½ C	236
Broccoli, cooked, drained	½ C	228
Chicken, white meat, fried	3 oz (90 g)	220
Melon, cantaloupe, raw	½ C	213
Tomato, red, raw	½ C	213
Apricots, canned, with juice	½ C	202
Carrots, raw	½ C	176

From U.S. Department of Agriculture: *National nutrient database for standard reference, SR20*, Washington, DC, updated September 2007, The Department. Available at http://www.nal.usda.gov/fnic/foodcomp/search/. Accessed November 18, 2007.

vitamin D metabolism. Restriction of dairy products may be necessary to reduce phosphorus and protein intake, so a calcium supplement (e.g., calcium carbonate or citrate) may be needed to achieve the recommended level of intake (see Table 16-1). Calcium citrate should not be used if the patient is receiving aluminum-containing phosphate binders, since it increases intestinal aluminum absorption (NKF, 2003a). Calcium-containing phosphate binders are also a good source of calcium; they should not be used in a hypercalcemic patient or a patient whose plasma parathyroid levels are below 150 pg/ml on two consecutive occasions (NKF, 2003a). Correction of metabolic acidosis also reduces bone loss (NKF, 2003a).

Vitamin-mineral supplementation. Supplements providing the Dietary Reference Intake (DRI) for water-soluble vitamins, copper, and zinc should be given to ensure no deficiencies result from dietary restrictions or losses in dialysis (NKF, 2000). An oral iron supplement may also be used if the individual is not receiving parenteral iron. Vitamin A levels should be assessed; if they are high, no supplements containing vitamin A should be used.

Iron, folic acid, and vitamin B_{12} intake must be adequate in the person receiving recombinant human erythropoietin (r-HuEPO) to allow for adequate RBC formation (see discussion of anemia that follows). If dietary intake is inadequate, then supplements should be used. Calcitriol, a synthetic form of 1,25-dihydroxyvitamin D_3, or related drugs, such as doxercalciferol, are prescribed to prevent renal osteodystrophy and hyperparathyroidism in individuals with kidney disease. Calcium intake of 800 to 1200 mg/day improves the effectiveness of the drugs, but serum calcium concentrations must be carefully monitored with the drug stopped if hypercalcemia occurs.

Individualized diet plan. It is important that each patient meets with a registered dietitian to have an individualized eating plan developed. An example of an individualized diet plan is shown in Table 16-4. The diet order in this case is for 45 g of protein (34 g of which should be HBV), 1000 mg of sodium, 1650 mg of potassium, 2650 kcal or more, and 720 ml of fluid per day.

Anemia. A hemoglobin target of 11 or 12 g/dl (or hematocrit of 33% to 36%) is recommended for both adults and children in CKD (NKF, 2007a). If there is no obvious source of blood loss, patients with anemia should undergo a complete evaluation, including RBC indices (mean cell volume), reticulocyte count, serum iron, total iron-binding capacity, percent transferrin saturation, serum ferritin, and test for occult blood in the stool (NKF, 2006).

- Differentiating among anemias
  - *Microcytic, hypochromic*: Iron deficiency is common, and it is associated with a microcytic, hypochromic (small RBCs, light in color) anemia, as is aluminum toxicity. Iron deficiency is associated with a low percent transferrin saturation and serum ferritin.
  - *Macrocytosis*: Folate or vitamin B_{12} deficiency is generally associated with macrocytosis (large, immature RBCs).

Table 16-4   Meal Plan of Man with CKD Not Receiving Dialysis

Menu	Pro (g)	Na (mg)	K (mg)	kcal
Breakfast				
Shredded wheat, ½ C	2	1	38	70
Frozen strawberries, ½ C	0.5	1.1	115	70
Sugar, 1 tsp	—	—	—	16
Half and half, ½ C	4	60	170	160
Cinnamon toast				
Low-protein bread, 1 slice	0.1	9	9	100
Margarine, 2 tsp	—	100	2	90
Sugar, 2 tsp	—	—	—	32
Snack				
Jellybeans, 1 oz	0.1	9	9	100
Lunch				
Shrimp salad				
Shrimp, 2 oz	13.8	60	90	150
Mayonnaise, 3 tsp	—	150	3	135
Lettuce, ¼ C shredded	0.5	4.5	57	13
Matzo, 1 piece	2	1	38	70
Margarine, 2 tsp	—	100	2	95
Cranberry juice, 1 C	0.1	9	9	100
With Polycose powder, 1 tbsp	—	6	—	31
Tangerine, 1 medium	0.5	1.5	115	40
Snack				
Hard candy, 1 oz	0.1	9	9	100
Dinner				
Grilled chicken, 2 oz	13.8	60	190	75
Rigatoni, low protein, ½ C	0.1	9	9	100
With margarine, 2 tsp	—	100	2	90
Stir-fried vegetables				
Mushrooms, ½ C	1	9	113	25
Zucchini, ½ C	1	9	113	25
Oil, 3 tsp	—	—	—	115
Hi-C, 1 C	0.1	9	9	100

Continued

Table 16-4   Meal Plan of Man with CKD Not Receiving
Dialysis—cont'd

Menu	Pro (g)	Na (mg)	K (mg)	kcal
Dinner				
With Polycose powder, 1 tbsp	—	6	—	31
Peaches, ½ C, canned, drained	0.7	3.5	215	75
Sugar mints, 37	0.1	9	9	100
Snack				
Low-protein toast, 2 slices	0.2	18	18	200
Margarine, 3 tsp	—	150	3	135
Honey, 1 tbsp	0.1	9	9	100
Milk, whole, ½ C	4	60	184	80
With Polycose powder, 1 tbsp	—	6	—	31
TOTALS	**44.8**	**979**	**1640**	**2664**

High-biologic-value (HBV) protein = 35.6 g; fluid = 720 ml.
CKD, Chronic kidney disease; *K,* potassium; *Na,* sodium; *Pro,* protein.

An increase in the reticulocyte count, as occurs with hemolytic conditions such as acute hemolytic-uremic syndrome,
also causes macrocytosis. If mean corpuscular volume
(MCV) is elevated, checking homocysteine (elevated in
folate deficiency) and methylmalonic acid (elevated in
vitamin B_{12} deficiency) levels will differentiate between
folate and vitamin B_{12} deficiency.

■ *Normocytic, normochromic*: Anemia of erythropoietin
(EPO) deficiency is usually associated with RBC of normal size and color. A normocytic, normochromic anemia
in a patient with serum creatinine of 2 mg/dl or greater (or
in one with a lower serum creatinine but marked muscle
wasting), in whom no other cause of anemia is present,
should be assumed to have deficiency of EPO resulting
from kidney disease. There is usually no need to measure
EPO (NKF, 2006).

■ Treating anemias (NKF, 2006)

- *Iron deficiency*: The initial treatment should be oral iron supplementation (200 mg elemental iron per day in adults; 2 to 3 mg/kg daily in children). The cause of the deficiency must also be sought (usually occult blood loss). If the anemia is corrected with iron supplements, the patient's iron status should then be monitored every 3 to 6 months to ensure that iron deficiency does not recur. If iron status improves but anemia persists, EPO deficiency is likely.
- *EPO deficiency*: An erythropoiesis stimulating agent (ESA; epoetin alfa or darbepoetin) can be initiated and titrated as necessary to maintain the hemoglobin in a target range of 10 to 12 g/dl, to avoid the need for transfusion. Hemoglobin concentrations greater than 12 g/dl have been associated with increased thrombotic events, and the FDA advises that the ESA be temporarily stopped if hemoglobin reaches that level (Center for Drug Research and Evaluation, 2008).
- *Iron supplementation*: Most patients will require iron supplementation to prevent anemia during ESA therapy. An oral supplement can be used initially, but parenteral iron supplementation will be needed if the patient is unable to maintain adequate iron status (transferrin saturation >20% and serum ferritin level >100 ng/ml) with the oral supplement.
- *Inadequate response to EPO and iron therapy*: If the patient is unable to maintain the hemoglobin in the target range with EPO treatment or requires r-HuEPO dosages of more than 300 units/kg/wk intravenously or more than 200 units/kg/wk subcutaneously (or an equivalent dose of a related product), in spite of adequate iron stores (transferrin saturation >20%, ferritin >100 ng/ml), carnitine deficiency may be present.

Carnitine. Carnitine is an essential cofactor in fatty acid metabolism, and fatty acids are important metabolic fuels for the cardiac and skeletal muscles. Carnitine is normally synthesized in the body, but it is also found in foods of animal origin. Dietary restrictions in patients with CKD can result in low dietary carnitine intakes. Synthesis may be low in infants, as well as in individuals with chronic liver and kidney diseases. Moreover, carnitine is lost during dialysis, and these losses contribute to dialysis-related carnitine disorder (DCD), characterized by low plasma free carnitine concentrations, an increase in the plasma ratio of acylcarnitine to free carnitine, anemia that is poorly responsive to treatment with r-HuEPO, severe hypotension during dialysis, cardiomyopathy, and skeletal muscle weakness (severe enough to interfere with quality of life).

The current recommendations of the NKF (Eknoyan et al., 2003) regarding DCD include the following:

- Measurement of carnitine and acylcarnitine concentrations is not necessary for diagnosis of the disorder or assessment of response to carnitine therapy. Carnitine supplementation is recommended for individuals who have the symptoms listed earlier (and for whom no other cause of the disorder can be identified).
- Treatment of DCD should consist of L-carnitine given intravenously at 20 mg/kg body weight following the dialysis procedure (to minimize losses). Insufficient data are available regarding the benefits and dosages to make any recommendation for oral therapy. D-Carnitine can be toxic. Over-the-counter preparations of carnitine may contain both D- and L-carnitine, and these should be avoided.
- Response to L-carnitine therapy should be evaluated every 3 months, with the dosage titrated as low as possible to achieve the desired response, and it should be discontinued in 9 to 12 months if no clinical improvement is apparent.

Dyslipidemia. Arteriosclerotic heart disease is common among individuals with CKD (NKF, 2003b). Dietary fat is a valuable energy source, but saturated fats raise serum cholesterol levels and should be limited to no more than approximately 7% of total energy intake. Cholesterol intake should be restricted to 200 mg/day. Individuals with hypercholesterolemia should use oils and soft margarines high in monounsaturated and polyunsaturated fats (those containing primarily liquid canola [rapeseed], olive, safflower, sunflower, corn, soybean, or cottonseed oils); lean meats, fish, or skinned poultry; and skim milk products. (See Chapter 14 for a more extensive discussion.) Unfortunately, hypercholesterolemia often continues even after renal transplant. Nutrition problems in the posttransplant patient are discussed in Chapter 10.

Simple carbohydrates—such as sugar, jam, syrup, hard candy, gumdrops, and jellybeans, are widely used as energy sources for the person who is not receiving dialysis, because they contribute little or no sodium, potassium, and protein. However, simple carbohydrates must be limited if hypertriglyceridemia occurs. To compensate, complex carbohydrates (breads, cereals, vegetables) can be used, up to the amount allowed by the protein restriction. Fat intake, with emphasis on monounsaturated fatty acids (found in olive, canola, and peanut oils, for example), can be increased to approximately 40% of energy intake and carbohydrate intake can be correspondingly decreased. Alcohol intake should be restricted (preferably to none or only an occasional drink, but in no case more than 1 or 2 drinks per day).

Constipation. The low fiber intake resulting from the need to limit whole grains, fruits, and vegetables to remain within the potassium and phosphorus restriction may contribute to constipation. Fluid restriction may worsen the problem. Regular use of phosphate-binding medications can contribute to constipation. To improve bowel function, obtain regular physical activity and restrict dietary phosphorus so that use of phosphate binders can be decreased.

Nutrition support. Anorexia resulting from uremia, medications, or depression; the restrictions of the renal diet; abdominal fullness from the peritoneal dialysis; infections or inflammation; metabolic acidosis that stimulates protein degradation; and electrolyte imbalances or circulatory instability associated with CKD or dialysis are all factors that can interact to impair nutritional status. Oral nutritional supplements are the first choice for the patient who cannot consume enough regular food to maintain an adequate nutritional status, and enteral tube feeding is preferred over total parenteral nutrition (TPN) if specialized nutrition support is needed (NKF, 2000; Cano et al., 2006). Specialized formulas for renal failure, with low protein, phosphorus, and electrolyte content, are available if needed by the patient not receiving dialysis (see Table 8-1). Usually, the dialyzed patient needs the higher protein and mineral content of a formula designed for general use. Some general-use formulas are available in concentrated forms (2 kcal/ml) for individuals needing fluid restriction.

Impaired growth is very common among children with CKD. Intensive dietary counseling, oral supplements, and enteral tube feeding can be used as needed to maximize nutrient intake. In addition, growth hormone is approved for use in children with short stature associated with CKD (NKF, 2000).

Nephrotic Syndrome

Nephrotic syndrome results from an altered permeability of the glomerular capillary membrane. It is characterized by albuminuria of more than 3 to 3.5 g/day in adults or 40 mg/hr/m^2 of body surface area in children, hypoalbuminemia (<2.5 g/dl), edema, and hyperlipidemia (elevated triglycerides and LDL cholesterol) (Behrman et al., 2004; Goldman and Ausiello, 2008). Nephrotic syndrome may be idiopathic or may result from conditions such as poststreptococcal glomerulonephritis, diabetes mellitus, systemic lupus erythematosus, or sickle cell disease. Obesity is a contributing factor in one type of nephrotic syndrome, focal segmental glomerulosclerosis (Appel, 2006; Goldman and Ausiello, 2008). Although nephrotic syndrome can occur at any age, it is 15 times more common in children than in adults. About 90% of children with the disorder have idiopathic nephrotic syndrome, with minimal change disease (glomeruli appear normal on biopsy) being the most common form (Behrman et al., 2004).

Treatment

Prednisone is the most common therapeutic agent (Behrman et al., 2004). Relapses are common in both children and adults, and cyclophospamide or cyclosporine is an option for treatment of repeated relapses or steroid-insensitive disease. Angiotensin-converting enzyme (ACE) inhibitors and angiotensin II receptor blockers can be used to reduce proteinuria in steroid-insensitive patients (Behrman et al., 2004). A sodium-restricted diet, antihypertensive agents, and diuretics are used in treatment of hypertension.

Nutrition Assessment and Care

Medical nutrition therapy in nephrotic syndrome is designed to maintain adequate nutritional status and to help control edema and hypertension. Assessment findings that are especially common or significant are summarized in Box 16-1, and nutrition assessment is described more fully in Chapter 2.

Intervention and education
Nutrition needs. A "no salt added" diet (see Box 14-3) helps to reduce edema and blood pressure (Roth et al., 2002). Some

nephrologists recommend a more stringent restriction of less than 2 g sodium/day (Appel, 2006). See Boxes 14-3 and 14-4 and Table 14-2 for information useful in educating the patient or caregivers about sodium restriction. As the edema and hypertension resolve, then the sodium intake can be liberalized.

A diet providing the Dietary Reference Intake (see Appendix A on Evolve) for protein, with emphasis on high-quality protein, is needed to provide amino acids for synthesis of albumin (ADA, 2002; Roth et al., 2002). A very-high–protein diet is not recommended, because it seems to increase proteinuria. Lean meats, poultry without skin, fish, egg whites, milk, yogurt, and reduced-sodium cheeses are good sources of high-quality protein.

As nephrotic syndrome resolves, the hyperlipidemia usually resolves with it (Roth et al., 2002). However, diet and lifestyle changes to control serum lipids are appropriate for virtually all individuals over 2 years of age, and therefore individuals with nephrotic syndrome can be encouraged to choose a diet consistent with the American Heart Association guidelines in Box 14-1. Since hypertriglyceridemia is common, carbohydrate intake should be limited, particularly intake of simple carbohydrates in items such as desserts, candy, and sugar-containing beverages. A diet with a moderate amount of fat (approximately 30% of energy intake) helps to reduce the amount of carbohydrate required. Saturated fat should be limited to no more than 7% of energy intake, and *trans* fat intake should be minimized to help reduce LDL cholesterol. Up to 10% of kcal can be from polyunsaturated fat (e.g., sunflower, corn, and soybean oils; oily fish; sunflower seeds and walnuts) and the remainder from monounsaturated fats (e.g., olive, peanut, canola, and safflower oils; pecans, hazelnuts, and almonds). If the hypertriglyceridemic patient drinks alcohol, it should be in minimal amounts (never more than 2 drinks/day for most men or 1/day for nonpregnant women and small men) (ATP III, 2002).

Corticosteroid use can lead to impaired glucose tolerance and hyperglycemia. Reducing intake of simple carbohydrates helps to reduce blood glucose levels. Complex carbohydrates such as whole grains and legumes provide energy while making less of a contribution to hyperglycemia. Dividing dietary carbohydrate into three or more meals or snacks daily, rather than consuming one or two large meals, also helps to reduce postprandial glucose concentrations.

Renal Calculi, or Nephrolithiasis

Calculi, or stones, can precipitate in any part of the urinary tract when the urine becomes supersaturated with the solute. The most important solutes, in terms of **nephrolithiasis**, are calcium, oxalate, and uric acid. As many as 90% of all stones contain calcium, with the majority being calcium oxalate (Borghi et al., 2006; Goldman and Ausiello, 2008). Risk factors for stone formation include renal tubular acidosis, primary hyperparathyroidism, Crohn disease, diabetes, obesity, and gout (Goldman and Ausiello, 2008).

Treatment

Many calculi pass through the urinary tract spontaneously, and therapy consists of analgesics to relieve the pain associated with calculi and treatment of any underlying causative factors, such as urinary tract infection, obstruction, or gout. Some stones that do not pass spontaneously can be fragmented through lithotripsy to make it possible for the smaller fragments to be excreted. Calculi that are very large, too hard to be fragmented, or in an inappropriate location for lithotripsy can be removed either endoscopically or surgically.

Nutrition Assessment and Care

Nutrition therapy can reduce the risk of recurrence of stones in some individuals. Assess the type and quantity of fluids usually consumed, and determine whether the patient has a history of previous stone formation. The composition of any stones excreted should be determined, because this provides a basis for determining whether dietary changes might be beneficial.

Intervention and education
Dietary measures to reduce recurrence of calculi. Measures to reduce stone formation, particularly the formation of calcium stones, include the following (Borghi et al., 2006; Goldman and Ausiello, 2008):

- Adequate fluid intake helps reduce the risk of precipitation of calculi. A reasonable goal is to consume adequate fluid in beverages, tube feedings, or intravenous infusions to produce 2 to 2.5 L of dilute urine daily.
- Consume several servings of fruits and vegetables daily, because this seems to decrease the risk of stone formation. This

effect may be related to the potassium and magnesium content of fruits and vegetables.

■ Encourage a calcium intake of 800 to 1200 mg daily, to decrease intestinal oxalate absorption. This amount is found in approximately 3 servings of milk or yogurt.

■ If calcium oxalate stones are formed, avoid the foods that are most likely to cause elevated urine oxalate: spinach, Swiss chard, and other deep green, leafy vegetables; rhubarb, beets (both leaves and roots); nuts; sesame and tahini; concentrated brans and all-bran cereals, chocolate soy milk, and miso. A detailed listing of the oxalate content of foods can be found at http://www.ohf.org/docs/Oxalate2008.pdf.

■ Vitamin C yields oxalate when it is metabolized, and large amounts raise urine oxalate concentrations. Intakes as high as 2 g/day should be avoided (Massey et al., 2005); it may be preferable for individuals at high risk for oxalate stones to limit vitamin C intake to 250 mg daily (Massey, 2003).

■ Limit nondairy animal protein (e.g., meat, poultry, seafood) intake unless there is a medical or physiologic need for more protein.

■ Limit sodium intake to no more than 3 g/day (see Box 14-3), since excessive amounts seem to increase calcium excretion.

■ If hypercalciuria is not present, then a high-calcium intake may be beneficial because calcium decreases oxalate absorption in the intestine. If the person has fat malabsorption, then a low-fat diet may be effective. Excessive calcium is lost in the feces during fat malabsorption because calcium becomes bound to fat that is not absorbed, and thus the calcium is also lost in feces. Fecal calcium loss permits enhanced oxalate absorption (Worcester, 2002).

■ Increase intake of dietary phytate from legumes, whole grains, and nuts if the stones do not contain oxalate.

Conclusion

The kidney plays an important role in maintaining adequate nutritional status by excreting the wastes of nutrient metabolism and synthesis of active erythropoietin and vitamin D. On the other hand, optimal nutrition is important for the health of the kidney. For example, protein restriction appears to delay the progression of renal disease (Fouque and Aparicio, 2007). The complex interaction between the kidney and nutrition must be considered in planning the care of all patients with kidney diseases.

REFERENCES

Adult Treatment Panel (ATP) III: *Third report of the national cholesterol education program (NCEP) expert panel on detection, evaluation, and treatment of high blood cholesterol in adults (adult treatment panel III),* Washington, DC, 2002, National Institutes of Health, National Heart, Lung and Blood Institute.

Afsar B et al: Malnutrition-inflammation score is a useful tool in peritoneal dialysis patients, *Perit Dial Int* 26(6):705, 2006.

American Dietetic Association (ADA): *Chronic kidney disease (non-dialysis) medical nutrition therapy protocol,* Chicago, 2002, The Association. Available at www.ngc.gov. Accessed at November 22, 2007.

Appel GB: Improved outcomes in nephrotic syndrome, *Cleve Clin J Med* 73(2):161, 2006.

Behrman RE, Kliegman RM, Jenson HB, editors: *Nelson textbook of pediatrics,* ed 17, Philadelphia, 2004, Saunders.

Borghi L et al: Dietary therapy in idiopathic nephrolithiasis, *Nutr Rev* 64(7 pt 1):301, 2006.

Cano N et al: ESPEN guidelines on enteral nutrition: adult renal failure, *Clin Nutr* 25(2):295, 2006.

Center for Drug Research and Evaluation: Information for healthcare professionals: erythropoiesis stimulating agents (ESA) [Aranesp (darbepoetin), Epogen (epoetin alfa), and Procrit (epoetin alfa)]. Available at http://www.fda.gov/cder/drug/InfoSheets/HCP/RHE200711HCP.htm. Accessed March 15, 2008.

Eknoyan G, Latos DL, Lindberg J: Practice recommendations for the use of L-carnitine in dialysis-related carnitine disorder: National Kidney Foundation Carnitine Consensus Conference, *Am J Kidney Dis* 41:868, 2003.

Fouque D, Aparicio M: Eleven reasons to control the protein intake of patients with chronic kidney disease, *Nat Clin Pract Nephrol* 3(7): 383, 2007.

Goldman L, Ausiello D, editors: *Cecil medicine,* ed 23, Philadelphia, 2008, Saunders.

Kalantar-Zadeh K et al: Appetite and inflammation, nutrition, anemia, and clinical outcome in hemodialysis patients, *Am J Clin Nutr* 80(2):299, 2004a.

Kalantar-Zadeh K et al: Comparing outcome predictability of markers of malnutrition-inflammation complex syndrome in haemodialysis patients, *Nephrol Dial Transplant* 19(6):1507, 2004b.

Massey LK: Dietary influences on urinary oxalate and risk of kidney stones, *Front Biosci* 8:s584, 2003.

Massey LK, Liebman M, Kynast-Gales SA: Ascorbate increases human oxaluria and kidney stone risk, *J Nutr* 135(7):1673, 2005.

National Kidney Foundation (NKF): K/DOQI clinical practice guidelines for bone metabolism and disease in chronic kidney disease, *Am J Kidney Dis* 43(4 suppl 2):S1, 2003a.

National Kidney Foundation (NKF): KDOQI clinical practice guidelines and clinical practice recommendations for anemia in chronic kidney disease, *Am J Kidney Dis* 47(5 suppl 3):S1, 2006.

National Kidney Foundation (NKF): K/DOQI clinical practice guidelines for management of dyslipidemias in patients with kidney disease, *Am J Kidney Dis* 41(4 suppl 3):I, 2003b.

National Kidney Foundation (NKF): K/DOQI clinical practice guidelines for nutrition in chronic renal failure, *Am J Kidney Dis* 35(6 suppl):S1, 2000.

National Kidney Foundation (NKF) Kidney Disease Outcome Initiative (K/DOQI): Clinical practice guidelines for chronic kidney disease: evaluation, classification, and stratification, *Am J Kidney Dis* 39(2 suppl 1):S1, 2002.

National Kidney Foundation (NKF) Disease Outcomes Quality Initiative (K/DOQI): KDOQI clinical practice guideline and clinical practice recommendations for anemia in chronic kidney disease: 2007 update of hemoglobin target, *Am J Kidney Dis* 50(3):471, 2007a.

National Kidney Foundation (NKF) Kidney Disease Outcome Quality Initiative: KDOQI clinical practice guidelines and clinical practice recommendations for diabetes and chronic kidney disease, *Am J Kidney Dis* 49(2 suppl 2): S12, 2007b.

Roth KS, Amaker BH, Chan JCM: Nephrotic syndrome: pathogenesis and management, *Pediatr Rev* 23(7):237, 2002.

Tjiong HL et al: Peritoneal dialysis with solutions containing amino acids plus glucose promotes protein synthesis during oral feeding, *Clin J Am Soc Nephrol* 2(1):74, 2007.

Worcester EM: Stones from bowel disease, *Endocrinol Metab Clin North Am* 31(4):979, 2002.

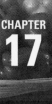

DIABETES MELLITUS

Diabetes mellitus is a disorder characterized by impaired carbohydrate, fat, and protein metabolism. Hyperglycemia and glucosuria commonly occur in untreated diabetes.

Overview of Diabetes

Diagnosis and Classification of Diabetes

Any one of the following criteria is sufficient for a diagnosis of diabetes in an adult (American Diabetes Association, 2008a):

- Symptoms of diabetes plus casual (any time of day without regard to time since the last meal) plasma glucose level of 200 mg/dl (11.1 mM) or higher. The classic symptoms of diabetes include polyuria, polydipsia, and unexplained weight loss.
- Fasting plasma glucose level of 126 mg/dl (7.0 mM) or higher. "Fasting" means no energy intake for at least 8 hours.
- Plasma glucose level of 200 mg/dl (11.1 mM) or higher 2 hours after an oral glucose tolerance test (a 75-g load of glucose taken orally).

Diabetes is classified according to its etiology, as described below (ADA, 2008a):

- **Type 1 diabetes** (previously known as *insulin-dependent diabetes*) is characterized by insulin deficiency that results from destruction of the beta cells of the pancreas. Most individuals with type 1 diabetes are normal weight or underweight at the time of diagnosis. Classic symptoms of untreated type 1 diabetes include polyuria, polydipsia (increased fluid intake), polyphagia (increased food intake), and weight loss. Insulin treatment is needed to survive.
- **Type 2 diabetes** (previously known as *non–insulin-dependent diabetes*) is characterized by insulin resistance, or decreased tissue uptake of glucose in response to insulin, along with an

insulin secretion defect that makes it impossible for the individual to release enough insulin to compensate for the insulin resistance. Type 2 diabetes is much more common than type 1 diabetes, accounting for about 90% to 95% of the diabetes in the United States and Canada. Eighty-three percent of adults with type 2 diabetes are overweight or obese (CDC, 2007).

■ **Other specific types of diabetes** are included in a broad category that encompasses genetic defects in pancreatic beta cell function (including maturity-onset diabetes of youth [MODY]); genetic defects in insulin action; diseases of the exocrine pancreas that damage the pancreas and thus impair beta cell function (e.g., pancreatitis, neoplasia, cystic fibrosis, hemochromatosis); endocrinopathies such as acromegaly; drug- or chemical-induced diabetes (e.g., glucocorticoids, injected pentamidine, thyroid hormone); and diabetes induced by infectious agents, uncommon immune-related illnesses, or genetic disorders.

■ **Gestational diabetes mellitus** is the term given to any glucose intolerance that first occurs or is recognized during pregnancy.

Prediabetes and Diabetes Prevention

Impaired fasting glucose (IFG) and impaired glucose tolerance (IGT) are considered prediabetes, or intermediate stages between the normal state and frank diabetes. People with IFG and IGT are at high risk for development of diabetes. These conditions are defined as follows (ADA, 2008a):

■ Impaired fasting glucose: fasting plasma glucose is 100 to 125 mg/dl (5.6 to 6.9 mmol/L).
■ Impaired glucose tolerance: 2-hour values in the oral glucose tolerance test (OGTT) are 140 mg/dl (7.8 mmol/L) or higher but below 200 mg/dl (11.1 mmol/L).

Diet and lifestyle interventions, including modest weight loss, a heart-healthy diet, regular physical activity, and possibly an increase in dietary fiber (Knowler et al., 2002; Krishnan et al., 2007; Lindström et al., 2006), hold promise for reducing the growing problem of diabetes.

Complications of Diabetes

Acute complications of type 1 diabetes include diabetic ketoacidosis (DKA) and hypoglycemia, and those of type 2 diabetes include hyperglycemic hyperosmolar nonketotic syndrome (HHNS) and infections such as pneumonia, cellulitis, bacteriuria, and vulvovaginitis. DKA results from insulin deficiency caused, for example, by new-onset diabetes (diagnosed when the patient develops DKA); too small a dosage; omission of doses; elevation of the insulin-antagonizing counterregulatory hormones (glucagon, catecholamines, cortisol, growth hormone), such as occurs during infection or trauma; use of drugs altering carbohydrate metabolism, such as glucocorticoids, thiazides, and second-generation antipsychotics; and cocaine use (Kitabchi and Nyenwe, 2006). In response to the insulin deficiency, hyperglycemia and glucosuria occur. Glucosuria leads to an osmotic diuresis with resulting dehydration and loss of electrolytes. The insulin deficit also allows increased lipolysis, or release of fatty acids from storage sites. Accelerated formation of ketones from the fatty acids results in ketosis (increased blood ketone levels because of increased production of ketones from fatty acids) and acidosis (because ketones are acidic). HHNS, on the other hand, is almost always precipitated by some stressor that increases blood glucose levels (surgery, trauma, burns, chronic disease, infection, drugs such as corticosteroids or diuretics, dialysis). HHNS results in marked hyperglycemia (often greater than 1000 mg/dl), elevation of serum osmolality, glucosuria, and dehydration. Ketosis is absent or only very mild. Although DKA is primarily seen in type 1 diabetes, it can occur in type 2, particularly among African-American and Hispanic individuals; similarly, HHNS occurs occasionally in type 1 (Kitabchi and Nyenwe, 2006).

The major chronic complications of diabetes are accelerated coronary heart disease, peripheral vascular disease, cerebrovascular disease, retinopathy, nephropathy, and neuropathy (Goldman and Ausiello, 2008).

Treatment

The chronic nature of the disease and the fact that optimal control is necessary to reduce the risk of complications mean that the patient and family must be able to understand and carry out the treatment with a great deal of independence. Planning of care begins with anthropometric measurements and a thorough health and diet history to assess the person's usual pattern of food intake and physical activity, nutrition needs and concerns, health and nutritional status, and educational needs (Box 17-1).

Box 17-1   Assessment of the Person with Diabetes

Anthropometric Data

Height
Weight
BMI
Waist circumference (adult)

Weight History

Maximal weight
History of weight loss/gain—amount, period of time, intentional/unintentional (If intentional weight loss occurred, how was it brought about? Was loss maintained or regained?)

Diet and Lifestyle History

Usual intake of food and beverages: amount, preparation methods, timing, alcohol use, sodium intake
Problems with intake: nausea, vomiting, swallowing disorder, bloating or discomfort, diarrhea
Food security issues: problems in shopping, purchasing, transporting, or preparing food
Use of supplements: vitamins, minerals, fiber, herbal and other complementary and alternative, other
Physical activity: type, intensity, frequency (include job related, housework, gardening, etc.)

Health History

Diabetes History

When diagnosed
Current diabetes symptoms: polyuria, polydipsia, polyphagia
History of hypoglycemia: frequency, severity
History of DKA or HHNS
Diabetes medication usage
Insulin: type, dosage, pattern of use
Oral hypoglycemic agents: type, dosage, schedule
Other diabetes therapies: GLP-1 receptor agonists, etc.

Continued

Box 17-1   Assessment of the Person with Diabetes—cont'd

Other Pertinent Health History

Smoking: ever smoked, currently smoke

Presence and duration of chronic illnesses or conditions: hypertension, hypercholesterolemia, atherosclerosis, kidney disease, retinopathy, neuropathy

Medication usage: type, dosage, and frequency

Antihypertensive agents, diuretics

Cholesterol-lowering therapy

Drugs that may cause hyperglycemia or hypoglycemia (see Table 17-4)

Over-the-counter

Herbal and other complementary and alternative

Laboratory Findings

Hemoglobin A_{1c}

Fasting plasma glucose

Daily record of plasma glucose concentrations from SMBG for the past month or more, if available

Serum total, LDL, and HDL cholesterol and triglycerides (adults)

Patient/Family Level of Understanding and Learning Needs

Diet and nutrition knowledge: basics of a healthy diet, optimal diet for prevention of coronary heart disease, level of interest and knowledge in carbohydrate counting or other advanced diet management techniques

Body weight regulation: appropriateness of current weight, weight goals, diet and lifestyle interventions for weight control

Medications for control of blood glucose and other related disorders such as hypertension: administration, side effects, goals of therapy

---

BMI, Body mass index; *DKA,* diabetic ketoacidosis; *GLP-1,* glucagon-like peptide–1; *HHNS,* hyperglycemic hyperosmolar nonketotic syndrome; *HDL,* high-density lipoprotein; *LDL,* low-density lipoprotein; *SMBG,* self-monitoring of blood glucose.

Treatment of diabetes hinges on an appropriate plan for diet, physical activity, and other lifestyle measures, as well as medications if necessary. Intensive management of diabetes to maintain blood glucose levels as near normal as possible reduces retinopathy, nephropathy, and neuropathy in both type 1 and type 2 diabetes (DCCT/EDIC, 2005; Genuth et al., 2003; Genuth, 2006). Further, the ADA has recommended treatment goals as outlined in Table 17-1, with a focus on maintaining near-normal glucose concentrations at all times while making allowances for the needs and preferences of the individual. Diabetes care is a team effort that usually involves several health professionals—one or more physicians, dietitians, nurses, and other professionals, such as a podiatrist and optometrist or ophthalmologist—as well as the patient and family members.

Diet and Lifestyle Approaches

Diet and lifestyle modifications are an essential component of the care of all people with diabetes. A registered dietitian (RD) who is knowledgeable in diabetes care is the best person to assist the individual and family in implementing the nutrition care plan. All health professionals on the team should be familiar with the principles of nutrition care in diabetes so that they can reinforce and provide information consistent with the instruction.

Medications

For intensive control of type 1 diabetes, continuous subcutaneous insulin infusion (CSII, or insulin pump therapy) or multiple daily insulin injections are needed. Insulin is available in four forms: (1) ultra–short-acting, (2) short-acting, (3) intermediate-acting, and (4) long-acting (Table 17-2). Intermediate-acting insulins are used less frequently than in the past, because basal-bolus therapy, which is favored now, is more easily achieved with the other insulin preparations. Basal insulin delivery maintains a constant, low insulin concentration throughout the day, to prevent the liver from releasing excessive amounts of glucose and also reduce the release of fat from adipose tissue. Boluses of ultra–short-acting or short-acting insulin are given with meals and snacks to provide sufficient insulin to promote tissue uptake of the carbohydrate in the food. CSII uses a continuous low-rate infusion of short- or ultra–short-acting insulin to maintain basal insulin levels; the patient is able to administer a bolus of insulin with meals or

Table 17-1   Summary of Recommendations for Adults
with Diabetes

Glycemic Control	
A_{1c}	$<7.0\%^*$
Preprandial capillary plasma glucose	90-130 mg/dl (5.0-7.2 mmol/L)
Peak postprandial capillary plasma glucose[†]	<180 mg/dl (<10.0 mmol/L)
Blood pressure	$<130/80$ mm Hg
Lipids[‡]	
LDL	<100 mg/dl (2.6 mmol/L)
Triglycerides	<150 mg/dl (<1.7 mmol/L)
HDL	>40 mg/dl (>1.0 mmol/L)[§]

Key Concepts in Setting Glycemic Goals

- A_{1c} is the primary target for glycemic control.
- Goals should be individualized.
- Certain populations (children, pregnant women, and elderly) require special considerations.
- More stringent glycemic goals (i.e., a normal A_{1c}, $<6\%$) may further reduce complications at the cost of increased hypoglycemia.
- Less intensive glycemic goals may be indicated in patients with severe or frequent hypoglycemia.
- Postprandial glucose may be targeted if A_{1c} goals are not met despite reaching preprandial glucose goals.

From the American Diabetes Association: Standards of medical care in diabetes—2007, *Diabetes Care* 30(suppl 1):S4, 2007. Used with permission.
A_{1c}, Hemoglobin A_{1c}; *HDL,* high-density lipoprotein; *LDL,* low-density lipoprotein.
[*]Where the nondiabetic range is 4.0%-6.0%.
[†]Postprandial glucose measurements should be made 1-2 hr after the beginning of the meal, generally peak levels in patients with diabetes.
[‡]Current National Cholesterol Education Program/Adult Treatment Panel III guidelines suggest that in patients with triglycerides ≥200 mg/dl, the "non-HDL cholesterol" (total cholesterol minus HDL) be utilized. The goal is ≤130 mg/dl.
[§]For women, it has been suggested that the HDL goal be increased by 10 mg/dl.

snacks by triggering the pump manually (Tamborlane et al., 2006). When using multiple daily injections, a long-acting insulin is given once or twice daily to maintain basal levels. Injections of ultra–short- or short-acting insulin are taken with meals and snacks. Because the risk of hypoglycemia is increased by intensive therapy, intensive management is not recommended for patients who are unwilling or unable to participate actively in their care. Data are insufficient regarding the effects of intensive control on children less than 13 years of age and adults over 65 years of age to make any recommendation for those age-groups (ADA, 2008c). Hypoglycemia may precipitate strokes or heart attacks if atherosclerosis is present, and thus older adults or others with

Table 17-2   Activity of Human Insulin and Insulin Analogues[*]

	Approximate Number of Hours After Injection		
Insulin	Onset	Peak	Duration
Ultra–Short-Acting			
Aspart	<0.25	1-3	4-6
Glulisine	<0.25	0.5-1.5	3-5
Lispro	<0.25	0.5-1.5	4-6
Short-Acting			
Regular	0.5-1	2-4	6-8
Intermediate-Acting			
NPH	1.5-5	4-12	14-18
Lente	2.5-5	4-12	16-20
Long-Acting			
Detemir	3-4	6-8[†]	18-24
Glargine	2-4	—[†]	20-24

Data from manufacturers' package inserts; Hirsch IB: Insulin analogues, *N Engl J Med* 352(2):174, 2005.

[*]The times of onset, peak activity, and duration may vary widely from individual to individual and at different times in the same individual. These times are guidelines only. Insulin analogues are modified insulin molecules.

[†]Insulin glargine has no peak of activity. The effect reaches a plateau after 3-4 hr. Detemir has a minimal peak effect. These long-acting insulins provide a basal level of insulin activity, and boluses of ultra–short- or short-acting insulin are given with meals and snacks to provide insulin action to dispose of the carbohydrate.

significant atherosclerosis need to be especially careful if they choose to use intensive therapy.

Type 2 diabetes progresses along a continuum, such that diet and lifestyle modifications may be sufficient to control blood glucose initially, but eventually one or more noninsulin hypoglycemic agents and/or insulin may need to be added to the regimen. The noninsulin therapeutic agents used are of several types (Table 17-3). Insulin sensitizers stimulate tissue glucose uptake, primarily in skeletal muscle, and decrease fasting blood sugar. Insulin secretagogues stimulate the pancreas to release insulin. Incretins are hormones released in increased amounts after eating; they stimulate insulin release, suppress glucagon secretion, delay gastric emptying, and reduce postprandial (postmeal) glucose concentrations. Inhibitors of the enzymes that digest starch help to reduce postprandial glucose concentrations. Pramlintide, a drug that mimics the action of amylin, a peptide released with insulin, causes delayed gastric emptying, suppression of glucagon secretion, and reduction in appetite (Cefalu et al., 2007).

Intensive control of blood glucose is strongly recommended because it has the potential to reduce the long-term complications of diabetes (Genuth et al., 2003; DCCT/EDIC, 2005; Genuth, 2006). Also, particularly for insulin-dependent individuals, it has the advantage of allowing increased flexibility in diabetes management. Meals and snacks can be eaten when desired, and there is no need to consume a predetermined amount of carbohydrate in a meal or snack. The dosage of ultra–short- or short-acting insulin can be adjusted by the individual or parent (or other caretaker) to suit the amount of carbohydrate consumed.

However, intensive control raises the risk of hypoglycemic episodes, the most feared short-term complication of diabetes (McNay et al., 2006); indeed, hypoglycemia is the major limiting factor in intensive control of blood glucose. Also, intensive glucose control has significantly increased the amount of weight gain in both type 1 and type 2 diabetes in most long-term studies carried out to date, which is an important concern because of the fact that both diabetes and overweight are risk factors for cardiovascular disease (Russell-Jones and Kahn, 2007). The reasons for the weight gain may include reduction of glucosuria with increased retention of calories; the anabolic effect of insulin on muscle and fat tissue; "defensive snacking" because of fear of hypoglycemia; increased food intake related to the increased flexibility of the basal-bolus

Table 17-3 Noninsulin Therapeutic Agents Used in Treatment of Type 2 Diabetes

Therapeutic Use/Specific Agents	Additional Benefits	Major Side Effects
Insulin Sensitizers		
Biguanide (metformin)	Appetite suppression	Nausea, abdominal pain, diarrhea*
Thiazolidinediones (rosiglitazone, pioglitazone)		Edema, weight gain, ? ↑ risk of cardiovascular events with rosiglitazone[†]
Stimulators of Insulin Secretion		
Meglitinides (repaglinide, nateglinide)	Restoration of first-phase insulin secretion[‡]	Hypoglycemia, weight gain
Sulfonylureas (e.g., glyburide, glipizide, glimepiride)		Hypoglycemia, weight gain
Incretins and Agents That Prolong Incretin Action		
GLP-1 receptor agonists (exenatide) [§]	Weight loss	Nausea
DPP-4 inhibitors (sitagliptin)	Weight neutral	Nasopharyngitis, upper respiratory infection; ↑ risk of hypoglycemia when given in combination with glimepiride

Continued

Table 17-3   Noninsulin Therapeutic Agents Used in Treatment of Type 2 Diabetes—cont'd

Therapeutic Use/Specific Agents	Additional Benefits	Major Side Effects
Inhibitors of Glucose Absorption		
α-Glucosidase inhibitors (acarbose, miglitol)*	Acarbose may ↓ CVD risk and hypertension	Flatulence, abdominal pain, diarrhea
Modifier of Insulin Action		
Amylin analogue (pramlintide)§	Modest weight loss	Nausea, hypoglycemia

Data from manufacturers' package inserts; Cefalu WT et al: Pharmacotherapy for the treatment of patients with type 2 diabetes mellitus: rationale and specific agents, *Clin Pharmacol Ther* 81(5):636, 2007.

CVD, Cardiovascular disease; *DPP-4*, dipeptidyl peptidase IV, the enzyme that degrades endogenous GLP-1; *GLP-1*, glucagon-like peptide–1.

*Side effects can be reduced by taking the drug with food and by gradually titrating the dose upward as tolerated.

†Patients receiving rosiglitazone should be informed of the possible increased risk of myocardial ischemia and heart failure. Insulin and nitrate drugs appear to increase the risk, and use of these drugs is not recommended for the patient taking rosiglitazone (http://www.fda.gov/cder/drug/InfoSheets/HCP/rosiglitazone-200707HCP.htm, updated 11/29/07, accessed 12/4/07).

§These agents require subcutaneous injection; all other drugs in the table can be administered orally.

‡Normal individuals release a short burst of insulin (the first-phase response) at the beginning of food intake, followed by a second phase that lasts as long as hyperglycemia is maintained. The first-phase response appears to be especially important in reducing hyperglycemia after a meal, and it is commonly lost early in development of type 2 diabetes (Leahy, 2005).

insulin regimen; stimulation of appetite by insulin signaling in the brain; and the unphysiologic route of insulin delivery into the subcutaneous tissue, which exposes the muscle and fat to higher concentrations of insulin than the normal route of insulin secretion into the hepatic portal vein (Hermansen and Mortensen, 2007). The disadvantages of intensive therapy should not be allowed to interfere with achieving optimal glucose control, however.

The new long-acting insulin analogues glargine (Lantus) and detemir (Levemir) are associated with less hypoglycemia, particularly at night, than NPH insulin (Ashwell et al., 2006; Hermansen and Mortensen, 2007). Also, insulin detemir appears not to stimulate weight gain as much as other forms of insulin (Russell-Jones and Kahn, 2007). The patient needs to be aware of the potential for weight gain with intensive therapy and strategies to overcome it, e.g., avoiding excessive snacking since there is less concern over hypoglycemia with insulins detemir and glargine.

Nutrition Assessment and Care

A thorough nutrition assessment should be performed as described in Chapter 2. Box 17-1 highlights common or especially serious findings in persons with diabetes.

Intervention and diabetes self-management education (DMSE)
Self-monitoring of blood glucose. Self-monitoring of blood glucose (SMBG) is an important tool of care. The frequency of monitoring depends on the individual's needs and goals, but SMBG is done a minimum of 3 times daily in type 1 diabetes (ADA, 2008c) and several times more if intensive therapy is used (discussed in more detail below). SMBG is recommended for patients with type 2 diabetes who are treated with insulin and is desirable for those treated with sulfonylureas and those who are not achieving their blood glucose goals. Whenever therapy is being modified, SMBG is recommended for both type 1 and type 2 diabetes (ADA, 2008c).

Medical nutrition therapy. The goals of therapy are as follows: (1) attain and maintain optimal metabolic outcomes, including blood pressure, glucose, and lipid levels, as close to normal as possible to prevent or reduce the risk for complications; (2) prevent and/or slow development of chronic complications of diabetes; (3) address individual needs, considering cultural, lifestyle, financial, and willingness to change; and (4) maintain the pleasure of eating by only limiting food choices when indicated by scientific evidence (ADA, 2008b). At its most basic, patient education includes wise food choices; portion control; and principles of a healthy lifestyle such as smoking cessation, physical activity, and moderation in alcohol intake, similar to the MyPyramid plan for healthy adults (http://diabetes.org/nutrition-and-recipes/nutrition/my-pyramid-response.jsp). For most individuals with diabetes, the educational program is more extensive and detailed, as described below.

Energy balance. Overweight and obesity increase insulin resistance and worsen glucose control (Leahy, 2005). In addition, overweight and obesity contribute to development of hypertension and cardiovascular disease in diabetic individuals, who are already at high risk for these problems (Buse et al., 2007). Even modest weight loss (5% to 7% of body weight) can reduce insulin resistance and improve control. Reduced energy and fat ($\approx$30% of total kcal) intake, combined with behavioral modification, regular moderate or vigorous physical activity, and lifestyle changes such as incorporating more physical movement into activities of daily living (e.g., park further from the door at the shopping mall) can achieve and maintain such a weight loss (ADA, 2008b). Very-low–carbohydrate diets (<130 g/day) are not recommended for people with diabetes because their long-term effects are not known (ADA, 2008c). Moreover, these diets tend to be higher in animal protein and fat than more balanced diets, and this might contribute to the development of cardiovascular disease.

Carbohydrate. Carbohydrate usually accounts for 50% or more of the energy consumed. Even when insulin is not used, carbohydrate (and other energy nutrients) should be spread as evenly as possible among the meals, and meals should be far enough apart (4 to 5 hours) to allow blood glucose to return to basal concentrations before each meal. Soluble fiber from oats, legumes, fruits, and vegetables may help to reduce serum lipid levels. At least 25 to 30 g of fiber daily is recommended for both diabetic and nondiabetic adults. Even higher fiber intakes (up to 38 g daily) are recommended for males 14 to 50 years of age, who have higher energy needs than other groups. Some foods have been identified as having a low **glycemic index**— that is, they cause less change in the blood glucose than a reference carbohydrate (usually white bread or pure glucose). White rice is a food of relatively high glycemic index, and legumes are low, for example. For individuals with diabetes, there may be a small advantage to choosing foods with low glycemic indexes most of the time (ADA, 2008c). A compilation of glycemic index data for various foods is available (Foster-Powell et al., 2002).

Learning to monitor carbohydrate intake in some consistent manner improves glucose control among people with diabetes. This can be done with carbohydrate counting, the use of exchange lists, or estimation based on experience; any of the three techniques can be used with good results (ADA, 2008c). **Carbohydrate counting** is a technique that focuses on the carbohydrate content of foods consumed. Carbohydrate is the main component of the diet that affects postprandial blood glucose levels and insulin requirements.

Depending on the skills and interest of the diabetic individual, carbohydrate counting can be a very simple or very complex technique. At its simplest, the dietitian teaches the person with diabetes to identify sources of carbohydrate in the diet, and they work together to make carbohydrate intake at a meal consistent from day to day. Keeping food records is encouraged to help the person recognize the relationship between carbohydrate intake and blood glucose levels. At an intermediate level the person further develops record-keeping skills, comparing blood glucose records with food intake records. The person learns to recognize patterns in blood glucose readings and to understand how they relate to food intake, physical activity, and diabetes medications. At its most complex level, carbohydrate counting is appropriate for people with type 1 diabetes who are receiving intensive insulin therapy. At this level the person with diabetes matches insulin dosages precisely with carbohydrate intake, decreasing or increasing the insulin dosage to allow consumption of less or more carbohydrate than usual (Warshaw and Kulkarni, 2004). In the *Choose Your Foods: Exchange Lists for Diabetes* (ADA, American Dietetic Association, 2007), foods are grouped according to similarities in their carbohydrate, protein, and fat content. An alternative resource, the *Exchange Lists for Weight Management* (ADA, American Dietetic Association, 2003), includes all the information from the 2003 *Exchange Lists for Meal Planning*, along with guidelines for controlling energy intake and increasing physical activity. This is useful for overweight individuals, whether or not they have diabetes.

In working with the person with diabetes to develop a meal plan, the dietitian considers the person's optimal energy intake (see Table 2-6 and Box 2-4). For children and pregnant and lactating women, the Dietary Reference Intake (DRI) (see Appendix A on Evolve) serves as a guideline. The desirable proportions of carbohydrate, protein, and fat in the diet are determined as described previously. Once these parameters are established, the number of exchanges (servings) from each group can be identified, and the exchanges can be assigned to specific meals and snacks so that the carbohydrate is spread evenly throughout the day. Starch, milk, and fruit exchanges contain approximately the same amount of carbohydrate (12 to 15 g/exchange) and can be substituted for one another.

Nonnutritive sweeteners (those containing negligible or no calories) include aspartame, acesulfame K, sucralose, and saccharin. These sweeteners can be consumed within the limits recommended by the U.S. Food and Drug Administration (ADA, 2008c). Individuals with phenylketonuria should not use aspartame (Nutrasweet). Nutritive sugar substitutes such as sugar alcohols (e.g., sorbitol) are sometimes used in products marketed to people with diabetes. They provide about one half the energy per gram as sugars do, but their energy contribution must be considered. Excessive amounts may cause diarrhea. The diabetic individual does not need to purchase special diabetic or dietetic foods but can choose from a wide variety of regular foods.

Protein. Adults with diabetes and normal renal function are believed to have protein needs similar to those of the general population. If chronic kidney disease develops, a protein intake no more than 0.8 to 1 g/kg/day is recommended in the early stages and no more than 0.8 g/kg/day in the later stages (ADA, 2008c).

Fat. A moderate amount of dietary fat (25% to 35% of total energy needs) helps to reduce the amount of carbohydrate in the diet and is consistent with a heart-healthy diet (Buse et al., 2007). Diabetes is a risk factor for dyslipidemias and coronary heart disease, and therefore monounsaturated and polyunsaturated fats should be emphasized. Saurated fats should provide less than 7% of the total energy intake, and *trans* fat intake should be minimal. Cholesterol intake should be limited to 300 mg/day for adults without hypercholesterolemia and 200 mg/day for those with elevated cholesterol (ATP III, 2002; Buse et al., 2007) (see Chapter 14). If serum triglyceride levels are elevated, steps to reduce them include a decrease in intake of sugars and other simple carbohydrates; a modest increase in intake of monounsaturated fat such as canola and olive oil to replace the carbohydrate calories if necessary; avoiding alcohol; and weight reduction (if overweight or obese). Omega-3 fat from oily fish such as salmon and sardines or fish oil supplements may be beneficial in diabetic individuals with very high triglycerides (Lichtenstein et al., 2006).

Alcohol. If adults choose to use alcohol, they should limit daily intake to no more than 2 drinks for men and 1 for women (1 drink ≥12 oz [360 ml] of beer, 5 oz [150 ml] of wine, or 1.5 oz [45 ml] of distilled spirits) (ADA, 2008c). Pregnant women, children, and people with a history of alcohol abuse should not consume alcohol, and individuals with pancreatitis or hypertriglyceridemia should avoid it as well. Hypertensive individuals should minimize their alcohol intake. Alcohol should be consumed with food, because drinking on an empty stomach raises the risk of hypoglycemia.

Vitamins, minerals, and sodium. No sound evidence suggests that individuals with diabetes have an increased need for vitamins, compared with nondiabetic adults. In addition, there is no evidence that supplements of chromium have any benefit for people with diabetes (ADA, 2008c).

Both hypertensive and nonhypertensive individuals with diabetes should attempt to reduce sodium intake to 1200 to 2300 mg/day (50 to 100 mmol/day), or approximately 3000 to 6000 mg salt (Buse et al., 2007). This requires that no salt be added to food and that efforts be made to choose food with the lowest sodium content possible (see Boxes 14-3 and 14-4). A diet rich in fresh or frozen (without salt added) vegetables and fruits that provides whole grains, low-fat or skim milk products, and limited amounts of unprocessed meats, poultry, and fish, such as the Dietary Approaches to Stop Hypertension (DASH) plan outlined in Table 14-1, can meet these guidelines.

Physical activity. At least 150 min/wk of moderate-intensity aerobic physical activity (50% to 70% of maximum heart rate) or at least 90 min/wk of vigorous aerobic exercise (>70% of maximum heart rate) is recommended to help improve glucose and weight control and reduce cardiovascular risk (Buse et al., 2007). The physical activity should be distributed over at least 3 days/wk and with no more than two 2 consecutive days without physical activity. If weight loss has been achieved, a minimum of 7 hours of moderate to vigorous exercise weekly will help to maintain the loss (Buse et al., 2007). Resistance training 3 times per week is also recommended (ADA, 2008c). The guidelines in Chapter 5 for becoming and remaining physically fit are appropriate for individuals with diabetes as long as they first have the approval of their physicians. Before beginning an exercise program, people with diabetes need to be assessed for retinopathy and peripheral or autonomic neuropathy so that their fitness regimens can be appropriately individualized. (Buse et al., 2007; ADA, 2008c).

Individuals with type 1 diabetes should monitor their blood glucose before and after exercise to determine whether insulin or food intake needs to be adjusted. The person should not exercise if ketosis is present (ADA, 2008c). If exercise is planned, the insulin dosage can be reduced to prevent hypoglycemia. If it is unplanned, extra carbohydrate will be needed (for a 70-kg person, the requirement is approximately 10 to 15 g of carbohydrate for every hour of moderate-intensity physical activity) (ADA, 2008b). One small apple, $\frac{1}{2}$ small banana, $\frac{1}{2}$ cup of regular soft drink, $\frac{1}{2}$ bagel, or 4 to 6 oz of fruit juice provides 10 to 15 g carbohydrate.

Pregnancy and lactation. The infant of a diabetic woman in poor control at the time of conception is at risk for fetal malformations or death. Additionally, infants of diabetic mothers are at increased risk of prematurity, respiratory distress syndrome, and macrosomia (excessive body size). Very good control of blood glucose during pregnancy reduces the risk of complications in the infant. To prevent congenital anomalies, it is best if intensive therapy begins before conception. Conception should not occur until a woman exhibits stable glycemic control, as evidenced by **hemoglobin A$_{1c}$ (Hb A$_{1c}$)** level. All women with potential for childbearing should consume at least 400 mcg folic acid per day from supplements or fortified foods in addition to consuming good food sources of folate (ADA, 2004b).

Both diabetes existing before pregnancy and gestational diabetes mellitus (GDM) increase the risk of fetal macrosomia, maternal hypertensive disorders, and need for cesarean delivery, as well as complications in the neonatal period, including hypoglycemia, hypocalcemia, and polycythemia. Good metabolic control reduces these risks, and the remainder of this section represents a summary of the most recent ADA position statements on GDM and diet during pregnancy (ADA, 2004a, 2008b). Daily SMBG is an important part of diabetic care in pregnancy. The goal is to maintain plasma glucose concentrations as follows: fasting, 105 mg/dl (5.8 mmol/L) or less; 1-hour postprandial, 155 mg/dl (8.6 mmol/L) or less; and 2-hour postprandial, 130 mg/dl (7.2 mmol/L) or less. A registered dietitian should counsel the woman about diet during pregnancy. For normal-weight women, no increase in energy intake is recommended during the first trimester of pregnancy; during the second and third trimesters, an increase of about 300 kcal (1255 kJ) daily over their prepregnant intake is usually adequate to support fetal growth. The diet should provide adequate energy and nutrients to promote optimal weight gain during pregnancy (see Chapter 3), but obese women with GDM have had improved glucose and triglyceride levels without an increase in ketone levels when following a moderately energy-restricted diet (approximately 25 kcal/kg actual body weight per day, or approximately 30% less than estimated energy needs). Limiting carbohydrate intake to 35% to 40% of energy intake improves maternal glucose concentrations and maternal and fetal outcomes. Adequate protein is usually provided by an intake of 0.75 g/kg/day plus an additional 10 g/day.

Regular meals and snacks are necessary to reduce the risk of hypoglycemia because of the fetus's continual requirement for nutrients. A bedtime snack helps to decrease the likelihood of hypoglycemia during sleep. Carbohydrate is divided into three small to moderate meals and two to four snacks daily; distributing it as evenly as possible throughout the day reduces the incidence of severe hyperglycemia. Physical activity can be encouraged as a means of improving control of blood glucose in women without medical or obstetric complications that would contraindicate it, although evidence is inadequate to make a firm recommendation about the type of exercise. Urine monitoring of ketones may be of benefit in determining the adequacy of energy intake and/or insulin dosages.

Breastfeeding should be encouraged, both because it can be associated with improved maternal postpartum weight loss and blood glucose control and because it has been shown to have emotional benefits for mother and infant and health benefits for the infant. An energy intake of approximately 200 kcal/day over pregnancy needs (but usually no more than about 1800 kcal/day) meets the needs of most women during the first 6 months of lactation.

Coping with acute illness. Individuals with diabetes must have anticipatory teaching about how to cope with sick days (e.g., acute viral illnesses):

- Continue to take insulin or other hypoglycemic medications.
- Check blood glucose and urine ketones frequently, every 2 to 4 hours or as indicated.
- Drink enough fluid to replace losses and maintain hydration. When vomiting, diarrhea, or fever is present, small amounts of liquids every 15 to 30 minutes help to prevent dehydration, replace electrolyte losses, and provide energy.
- Consume approximately 45 to 50 g of carbohydrate (adults), or approximately three carbohydrate choices (Box 17-2) every 3 to 4 hours.
- Notify the health care provider if it is impossible to take and retain carbohydrate-containing foods and fluids for 4 hours or more, if blood glucose is difficult to control or ketonuria is present, if persistent diarrhea occurs, if severe abdominal pain is present, or if the illness lasts more than 24 hours.

Minimizing acute complications
Hypoglycemia. Hypoglycemia is most common in people treated with insulin but can also occur with oral hypoglycemic therapy.

Box 17-2   Foods and Fluids for Sick Days*

½ Cup (120 ml) regular gelatin dessert
½ Cup (120 ml) fat-free, light, or regular ice cream
½ Cup (120 ml) sherbet or sorbet
1 Frozen fruit juice bar
6 Saltine crackers
4 Slices Melba toast
1 Cup (240 ml) tomato, vegetable, chicken noodle, or cream soup
½ Cup (120 ml) sugar-free (or ¼ cup regular) pudding
¾ Cup (180 ml) regular ginger ale
½ Cup (120 ml) regular cola or lemon-lime soda
½ Cup (120 ml) orange juice

---

*Each serving provides approximately 15 g of carbohydrate.

Instruction should be planned to help the person (and significant others, as appropriate):

- Be aware of and avoid common precipitating factors: failing to eat regularly, vomiting or poor food intake during acute illness, prolonged or intense physical activity without a compensatory increase in carbohydrate intake or decrease in insulin dosage, alcohol intake, and use of medications that make hypoglycemic episodes more frequent or severe (Table 17-4).
- Recognize signs and symptoms of hypoglycemia: hunger, irritability, headache, shakiness, sweating, and altered neurologic status ranging from drowsiness to unconsciousness and convulsions. Repeated episodes of hypoglycemia can cause symptom unawareness. A previous episode of hypoglycemia also impairs the body's normal release of counterregulatory hormones such as epinephrine during subsequent episodes of hypoglycemia (Cryer, 2005). Recurrent hypoglycemia is to be avoided and the treatment plan may need to be adjusted if hypoglycemic episodes are common (ADA, 2008c).
- Test blood glucose regularly and any time signs of hypoglycemia occur.
- Correct hypoglycemia (blood glucose <70 mg/dl [<3.8 mmol/L]) if it occurs. If the person is conscious, approximately 15 to 20 g of glucose (available in a gel or in tablets) is the preferred treatment, but any carbohydrate that provides glucose can be used (ADA, 2008c). Fifteen grams of carbohydrate is found in 1.5 tbsp of raisins, 3 oz (90 ml) of apple juice, 3.3 oz (100 ml) of regular cola beverage, or 3 jellybeans or gumdrops. Fat can slow gastric emptying, and therefore consuming fat with the carbohydrate (e.g., a chocolate bar) may delay recovery from hypoglycemia. The blood glucose response to carbohydrate intake will vary, so blood sugar should be retested in 15 to 60 minutes and more carbohydrate should be consumed if blood sugar is still low (ADA, 2008b, 2008c). For the unconscious or convulsing individual, glucagon, 0.5 to 1 mg, will reverse hypoglycemia. Once conscious, the person should eat a carbohydrate-containing meal or large snack in order to avoid a repeated episode of hypoglycemia.
- Wear a Medic-Alert bracelet so that treatment can be given if the individual becomes confused or unconscious.

Table 17-4   Selected Drugs That Can Alter Glucose Control

	Indication/Use
Drugs That Can Cause or Contribute to Hyperglycemia	
Atypical antipsychotics (clozapine, olanzapine, risperidone)	Schizophrenia, psychosis
β-Adrenergic receptor agonists (e.g., albuterol, formoterol, salmeterol)	Bronchodilation, asthma
Glucocorticoids (e.g., dexamethasone, hydrocortisone, prednisolone, prednisone)	Adrenocortical deficiency, antiinflammatory, immune modifier
Niacin (pharmacologic doses)	Elevated serum triglycerides, low HDL cholesterol
Pentamidine (long-term effect)	Protozoal infection
Phenytoin	Seizures
Protease inhibitors (e.g., retinavir, nelfinavir, saquinavir)	HIV infection
Thiazide diuretics (e.g., chlorothiazide, hydrochlorothiazide)	Hypertension
Drugs That Can Cause or Contribute to Hypoglycemia	
Angiotensin-converting enzyme (ACE) inhibitors (e.g., captopril, enalapril, ramipril)	Hypertension
β-Adrenergic receptor antagonists (e.g., atenolol, propanolol, metoprolol)	Angina, cardiac dysrhythmia, hypertension
Ethanol	
Pentamidine (acute effect)	Protozoal infection
Salicylates (aspirin and aspirin-containing drugs)	Mild to moderate pain, fever, rheumatoid arthritis

Data from manufacturers' package inserts; drug monographs by Gold Standard Inc., 2007. Available at at www.accessmedicine.com. Accessed December 5, 2007.
HDL, High-density lipoprotein; *HIV,* human immunodeficiency virus.

Diabetic ketoacidosis. Diabetic ketoacidosis occurs primarily in individuals with type 1 diabetes. Instruction should include the following:

- Be aware of precipitating factors, such as acute infectious illnesses or failure to take the prescribed dosage of insulin or oral hypoglycemic agents.
- Continue to take insulin during acute illnesses.
- Recognize the signs and symptoms, such as elevated blood glucose, thirst, warm dry skin, nausea and vomiting, "fruity"-smelling breath, pain in abdomen, drowsiness, and polyuria.
- Check blood glucose if the symptoms occur, and obtain medical treatment if blood glucose is excessively elevated.

Hyperglycemic hyperosmolar nonketotic syndrome. HHNS is more common in the individual with type 2 diabetes. Instruction should include the following:

- Be aware of precipitating factors, such as infections or other stress.
- Recognize the symptoms, such as excessive thirst, polyuria, dehydration, shallow respirations, and altered sensorium.
- Check blood glucose if symptoms occur, and obtain medical attention if the blood glucose level is excessive.

Diabetic gastroparesis. **Gastroparesis**, or impaired gastric emptying, is a relatively common problem, perhaps related to neuropathy. The symptoms may include bloating, early satiety, nausea, and vomiting. Variability in gastric emptying may make glucose levels more labile and difficult to control. Metoclopramide and other prokinetic agents may be used to stimulate gastric emptying (Goldman and Ausiello, 2008). Medical nutrition therapy includes consumption of small, frequent meals, which may be better tolerated than large meals if early satiety is a problem. Food should be chewed thoroughly. People with gastroparesis are at risk for formation of gastric bezoars (hardened gastrointestinal contents, often containing food fibers), and individuals with very severe gastroparesis may find it necessary to decrease the intake of insoluble fiber (e.g., wheat bran, whole wheat, brown rice). Decreasing fat intake may be of benefit, since fat in the stomach slows gastric emptying. Maintaining an upright posture for at least 1 to 2 hours after a meal allows gravity to facilitate gastric emptying (Abell et al., 2006).

Celiac disease. Celiac disease, or gluten-sensitive enteropathy, is several times more likely to occur in individuals with type 1 diabetes as in the general population (Ludvigsson et al., 2006). Unexplained abdominal discomfort, diarrhea, and weight loss or poor growth occur in celiac disease. The diagnosis and medical nutrition therapy of this disorder are described in Chapter 11.

Eating disorders. Bulimia nervosa is more common among females with type 1 diabetes than in nondiabetic individuals (Mannucci et al., 2005). Skipping insulin doses and self-induced vomiting are two practices reported by young women with type 1 diabetes. Screening of individuals with diabetes for eating disorders should be part of the initial and ongoing assessment.

Conclusion

The prevalence of diabetes, particularly type 2 diabetes, is steadily increasing (CDC, 2007). The overweight and obese, people with a family history of type 2 diabetes, and women with GDM are particularly likely to develop type 2 diabetes. Lifestyle interventions, including a healthy diet, modest weight loss, and regular moderate to vigorous physical activity, hold promise for prevention of diabetes. Widespread public education about these interventions and public measures to promote physical activity and wise food choices are essential to promote adoption of these simple but effective measures.

REFERENCES

Abell TL et al: Treatment of gastroparesis: a multidisciplinary clinical review, *Neurogastroenterol Motil* 18(4):263, 2006.

Adult Treatment Panel (ATP) III: *Third report of the national cholesterol education program (NCEP) expert panel on detection, evaluation, and treatment of high blood cholesterol in adults (adult treatment panel III)*, Washington, DC, 2002, National Institutes of Health, National Heart, Lung and Blood Institute.

American Diabetes Association: Diagnosis and classification of diabetes mellitus, *Diabetes Care* 31(suppl 1):S55, 2008a.

American Diabetes Association: Gestational diabetes mellitus, *Diabetes Care* 27(suppl 1):88, 2004a.

American Diabetes Association: Nutrition recommendations and interventions for diabetes, *Diabetes Care* 31(suppl 1):S61, 2008b.

American Diabetes Association: Preconception care of women with diabetes, *Diabetes Care* 27(suppl 1):76S, 2004b.

American Diabetes Association: Standards of medical care in diabetes—2008, *Diabetes Care* 31(suppl 1):S12, 2008c.

American Diabetes Association, American Dietetic Association: *Choose your foods: exchange lists for diabetes*, Alexandria, Va, and Chicago, 2007, The Associations.

American Diabetes Association, American Dietetic Association: *Exchange lists for weight management*, Alexandria, Va, and Chicago, 2003, The Associations.

Ashwell SG et al: Improved glycaemic control with insulin glargine plus insulin lispro: a multicentre, randomized, cross-over trial in people with type 1 diabetes, *Diabet Med* 23(3):285, 2006.

Buse JB et al: Primary prevention of cardiovascular diseases in people with diabetes mellitus: a scientific statement from the American Heart Association and the American Diabetes Association, *Circulation* 115(1):114, 2007.

Cefalu WT, Waldman S, Ryder S: Pharmacotherapy for the treatment of patients with type 2 diabetes mellitus: rationale and specific agents, *Clin Pharmacol Ther* 81(5):636, 2007.

Centers for Disease Control and Prevention (CDC): Age-adjusted rates of current smoking, overweight, and obesity per 100 adults with diabetes, United States, 1994-2004. Available at http://www.cdc.gov/diabetes/statistics/comp/fig7_smoking.htm. Accessed December 3, 2007.

Cryer PE: Mechanisms of hypoglycemia-associated autonomic failure and its component syndromes in diabetes, *Diabetes* 54(12):3592, 2005.

Diabetes Control and Complications Trial/Epidemiology of Diabetes Interventions and Complications Study Research Group (DCCT/EDIC): Intensive diabetes treatment and cardiovascular disease in patients with type 1 diabetes, *N Engl J Med* 353(25):2643, 2005.

Foster-Powell K, Holt SH, Brand-Miller JC: International table of glycemic index and glycemic load values: 2002, *Am J Clin Nutr* 76(1):5, 2002.

Genuth S: Insights from the Diabetes Control and Complications Trial/Epidemiology of Diabetes Interventions and Complications study on the use of intensive glycemic treatment to reduce the risk of complications of type 1 diabetes, *Endocr Pract* 12(suppl 1):34, 2006.

Genuth S et al: Implications of the United Kingdom prospective diabetes study, *Diabetes Care* 26(suppl 1):S28, 2003.

Goldman L, Ausiello D, editors: *Cecil medicine,* ed 23, Philadelphia, 2008, Saunders.

Hermansen K, Mortensen LS: Bodyweight changes associated with antihyperglycaemic agents in type 2 diabetes mellitus, *Drug Saf* 30(12):1127, 2007.

Kitabchi AE, Nyenwe EA: Hyperglycemic crises in diabetes mellitus: diabetic ketoacidosis and hyperglycemic hyperosmolar state, *Endocrinol Metab Clin North Am* 35(4):725, 2006.

Knowler WC et al: Reduction in the incidence of type 2 diabetes with lifestyle intervention or metformin, *N Engl J Med* 346(6):393, 2002.

Krishnan S et al: Glycemic index, glycemic load, and cereal fiber intake and risk of type 2 diabetes in US black women, *Arch Intern Med* 167(21):2304, 2007.

Leahy JL: Pathogenesis of type 2 diabetes mellitus, *Arch Med Res* 36(3):197, 2005.

Lichtenstein AH et al: Diet and lifestyle recommendations revision 2006. a scientific statement from the American Heart Association Nutrition Committee, *Circulation* 114(1):82, 2006.

Lindström J et al: Sustained reduction in the incidence of type 2 diabetes by lifestyle intervention: follow-up of the Finnish Diabetes Prevention Study, *Lancet* 368(9548):1673, 2006.

Ludvigsson JF et al: Celiac disease and risk of subsequent type 1 diabetes: a general population cohort study of children and adolescents, *Diabetes Care* 29(11):2483, 2006.

Mannucci E et al: Eating disorders in patients with type 1 diabetes: a meta-analysis, *J Endocrinol Invest* 28(5):417, 2005.

McNay EC et al: Cognitive and neural hippocampal effects of long-term moderate recurrent hypoglycemia, *Diabetes* 55(4):1088, 2006.

Russell-Jones D, Kahn R: Insulin-associated weight gain in diabetes—causes, effects and coping strategies, *Diabetes Obes Metab* 9:799, 2007.

Tamborlane WV et al: The renaissance of insulin pump treatment in childhood type 1 diabetes, *Rev Endocr Metab Disord* 7(3):205, 2006.

Warshaw HS, Kulkarni K: *Complete guide to carb counting,* ed 2, Alexandria, Va, 2004, American Diabetes Association.

ALCOHOL-RELATED, MENTAL, AND NEUROLOGIC DISORDERS

Alcohol Abuse and Alcoholism

Alcohol abuse can be defined as heavy drinking with an increasing tolerance for ethanol but no withdrawal symptoms when drinking stops. **Alcoholism** refers to a strong craving for ethanol, associated with increasing tolerance to alcohol's intoxicating effects and symptoms of withdrawal when drinking is discontinued. Approximately two thirds of adults in the United States drink alcohol, with about 10% of those who drink or 7% of the total adult population reporting that they are heavy drinkers (NIAAA, 2007). Both genetic and environmental factors appear to contribute to development of alcoholism and alcohol abuse.

The effect of alcohol on body weight has been a controversial issue. Ethanol is energy rich, containing 7.1 kcal/g (Table 18-1). Approximately 75% of this energy in alcohol is usable when alcohol is metabolized by means of the alcohol dehydrogenase pathway, which is responsible for most ethanol metabolism when drinking is light to moderate. A second alcohol-metabolizing pathway, the microsomal ethanol oxidizing system (MEOS), is inducible, meaning that its activity increases with heavy drinking. Less than 50% of the energy contained in alcohol is available to the body when it is metabolized by means of the MEOS (Lieber, 2005). Heavy drinkers have been found to have lower body mass indexes (BMIs) than people who drank moderately (Suter, 2005; Kim et al., 2007). On the other hand, moderate drinking is associated with weight gain, particularly in people consuming a high-fat diet, those who are obese, and those with a family history of obesity (Suter, 2005).

Steatosis, or fatty liver, occurs in alcoholic liver disease because metabolism of alcohol through the alcohol dehydrogenase pathway favors increased formation and decreased metabolism of fatty acids. Alcohol metabolism by way of the MEOS generates oxidative stress. Together, the accumulation of fat in the liver and the oxidative

473

Table 18-1   Approximate Alcohol and Kilocalorie Content of Some Common Alcohol Beverages

Beverage and Serving Size	Alcohol (g/Serving)	kcal/Serving
Beer, Ale, and Malt Liquor		
Beer, 12 fl oz	13.5	153
Beer, light, 12 fl oz	11	103
Beer, no-alcohol, 12 fl oz	1.5	90
Malt liquor or ale, 12 fl oz	15	150
Cocktails		
Daiquiri, 2 fl oz	15	112
Martini, 2.3 fl oz	19	135
Piña colada, 4.5 fl oz	13	245
Whiskey sour, 3.5 fl oz	14	158
Distilled Spirits (Gin, Rum, Vodka, Whiskey), 1.5–fl oz Jigger		
80 proof	14	97
90 proof	16	110
100 proof	18	124
Wines		
Dessert, sweet, 3.5 fl oz	21	165
Red, 5 fl oz	15	127
White, 5 fl oz	13	172

Data from U.S. Department of Agriculture: *National nutrient database for standard reference, SR20*, Washington, DC, updated September 2007, The Department. Available at http://www.nal.usda.gov/fnic/foodcomp/search/. Accessed January 10, 2008. *fl oz*, Fluid ounce (approximately 30 ml).

stress lead to release of cytokines and inflammatory changes in the liver. These inflammatory changes stimulate fibrosis, or replacement of normal liver tissue with connective tissue, contributing to cirrhosis (Lieber, 2004). Alcohol liver disease occurs even among individuals with adequate diets (Lieber, 2004). In addition to fatty liver and cirrhosis, heavy alcohol use can contribute to metabolic complications such as hypoglycemia, lactic acidosis, hyperuricemia (contributing to gout), hypertriglyceridemia, and ketoacidosis.

Wernicke encephalopathy is an acute neuropsychiatric disorder resulting from thiamin deficiency that is relatively common among alcoholic individuals with inadequate diets. Signs and symptoms include abnormal ocular motility (ophthalmoplegia and nystagmus), ataxia, and mental status changes. Korsakoff syndrome, characterized by severe memory deficits, is a separate disorder but can occur along with Wernicke encephalopathy. Genetic susceptibility and environmental factors appear to contribute to the development of Wernicke-Korsakoff disease (Sechi and Serra, 2007).

Treatment

Comprehensive therapy for alcohol dependence includes individual or group counseling, usually involving family members and/or close friends, and a nutritious diet. Prolonged follow-up (e.g., through participation in a group such as Alcoholics Anonymous) is necessary for most recovering alcoholics. Disulfiram, naltrexone, and acamprosate are three drugs that are approved by the FDA for promotion of alcohol abstinence; they are most effective as adjuncts to psychologic treatment (Goldman and Ausiello, 2008). Benzodiazapines such as diazepam or lorazepam may be used to reduce alcohol withdrawal symptoms.

Nutrition Assessment and Care

A thorough nutrition assessment should be performed as described in Chapter 2. Box 18-1 highlights common or especially serious findings in alcohol abuse and alcoholism. Heavy alcohol use has adverse effects on nutrition because it may displace other, more nutritious, foods in the diet; alcoholics who develop cirrhosis of the liver consume about one half of their calories in the form of alcohol (Lieber, 2004). Not all alcoholics have inadequate diets, however. More affluent heavy drinkers may have dietary nutrient intakes that are very similar to those in moderate drinkers and abstainers (Bergheim et al., 2003). However, circulating concentrations of nutrients including retinol (vitamin A), carotenoids including lycopene and carotene, vitamin C, zinc, and selenium may be lower, suggesting a difference in metabolism in these nutrients (Bergheim et al., 2003).

Chronic alcohol abuse is associated with low levels of thiamin, niacin, pyridoxine, and vitamin B_{12}, as well as impaired utilization of folate and vitamins (Goldman and Ausiello, 2008). In addition, zinc levels may be low as a result of increased urinary excretion (Bergheim et al., 2005). Organ damage associated with alcohol abuse—including hepatitis, hepatic cirrhosis, and pancreatitis—interferes with absorption of fat, fat-soluble vitamins, and minerals

Box 18-1   Assessment in Alcohol Abuse and Alcoholism

Protein-Energy Malnutrition (PEM) or Protein-Calorie Malnutrition (PCM)

History

Inadequate intake or impaired absorption of nutrients related to chronic alcohol or other drug abuse; anorexia, nausea, or vomiting related to alcoholic liver disease

Physical examination

Hepatomegaly related to malnutrition and/or toxic effects of alcohol; ascites, edema; muscle wasting; triceps skinfold <5th percentile; BMI <18.5 (↓ body weight and BMI may be masked by presence of ascites and edema)

Laboratory analysis

↓ Serum albumin, transferrin, or prealbumin (↓ levels may indicate liver failure instead of or in addition to malnutrition); ↓ creatinine-height index

Overweight/Obesity

History

Excessive intake of energy from alcohol and dietary intake

Physical examination

BMI >25; triceps skinfold >95th percentile

Vitamin Deficiencies

B Complex, Especially B_1, B_6, Folate

History

Alcohol abuse; excessive ethanol or carbohydrate intake without adequate vitamins

Physical examination

Peripheral neuropathy; dermatitis; glossitis, cheilosis; edema, congestive heart failure; confusion, ataxia, nystagmus, memory loss

---

Box 18-1   Assessment in Alcohol Abuse and
Alcoholism—cont'd

Laboratory analysis

↓ Hct, ↑MCV, ↓ serum or RBC folate (NOTE: Laboratory assessment of vitamins B_1 and B_6 is rarely done; these vitamins have low toxicity; large doses are given, and response is evaluated clinically.)

(Lieber, 2004). Gastritis related to alcohol abuse may result in iron deficiency anemia from blood loss. Goals of medical nutrition therapy are to support the individual in avoiding alcohol and to correct nutritional deficits.

Intervention and education

Promoting hepatic regeneration and correcting nutritional deficits. The most important dietary change is abstinence from alcohol to allow the liver to heal. A nutritious diet adequate in energy, protein, and micronutrients can promote hepatic regeneration. The MyPyramid or Dietary Approaches to Stop Hypertension (DASH) diet plans (see Chapter 14) can be used in patient education. If esophageal varices are present, foods that are soft in texture reduce the risk of bleeding varices. Medical nutrition therapy of hepatitis, hepatic encephalopathy, and steatorrhea related to alcohol abuse is described in Chapter 11. If ascites are present, then a sodium restriction can help relieve the fluid retention (see Boxes 14-3 and 14-4).

In the severely malnourished alcoholic, especially if Wernicke encephalopathy or Korsakoff syndrome is suspected, thiamin is given initially in large doses (50 to 100 mg daily) (Goldman and Ausiello, 2008). Because toxicity of thiamin is generally low, blood testing for thiamin status (enzymes dependent on thiamin) is rarely done. Oral thiamin supplementation is usually given for a period of weeks to months, until cardiovascular and neurologic symptoms have resolved or it is clear there will be no further improvement. The other B vitamins (particularly folic acid and vitamin B_6), zinc, and magnesium are administered orally at dosages 2 to 3 times the Dietary Reference Intake (DRI) for several weeks to replenish the tissue stores of these nutrients. Vitamin A levels in the liver are likely to be low in alcoholic liver disease, but vitamin A should be given only cautiously, particularly if the patient has not stopped drinking. Vitamin A can be toxic, and alcohol increases the likelihood of toxicity in the liver (Lieber, 2004).

Disorders of Mental Health

Psychiatric disorders and their treatment can have important impacts on nutritional status. In the majority of instances, nutritional deficiencies have little or no role in causing psychiatric illness. One exception to this rule is the changes in mentation, depression, and psychoses that may occur in vitamin B_{12} deficiency.

Nutrition Assessment and Care

The goal of care is for the person to be able to cope with nutrition-related symptoms of mental health impairment and its therapy. Chapter 2 describes nutrition assessment in detail, and Box 18-2 outlines common nutritional considerations in the patient with disruptions of mental health.

Intervention and education. Nutrition plays an important supportive role in the care of the patient with a mental disorder. Some of the more common nutrition problems, along with diet and lifestyle approaches to their management, are summarized in Box 18-3.

Obesity is increasingly common among people with mental health disorders, as it is in the general population. This may be related to the disease itself (e.g., a decrease in activity in major depression) and also to medications prescribed. The "atypical" or second-generation antipsychotics in wide use are associated with weight gain, often substantial amounts (e.g., an average of 7.7 kg [16.9 lb] within 6 months in one trial) (Henderson, 2007) (Box 18-4). Additional side effects of these drugs include hyperlipidemia and hyperglycemia. Clozapine (Clozaril) and olanzapine (Zyprexa), in particular, have been associated with insulin resistance and development of type 2 diabetes, whereas metabolic side effects and weight gain are less common with newer drugs, such as risperidone (Risperdal) and aripiprazole (Abilify) (Henderson, 2007). Patients taking atypical antipsychotics can benefit from anticipatory guidance regarding the need to increase physical activity and reduce energy intake to reduce weight gain (Milano et al., 2007).

Box 18-2   Assessment of Common Nutrition-Related
Problems in Neural and Mental Health Disorders

Constipation

Possibly Related to:

- Decreased physical activity
- Medications such as quetiapine (Seroquel) and other atypical antipsychotics; imipramine (Tofranil) and other tricyclic antidepressants; benztropine (Cogentin), trihexyphenidyl (Artane), and other anticholinergics

Evidenced by:

- Infrequent bowel movements and passage of hard, dry stool

Decreased Bone Mineral Density

Possibly Related to:

- Use of SSRIs, which may alter bone metabolism
- Decreased physical activity related to depression or drowsiness from medications
- Weight loss because of anorexia
- Chronic disease contributing to both depression and bone mineral loss, e.g., diabetes, CKD, COPD
- Smoking or heavy alcohol use
- Diet inadequate in vitamin D and/or calcium because of avoidance of dairy products
- Inadequate sun exposure for vitamin D formation because of far northern or southern latitude, little time outside, use of suncreen, covering of skin with clothing, and/or dark skin pigmentation
- Bone mineral loss caused by corticosteroid therapy

Evidenced by:

- DEXA or equivalent testing

Hyperlipidemia and/or Hyperglycemia

Possibly Related to:

- Use of atypical antipsychotics with exacerbation of insulin resistance and the metabolic syndrome
- Overweight or obesity
- Ketogenic diet

Continued

Box 18-2   Assessment of Common Nutrition-Related Problems in Neural and Mental Health Disorders—cont'd

Evidenced by:

- ↑ Serum total cholesterol, LDL cholesterol, and/or triglycerides; ↓ HDL cholesterol; ↑ fasting or postprandial plasma glucose

Overweight or Obesity

Possibly Related to:

- Use of atypical antipsychotics
- Sedentary lifestyle; decreased activity related to depression or drowsiness from medications
- Excessive intake of kcal-containing beverages related to dry mouth (side effect of anticholinergic and some antipsychotic medications)

Evidenced by:

- BMI >25 (adults) or >85th percentile for age and gender (children), triceps skinfold >85th percentile for age and gender

Underweight or Weight Loss

Possibly Related to:

- Inadequate intake caused by:
  - Restricted or unpalatable diet (e.g., ketogenic diet)
  - Dysphagia or other feeding/swallowing difficulties, delayed gastric emptying with tricyclic antidepressants, severe constipation
  - Inadequate intake caused by tremors or poor coordination with difficulty feeding self
  - Dementia or memory loss (refusing or forgetting to eat)
  - Medications causing anorexia or weight loss, e.g., topiramate (Topamax), bupropion (Wellbutrin)

Evidenced by:

- Unplanned weight loss of ≥10% in 6 months or 5% in 1 month
- BMI <18.5 (adults) or <5th percentile for age and gender (children)
- ↓ Serum albumin, transferrin, or prealbumin if protein-calorie malnutrition is present (may also be caused by alcoholic or other liver disease)

Box 18-2   Assessment of Common Nutrition-Related Problems in Neural and Mental Health Disorders—cont'd

Vitamin B$_{12}$ Deficit

Possibly Related to:

- Inadequate intake from avoidance of animal products because of strict vegetarian diet, poverty, difficulty chewing or dysphagia, etc.
- Age-related decrease in gastric acid and/or intrinsic factor production or autoimmune destruction of intrinsic factor–producing cells (pernicious anemia)
- Inadequate pancreatic enzymes for removal of R protein attached to vitamin B$_{12}$ because of pancreatitis
- Inadequate absorption related to ileal disease or resection
- Inactivation of vitamin B$_{12}$ related to nitrous oxide exposure during dental or surgical procedures or recreational use (abuse) (Singer et al., 2008)

Evidenced by:

- Numerous possible signs and symptoms including but not limited to loss of position sense, ataxia, loss of bladder and bowel control, optic neuritis, dementia, psychoses, mood disturbances
- Macrocytic (megaloblastic) anemia with ↑ MCV and ↑ methylmalonic acid concentrations

BMI, Body mass index; *CKD,* chronic kidney disease; *COPD,* chronic obstructive pulmonary disease; *DEXA (or DXA),* dual energy x-ray absorptiometry; *HDL,* high-density lipoprotein; *LDL,* low-density lipoprotein; *MCV,* mean corpuscular volume; *SSRIs,* selective serotonin reuptake inhibitors, e.g., fluoxetine (Prozac), sertraline (Zoloft), and escitalopram (Lexapro).

A decrease in bone mineral density and vulnerability to fractures are prevalent among individuals with depression. This may be related to treatment with selective serotonin reuptake inhibitors (SSRIs) (Diem et al., 2007b; Haney et al., 2007). It has also been suggested that depression itself, perhaps by altering the body's hormonal environment, might contribute to bone loss (Sogaard et al., 2005; Diem et al., 2007a). Moderately intense weight-bearing exercise most days of the week and a diet adequate in calcium and vitamin D (see Appendix B on Evolve) can help to reduce bone loss.

Box 18-3   Diet and Lifestyle Approaches to Common
Nutrition Problems in Patients with Neuropsychiatric
Disorders

Constipation

- Increase intake of fiber-containing foods.
  - Bran, whole-grain cereals and breads, legumes, vegetables, and fresh and dried fruits are good sources (see Appendix C on Evolve).
  - Set a goal of 30 g fiber or more daily.
  - Use fiber-containing formulas if enteral tube feedings are necessary.
- Maintain a liberal fluid intake (30 to 50 ml/kg [14 to 23 ml/lb] for adults, unless contraindicated) to encourage formation of soft, bulky stools.
- Consume dried plums (prunes) or prune juice regularly for the natural laxative properties.
- Participate in regular physical activity (preferably at least 30 minutes daily) as tolerated to stimulate gastrointestinal motility.

Decreased Bone Mineral Density

- Participate in daily weight-bearing exercise.
- If underweight, consume small, frequent meals and snacks of energy-dense foods or use balanced liquid supplements between meals.
- Stop smoking.
- Consume alcohol moderately if at all (no more than 1 drink daily for women or 2 for men) (Sampson, 2002).
- Consume adequate vitamin D and calcium through dietary intake or use of appropriate supplements.

Dysphagia or Difficulty Swallowing

- Try thickened liquids. Thin liquids such as water, coffee, or tea are often among the most difficult items to swallow.
  - Shakes, commercial supplements (see Table 8-1), or beverages thickened with infant cereals, cornstarch, or instant potatoes may be easier to swallow.
  - Sherbet, sorbet, fruit ices, and frozen yogurt or ice cream can be used to supply some of the individual's fluid needs if they do not result in excessive energy intake.

Box 18-3   Diet and Lifestyle Approaches to Common
Nutrition Problems in Patients with Neuropsychiatric
Disorders—cont'd

- Commercial thickened water, coffee, and juices, as well as thickeners to be added to regular foods and beverages, are available (Hormel HealthLabs, Novartis Nutrition); different levels of thickening can be achieved, depending on the patient's needs.
- Avoid dry, hard foods.
  - Use soft, moist foods such as casseroles, meats and vegetables with gravies and sauces, mashed potatoes, applesauce, and cooked cereals.
- Avoid slick foods such as gelatin or pasta salad if these appear to cause difficulty.
- Maintain an upright position during and for at least 30 minutes after meals.
- Keep the chin positioned slightly downward.
- Consult speech or physical therapists for suggestions on techniques to improve swallowing effectiveness.
- Do not rush while eating.
- Avoid eating alone, if possible.
- Consider percutaneous endoscopic gastrostomy (PEG) or other enteral tube feeding techniques if necessary to deliver nutrients safely.

Overweight and Obesity

- Participate in moderate to vigorous physical activity for 30 to 60 minutes or more daily at least 5 days per week if possible.
- Decrease energy intake (about 500 kcal less than usual daily intake); choose low-energy but nutrient-rich foods for meals and snacks: increase intake of raw or lightly cooked vegetables, fruits, skim and low-fat milk products, and whole grains; decrease intake of fatty foods, whole milk and milk products made with whole milk or cream, and typical dessert and snack items.
- Drink water or chew sugar-free gum, rather than drinking sugared or other high-calorie beverages, to relieve dry mouth.

Continued

Box 18-3   Diet and Lifestyle Approaches to Common Nutrition Problems in Patients with Neuropsychiatric Disorders—cont'd

Underweight

- Consume small, frequent meals and snacks.
- Drink kcal-containing beverages, such as milk or juice, rather than plain water most of the time.
- Choose kcal-dense foods in place of those lower in energy, e.g., fruit yogurt rather than a rice cake for a snack, marinated bean salad rather than leafy greens.

Box 18-4   Drugs Frequently Associated with Weight Gain

Atypical Antipsychotics

Clozapine (Clozaril)*
Olanzapine (Zyprexa)*
Quetiapine (Seroquel)
Risperidone (Risperdal)
Ziprasidone (Geodon)
Aripiprazole (Abilify)

Antimania and/or Anticonvulsants

Divalproex/valproic acid (Depakote, Depakene)
Lithium (Eskalith)
Gabapentin (Neurontin)
Carbamazepine (Tegretol)

Antidepressants

Mirtazapine (Remeron)*
Amitriptyline (Elavil, Tryptanol)
Imipramine (Tofranil)
Nortriptyline (Aventyl)
Desipramine (Norpramin)

Data from manufacturers' package inserts and Gold Standard Inc., 2007. Available at www.accessmedicine.com. Accessed December 5, 2007.
*Especially likely to cause weight gain. Within groups, drugs are ordered top to bottom according to the approximate likelihood and amount of weight gain expected.

Neurologic Disorders
Seizure Disorders

Numerous types of seizure disorders (generally referred to as epilepsy) occur. Partial seizures affect only one cerebral hemisphere so that consciousness is maintained but some cognitive functions such as speech are transiently lost. Generalized seizures affect the brain as a whole, and consciousness is lost, but the loss of consciousness may be so brief that it is barely noticeable. Signs of seizure disorders range from subtle (a blank stare or a brief twitching of the mouth or eyelids) to severe (tonic-clonic seizures, with alternate sustained contraction and relaxation of the muscles). Seizure disorders may occur as a result of hypoxia or central nervous system trauma, stroke, neoplasms, infections, congenital disorders, and degenerative diseases such as Alzheimer. A variety of metabolic disorders (hypoglycemia, hypocalcemia, hypomagnesemia, medication side effects) can cause seizures; in these cases, correcting the underlying disorder is the primary treatment. A significant percentage of convulsive disorders are idiopathic, with no known cause (Goldman and Ausiello, 2008).

Treatment

Correction of the cause of the seizures (e.g., hypoglycemia) is the primary intervention, if possible. For seizures where this is not possible, anticonvulsant medications are the major means of treatment. Anticonvulsants used include carbamazepine (Tegretol, Carbatrol, and others), hydantoins (phenytoin [Dilantin]), ethosuximide (Zarontin), valproic acid (Depakene, etc.), benzodizapines (clonazepam [Klonopin]), phenobarbital, the γ-aminobutyric acid (GABA) receptor agonist gabapentin (Neurontin), lamotrigine (Lamictal), levetiracetam (Keppra), and topiramate (Topamax). For patients who are inadequately controlled by medications, surgery to remove the cerebral region involved with the seizures, if it can be identified, can be curative. Electrical stimulation of the vagus nerve in the neck has also been effective in some cases (Goldman and Ausiello, 2008).

Nutrition assessment and care

Chapter 2 describes nutrition assessment in detail, and common assessment findings in seizure disorders are summarized in Box 18-2. Long-term use of anticonvulsant medications increases the risk of drug-nutrient interactions and may impair nutritional status.

Intervention and education

Anticonvulsant medications. Many commonly used anticonvulsants—including phenytoin, phenobarbital, and primidone—accelerate the turnover of vitamin D and can contribute to poor bone mineralization (osteomalacia). Intake of the anticonvulsants and calcium at the same time impairs the absorption of both the drug and the nutrient. Vitamin D and calcium supplements may be needed by people who take these medications, but they should not be taken at the same time as the medications.

Ketogenic diet. High levels of blood ketones produced from the metabolism of fat appear to decrease seizure activity. A diet that stimulates ketone production (a **ketogenic diet**, generally 80% of energy from fat, 15% from protein, and 5% from carbohydrate) is used by selected individuals who exhibit a poor response to anticonvulsant medications. Nearly 30% of children on the diet were found to be free of seizures or have at least a 90% reduction in seizures, and many were able to discontinue or reduce use of medications (Freeman et al., 2007a). The high fat intake is unpalatable to some individuals, and the strict diet can be a burden. Potential side effects include uric acid kidney stones and hypocalcemia. In addition, the diet can result in poor growth, especially in young children, who must be especially carefully monitored for growth delays. Hypercholesterolemia is common, and there is a concern about promotion of arteriosclerotic heart disease. Soft (tub or squeeze bottle) margarine and polyunsaturated and monounsaturated oils, such as corn, soybean, safflower, sunflower, canola, and olive oil, can be substituted for butter and cream if serum cholesterol becomes excessive. The ketogenic diet is contraindicated in a few metabolic disorders involving fat metabolism, such as pyruvate-carboxylase deficiency, defects of fatty acid oxidation, and carnitine deficiency (Kossoff, 2004).

In the classic diet the ratio of dietary fat to the combined carbohydrate and protein intake is between 3:1 and 4:1 (3 to 4 g of fat for every gram of carbohydrate plus protein). The diet commonly includes a protein allowance of 1.2 g/kg desirable body weight for children under 2 years of age and 1 g for children between 2 and 19 years. To promote ketosis, energy intake is limited to approximately 75 kcal/kg/day for children ages 1 to 3 years, 68 kcal/kg/day for children ages 4 to 6 years, and 60 kcal/kg/day for children ages 7 to 10 years. (For more information, consult Freeman et al., [2007b].) A downloadable ketogenic diet meal planner is available at www.stanford.edu/group/ketodiet. The ketogenic diet is usually low in vitamins C, A, and B complex and in iron, zinc, and calcium. A daily supplement providing the DRI for the person's age is advisable. Many medications, including vitamin and mineral supplements, contain carbohydrates, which must be considered in calculating the diet; see McGhee and Katyal (2001) for a compilation.

Traditionally, fluids are restricted to approximately 600 to 1200 ml/day, with no more than 120 ml taken in a 2-hour period, to prevent expansion of plasma volume with dilution of the ketones. It is not clear that this is necessary, and a more liberal fluid allowance might reduce the risk of kidney stones (Freeman et al., 2007a).

The Atkins diet for weight reduction can also cause ketosis and is less restrictive, containing approximately 60% fat, 30% protein, and 10% fat, making it possible for the individual to eat away from home, e.g., at a school cafeteria. Its use in seizure disorders is under study (Freeman et al., 2007a).

Cerebral Palsy

Cerebral palsy (CP) is a disability characterized by motor incoordination that results from a problem in early brain development (Behrman et al., 2004). CP is often associated with developmental, speech, cognitive, visual, and hearing defects. Children with the disorder may display spastic symptoms (hypertonic muscles with jerky movements) or athetoid symptoms (hypotonic infants that may become increasingly rigid with age) (Behrman et al., 2004).

Treatment

Physical therapy and judicious use of devices such as computers that make communication by nonverbal individuals possible can help people with CP achieve their maximum potential. Dantrolene sodium (Dantrium), the benzodiazepines (e.g., Valium, Ativan), and baclofen (Lioresal) have been used to treat spasticity. For severe spasticity, surgical procedures for muscle release or lengthening can be used to relieve contractures and improve movement. Botulinum toxin injections have also been used to relieve spasticity (Behrman et al., 2004).

Nutrition assessment and care

Chapter 2 describes nutrition assessment in detail, and common assessment findings in cerebral palsy are summarized in Box 18-2. Goals of care are to maintain adequate intake of nutrients and to prevent obesity, which further impairs mobility in individuals with CP.

Intervention and education
Chewing and swallowing problems. Provision of adequate nutrients may be difficult because of neuromuscular impairments and persistence of primitive reflexes. To minimize these problems, follow these guidelines:

- Individuals with CP should be placed in good anatomic position for feeding. Those with spastic CP are especially likely to hyperextend their necks, which makes swallowing difficult. Positioning them with back straight and hips and knees flexed reduces hyperextension. Separating the legs promotes stability.
- Underweight is a common problem, largely because of difficulty ingesting food. Athetoid CP, in particular, may be associated with a tongue thrust that pushes food out of the mouth (Behrman et al., 2004). Parents and caregivers may spend hours daily feeding an individual with CP. Because of the prolonged mealtimes, provision of snacks is often not effective in increasing intake. Thus increasing the energy content of foods eaten at mealtimes is the best alternative. Skim milk powder, margarine, oils, or modular ingredients (see Chapter 8) can be added to foods to increase energy density. Gastrostomy feedings are beneficial for many children who cannot eat enough to maintain their nutritional status and obtain adequate nutrients to support growth (Samson-Fang et al., 2003; Sullivan et al., 2005).
- Additional suggestions can be found in Box 18-3.

Promoting self-feeding. To make it easier for people with CP to feed themselves, follow these suggestions:

- Use plates with rims to allow food to be scooped up by pushing it against the rim.
- Use specially made silverware with thick handles or insert the spoon or fork handle into a rolled washcloth to make it easier to grip (van Roon and Steenbergen, 2006).
- Prevent scooting of plates or bowls by putting suction cups, such as those used for soap holders, under them.

Preventing or correcting obesity. Individuals who are very inactive, such as those with severe motor impairments who use a wheelchair, may become overweight or obese. The following guidelines help to prevent or alleviate this problem:

- Try reducing fat in the diet. Choose lean meat and skinless poultry; use skim or low-fat milk and dairy products made with skim or low-fat milk; limit intake of fried or fatty foods; serve pastries, doughnuts, and high-fat cookies and cakes rarely; use butter or margarine sparingly; use low-fat or fat-free salad dressings.
- Serve unsweetened beverages or those sweetened with sugar substitutes. Beverages consumed before or with meals help the person feel full faster.
- Increase intake of whole grains and fresh fruits and vegetables, which are bulky and help the individual to feel full more quickly.
- If gastrostomy feedings are used, assess weight gain and fat mass regularly because it is easy to overfeed individuals with CP, which makes the role of the caregiver much more difficult (Sullivan et al., 2006).
- Increase activity to the extent possible, encouraging activities that improve both cardiorespiratory fitness and muscular strength (Fowler et al., 2007).

Preventing or correcting constipation. See Box 18-3 for measures to relieve constipation.

Amyotrophic Lateral Sclerosis

Amyotrophic lateral sclerosis (ALS) is a progressive degenerative neurologic disease that results in atrophy of the muscles. Bulbar signs (difficulty chewing, swallowing, and speaking) may be among the earliest signs, or they may occur concomitant with weakness of the extremities and trunk muscles (Goldman and Ausiello, 2008).

Treatment

Although there is no cure for ALS, riluzole (Rilutek), a neuroprotective drug, extends survival or delays the time until tracheotomy is needed. This drug has numerous gastrointestinal side effects, including nausea, vomiting, dyspepsia, anorexia, and diarrhea. Physical therapy can help maintain as much muscle mass as possible as the disease progresses. A multidisciplinary approach is invaluable in dealing with the many problems involved in care, including depression, excessive drooling, dysphagia, and respiratory difficulties. A speech therapist can assist with interpretation of barium swallow testing and determination of the time when it may be unsafe to feed the patient orally.

Nutrition assessment and care

Chapter 2 describes nutrition assessment in detail, and common assessment findings in ALS are summarized in Box 18-2. Weight loss is inevitable because of muscle wasting. Nutritional deficits, however, accelerate loss. When weight loss in 6 months is greater than 10% of the usual body weight, energy deficits should be suspected. Chair or bed scales are often necessary to obtain weights. BMI may not be very useful in people with ALS because of the effects of muscle wasting on their body composition. Bioelectrical impedance has been used to assess lean body mass in individuals with ALS. Goals of care are to prevent nutritional deficits and maintain feeding safety, i.e., prevent choking or pulmonary aspiration.

Intervention and education.   These measures can assist the person with ALS and caregivers in maintaining an adequate diet:

- Small, frequent feedings are less tiring than a few larger meals.
- Eating utensils with enlarged handles or with loops to fit over the hands reduce dropping of utensils.
- Protein foods may be difficult to chew, especially if dry. Good protein sources are tender, chopped meats and poultry; moist casseroles made with meat, fish, or poultry; cheese and cottage cheese; yogurt; and poached, soft-cooked, or scrambled eggs. Gravies and sauces served with meats make chewing and swallowing easier.
- Commercial supplements (high-protein puddings and beverages and/or modular ingredients to be added to other foods) can be used if intake from a diet of regular foods is inadequate.
- Box 18-3 includes suggestions for dealing with dysphagia. Many individuals with ALS require gastrostomy feedings when their swallowing ability deteriorates to the point that pulmonary aspiration is very likely.
- Inactivity and muscle weakness contribute to constipation. See Box 18-3 for measures to address this problem.

Multiple Sclerosis

Multiple sclerosis (MS), a disease of the central nervous system, affects the myelinated nerve fibers and the muscles they innervate. Patches of the myelin surrounding the nerves degenerate, and the myelin is replaced by scars. The course of MS is described as relapsing remitting (with exacerbations followed by full or partial remission of symptoms), secondary progressive (beginning with the relapsing remitting form of the disorder, followed in 20 to 40 years by at least 6 months of progressive worsening with no remission), and primary progressive (in which there is progressive worsening over at least 1 year with no sign of remission). The cause is not known, although autoimmunity, infectious triggers, environmental factors, and genetic predisposition have all been suggested to play a role (Goldman and Ausiello, 2008).

Treatment

Although there is no cure for MS, immunomodulators, such as interferon beta-1a and -1b (Avonex, Rebif, Betaserone), and immunosuppressives, such as glatiramer acetate (Copaxone), are used to reduce the likelihood of acute exacerbations of the disease. Steroids are frequently used for their antiinflammatory properties in acute exacerbations of the disease. Mitoxantrone (Novantrone), an antineoplastic agent, improves neurologic function and reduces relapses in selected patients with secondary (chronic) progressive, progressive relapsing, or worsening relapsing remitting forms of the disease (Goldman and Ausiello, 2008). These drugs may have nutritional impacts, such as nausea, vomiting, diarrhea, and stomatitis. Natalizumab, a monoclonal antibody, is approved for use in carefully selected patients under close supervision. Numerous medications are used for palliation of symptoms. Muscle spasms are a common problem that may be alleviated by baclofen or tizanidine (Zanaflex). Stretching exercises and physical therapy may be beneficial. Urinary retention, which contributes to urinary tract infections, is another frequently encountered symptom, which can be treated with anticholinergic agents, such as oxybutynin (Ditropan) or propantheline (Pro-Banthine). Pain and paroxysmal spasms may be treated with anticonvulsants, such as gabapentin (Gabarone), pregabalin (Lyrica), or carbamazepine (Tegretol), or tricyclic antidepressants, such as amitriptyline (Elavil). Even small increases in environmental temperature may worsen symptoms, and thus cool showers or air conditioning may be effective in promoting comfort (Goldman and Ausiello, 2008).

Nutrition assessment and care

Chapter 2 describes nutrition assessment in detail, and common assessment findings in MS are summarized in Box 18-2.

Intervention and education

Fat and micronutrient intake. Many individuals with MS use complementary and alternative treatments for treatment of MS or relief of the symptoms associated with it. Epidemiologic data suggest that diets high in saturated fat and low in vitamin D are associated with development of MS. Therefore increasing polyunsaturated fatty acid (PUFA) intake and using vitamin D supplements are popular therapies. A meta-analysis of studies of PUFA supplementation in MS (either omega-3 fatty acids, such as in fish oils, or omega-6 fatty acids from plant sources) determined that it had no major effect on disease progression (Farinotti et al., 2007). The same meta-analysis indicated that it was impossible to separate the effects of vitamin D from other interventions in the clinical trials available to date (Farinotti et al., 2007). The Swank diet, a very–low-fat diet supplemented with vegetable and cod liver oil, has been recommended for MS, but no randomized, controlled trials of this regimen have been done (Schwarz and Leweling, 2005).

Many individuals with MS take antioxidant supplements such as vitamins E and C and selenium, since some data suggest that oxidative stress contributes to development of MS (Schwarz and Leweling, 2005). Evidence is insufficient that antioxidant intake improves symptoms (Schwarz and Leweling, 2005), but a diet rich in antioxidant micronutrients is generally rich in other nutrients as well, and thus it can be encouraged. A supplement providing the DRI for antioxidants is unlikely to cause harm, but large doses of micronutrients do not offer any known advantage and could have toxicity.

Constipation. Constipation is reported by more than 30% of people with MS (Goldman and Ausiello, 2008). Generalized muscle weakness, immobility, low fiber intake, and constipating medications probably are etiologic factors. Measures to help prevent or correct constipation can be found in Box 18-3.

Osteoporosis. Osteoporosis is common among individuals with MS, and a diet adequate in calcium and vitamin D is needed to reduce the risk (Schwarz and Leweling, 2005).

Parkinsonism (Parkinson Disease)

Parkinsonism is a progressive neuromuscular disorder characterized by a low content of dopamine in the basal ganglia of the central nervous system. This results in tremor, rigidity, a characteristic "pill rolling" movement of the fingers, and hypoactivity. The cause is not known, but it has been speculated that oxidative damage from free radicals in the central nervous system may be involved. Two genes have been linked to parkinsonism, and it has been suggested that there is a genetic-environmental cause for this disorder—that is, a genetic susceptibility to develop the disease on exposure to environmental factors, which might include toxins, smoking, or head trauma.

Treatment

The monoamine oxidase inhibitor (MAOI) selegiline (Carbex) may have a neuroprotective effect. Dopamine receptor agonists, such as pramipexole (Mirapex), ropinirole (Requip), and pergolide (Permax), may be used to increase central nervous system dopamine activity, but they can cause sleepiness and increase impulse control disorders, such as compulsive gambling and shopping. Levodopa (Larodopa), a precursor of dopamine, or a combination of levodopa and carbidopa (Sinemet) is used to treat parkinsonism when the other drugs no longer control the symptoms. However, levodopa becomes less effective over time. Use of the MAOI rasagiline (Azilect) or entacapone (Comtan, an inhibitor of the primary enzyme that metabolizes dopamine) improves the effectiveness of levodopa therapy. Common nutrition-related side effects of levodopa and the drugs used as adjuncts to it are nausea, vomiting, anorexia, and dry mouth. Anticholinergic agents, such as procyclidine (Kemadrin), benztropine mesylate (Cogentin), and trihexyphenidyl (Artane), may relieve excessive salivation and reduce the rigidity associated with the disease. The anticholinergics can cause the mouth to be excessively dry, increasing feeding problems; taking these drugs after meals may reduce difficulties in chewing and swallowing (Goldman and Ausiello, 2008).

Nutrition assessment and care

Chapter 2 describes nutrition assessment in detail, and common assessment findings in parkinsonism are summarized in Box 18-2. People with Parkinson disease may experience weight loss because the tremors and involuntary movements increase energy expenditure and may make it difficult for them to feed themselves adequately. Parkinson disease may also impair the ability to swallow, interfering with intake of foods and beverages. In addition, levodopa has significant drug-nutrient interactions that must be understood to maximize the benefits of the medication.

Intervention and education
Preventing or correcting weight loss

- Monitor weight regularly.
- If tremor is pronounced, choose foods that are easy to get to the mouth (sandwiches and other foods eaten with the hands, or foods that can be impaled with a fork such as chunks of fruit or vegetables). Soups or other foods that must be balanced on a utensil are difficult and embarrassing for the person with a tremor to consume.
- Keep foods warm and palatable for slow eaters by using insulated dishes or a warming tray.
- Avoid interruptions (e.g., medication administration) during meals and snacks. Any distraction can cause the elderly person with parkinsonism to lose focus on eating and have difficulty starting again.
- Plate guards (high rims around the plate) may be needed to help affected people scoop up food and bring it to their mouths.
- Avoid especially tough, hard, and chewy foods.

Optimizing drug therapy

- Take levodopa at least 30 minutes before or 60 minutes after a meal. If the drug causes nausea, it can be taken with a small, low-protein snack, such as a cracker. Food, particularly protein, consumed at the same time as levodopa impairs its action. Nausea usually diminishes as the person adjusts to the drug, and it can then be taken on an empty stomach.
- Avoid taking iron supplements at the same time as levodopa, because iron can impair levodopa absorption.
- After several years of levodopa therapy, individuals may become less responsive to the drug. If this occurs, the first step should be to assess protein intake. The North American diet often includes twice the DRI for protein, which may reduce effectiveness of levodopa. It may be necessary to change the diet pattern to improve the drug action:

- If protein intake is high, reduce it to no more than the DRI (see Appendix A on Evolve). Meat, fish, and poultry servings should total no more than approximately 5 or 6 oz/day. (Three oz is approximately the size of a deck of cards.) Two or three servings of milk products will provide most of the remaining protein.

Constipation. The disease itself or medications used may result in constipation. Consult Box 18-3 for measures to relieve constipation.

Stroke

Stroke, or cerebrovascular accident, refers to neurologic symptoms resulting from the interruption of blood flow to the brain. Stroke can result from ischemia (diminished blood flow usually related to blood vessel occlusion; about 85% of strokes) or hemorrhage (subarachnoid or intracerebral). Symptoms vary, depending on the extent and location of the stroke. Some individuals experience hemiplegia, or paralysis of one side of the body; visual field defects (e.g., hemianopia, or failure to see half of the visual field); apraxia (inability to perform a known task in response to verbal instructions); and dysphagia. Cerebral edema, increasing the intracranial pressure and damage to the brain, can develop with all types of stroke (Goldman and Ausiello, 2008).

Treatment

Pharmacologic therapy is aimed at decreasing or preventing extension of the damage. Use of recombinant tissue plasminogen activator (rt-PA) or another thrombolytic agent within 3 hours of the stroke has been effective in minimizing the effect of ischemic stroke. Steroids or osmotic agents such as mannitol may be used to reduce cerebral edema. Blood pressure is cautiously reduced if high, to avoid reducing cerebral circulation further (Goldman and Ausiello, 2008).

Nutrition assessment and care

Assessment is summarized in Box 18-2. The extent and location of the stroke will determine the severity and exact type of problems experienced. Thorough assessment to provide the basis for an individualized plan of care is thus essential.

Intervention and education
Prevention of stroke. Avoiding hypertension is an important measure in reducing the risk of stroke. Maintaining or achieving a

healthy body weight, participating in moderately vigorous physical activity for 30 minutes or more almost every day, avoiding excessive alcohol intake, ceasing smoking (if applicable), and consuming a low to moderate sodium intake reduce the likelihood of high blood pressure (Goldstein et al., 2006).

Epidemiologic evidence indicates that the risk of stroke, particularly in people with hypertension, is lessened by a diet rich in potassium, magnesium, calcium, and fiber (Ding and Mozaffarian, 2006). Also, high blood levels of the amino acid homocysteine have been found to be predictors of cardiovascular diseases, including stroke, and homocysteine concentrations have been found to be lowest in people with the highest serum concentrations of folic acid, vitamin B_6, and vitamin B_{12} (Selhub, 2006). There is little evidence that any of these nutrients by themselves (i.e., taken in the form of a supplement) would aid in prevention of strokes. It may be that they are simply markers of a nutritious diet and a healthful lifestyle. It appears, however, that a diet rich in fruits and vegetables and whole grains—which would provide good sources of fiber, minerals, folate, and other B vitamins—might reduce the likelihood of stroke (Goldstein et al., 2006).

Coping with feeding difficulties after stroke
Hemiplegia

- Anticipate more difficulty in self-feeding if the dominant hand is affected.
- Provide unobtrusive help in opening packages of utensils or condiments, cutting or buttering foods, or feeding the person, if necessary.
- Check for "pocketing" of food in the cheek on the affected side during meals, which occurs because the individual cannot sense that the food is there.
- Provide good mouth care after meals. Teach the patient or home caregivers to do this before discharge.

Visual field defects. The individual may fail to eat half the food on the tray because of not seeing it. Teach the individual to compensate by scanning, or routinely turning the head and moving the eyes toward the affected side.

Dysphagia. Muscle weakness or incoordination, impaired gag or swallowing reflexes, and impaired cough contribute to dysphagia.

Dysphagia in turn reduces the adequacy of nutrient intake and increases the likelihood of pulmonary aspiration (see Box 18-3).

Alzheimer Disease and Dementia

Alzheimer disease (AD) is the most common cause of dementia, or progressive loss of mental function because of an organic cause. The cause is not definitely known, but the most common findings in the brains of individuals with AD are cerebral atrophy, senile plaques, and neurofibrillary tangles, as well as low levels of the neurotransmitter acetylcholine. Genetic factors are believed to be involved in many cases of AD. Oxidative damage to the neurons has also been suggested as a likely cause. Affected people experience memory loss, shortened attention span, expressive and receptive language disorders, apraxia (inability to perform a task in response to verbal commands), loss of reasoning skills, and intolerance of frustration (Goldman and Ausiello, 2008).

Treatment

A cure for AD is unavailable at this time, but some medications can improve symptoms. Cholinesterase inhibitors, such as donepezil (Aricept), rivastigmine (Exelon), galantamine (Razadyne), and memantine (Namenda), can help to improve behavior and memory in some individuals. Memantine is an antagonist at the central nervous system N-methyl-D-aspartate (NMDA) receptors, which must be stimulated to allow learning and memory to occur. *Gingko biloba,* an extract derived from the gingko tree, has antioxidant and anticholinesterase properties and is sometimes used for individuals with AD. Antipsychotropic medications may be needed to control the agitation experienced by some individuals with more advanced AD.

Nutrition assessment and care

Chapter 2 describes nutrition assessment in detail, and common assessment findings in AD are summarized in Box 18-2. Progressive loss of self-care skills affects food intake and nutritional status. Weight loss and underweight are common in individuals with AD (Belmin, 2007).

Intervention and education. Nutrition interventions are designed to encourage an adequate intake in order to maintain weight and strength, lessen morbidity (e.g., decubitus ulcers, pneumonia), and optimize comfort.

The following list summarizes nutrition management of some of the more common problems experienced by the individual with AD:

- *Memory loss*: The individual may forget to eat or to finish a meal. Provide verbal and nonverbal cues that it is mealtime (e.g., announce the meal to the person; put utensils in the person's hand). Eating in a group setting may improve intake because the individual observes models of eating behavior.
- *Poor swallowing*: Swallowing difficulties increase the risk of pulmonary aspiration. See Box 18-3 for suggestions for improving swallowing.
- *Inadequate intake*: Inadequate consumption is common even in the individual with no swallowing problems. Provide adequate time for the individual to eat, and avoid distractions during mealtimes. Many affected people experience "sundowning," or restlessness and agitation in the evening, and food intake is poor at this time. Maximize intake at meals when cognitive abilities are better. The affected person may need to be fed. Use diversions (cheerful conversation, touching, holding hands) to redirect behavior if the person is combative or resistive when being fed.

Conclusion

Most neural and mental diseases do not result from any dietary deficiency or problem. The neuropsychiatric syndrome associated with vitamin B_{12} deficiency and Wernicke encephalopathy and Korsakoff syndrome resulting from thiamin deficiency are exceptions to this rule. Even though nutrition does not appear to play a major role in the etiology of most neural and mental health disruptions, it is an important adjunctive treatment and can help to relieve many symptoms. An individualized plan of care should be a part of the treatment of all individuals with disruptions of mental or neurologic health.

REFERENCES

Behrman RE, Kliegman RM, Jensen HB, editors: *Nelson textbook of pediatrics*, ed 17, Philadelphia, 2004, Saunders.

Belmin J: Practical guidelines for the diagnosis and management of weight loss in Alzheimer's disease: a consensus from appropriateness ratings of a large expert panel, *J Nutr Health Aging* 11(1):33, 2007.

Bergheim I, McClain CJ, Arteel GE: Treatment of alcoholic liver disease, *Dig Dis* 23(3-4):275, 2005.

Bergheim I et al: Nutritional deficiencies in German middle-class male alcohol consumers: relation to dietary intake and severity of liver disease, *Eur J Clin Nutr* 57(3):431, 2003.

Diem SJ et al: Depressive symptoms and rates of bone loss at the hip in older women, *J Am Geriatr Soc* 55(6):824, 2007a.

Diem SJ et al: Use of antidepressants and rates of hip bone loss in older women: the study of osteoporotic fractures, *Arch Intern Med* 167(12):1240, 2007b.

Ding EL, Mozaffarian D: Optimal dietary habits for the prevention of stroke, *Semin Neurol* 26(1):11, 2006.

Farinotti M et al: Dietary interventions for multiple sclerosis, *Cochrane Database Syst Rev* (1):CD004192, 2007.

Fowler EG et al: Promotion of physical fitness and prevention of secondary conditions for children with cerebral palsy: section on pediatrics research summit proceedings, *Phys Ther* 87(11):1495, 2007.

Freeman JM, Kossoff EH, Hartman AL: The ketogenic diet: one decade later, *Pediatrics* 119(3):535, 2007a.

Freeman JM et al: *The ketogenic diet: a treatment for children and others with epilepsy,* ed 4, New York, 2007b, Demos Medical Publishing.

Goldman L, Ausiello D, editors: *Cecil medicine*, ed 23, Philadelphia, 2008, Saunders.

Goldstein LB et al: Primary prevention of ischemic stroke: a guideline from the American Heart Association/American Stroke Association Stroke Council, *Circulation* 113(24):e873, 2006.

Haney EM et al: Association of low bone mineral density with selective serotonin reuptake inhibitor use by older men, *Arch Intern Med* 167(12):1246, 2007.

Henderson DC: Weight gain with atypical antipsychotics: evidence and insights, *J Clin Psychiatry* 68(suppl 12):18, 2007.

Kim SY et al: Alcohol consumption and fatty acid intakes in the 2001-2002 National Health and Nutrition Examination Survey, *Alcohol Clin Exp Res* 31(8):1407, 2007.

Kossoff EH: More fat and fewer seizures: dietary therapies for epilepsy, *Lancet Neurol* 3(7):415, 2004.

Lieber CS: Alcoholic fatty liver: its pathogenesis and mechanism of progression to inflammation and fibrosis, *Alcohol* 34(1):9, 2004.

Lieber CS: Metabolism of alcohol, *Clin Liver Dis* 9(1):1, 2005.

McGhee B, Katyal N: Avoid unnecessary drug-related carbohydrates for patients consuming the ketogenic diet, *J Am Diet Assoc* 101(1):87, 2001.

Milano W et al: Appropriate intervention strategies for weight gain induced by olanzapine: a randomized controlled study, *Adv Ther* 24(1):123, 2007.

National Institue on Alcohol Abuse and Alcoholism (NIAAA): Data/ statistical tables. Available at http://www.niaaa.nih.gov/Resources/ DatabaseResources/QuickFacts/. Accessed December 7, 2007.

Sampson HW: Alcohol and other factors affecting osteoporosis risk in women, *Alcohol Res Health* 26(4):292, 2002.

Samson-Fang L, Butler C, O'Donnell M: Effects of gastrostomy feeding in children with cerebral palsy: an AACPDM evidence report, *Dev Med Child Neurol* 45(6):415, 2003.

Schwarz S, Leweling H: Multiple sclerosis and nutrition, *Mult Scler* 11(1):24, 2005.

Sechi G, Serra A: Wernicke's encephalopathy: new clinical settings and recent advances in diagnosis and management, *Lancet Neurol* 6(5):442, 2007.

Selhub J: The many facets of hyperhomocysteinemia: studies from the Framingham cohorts, *J Nutr* 136(6 suppl):1726S, 2006.

Singer MA et al: Reversible nitrous oxide-induced myeloneuropathy with pernicious anemia: case report and literature review, *Muscle Nerve* 37:125, 2008.

Sogaard AJ et al: Long-term mental distress, bone mineral density and non-vertebral fractures: the Tromso Study, *Osteoporos Int* 16(8):887, 2005.

Sullivan PB et al: Gastrostomy feeding in cerebral palsy: too much of a good thing? *Dev Med Child Neurol* 48(11):877, 2006.

Sullivan PB et al: Gastrostomy tube feeding in children with cerebral palsy: a prospective, longitudinal study, *Dev Med Child Neurol* 47(2):77, 2005.

Suter PM: Is alcohol consumption a risk factor for weight gain and obesity? *Crit Rev Clin Lab Sci* 42(3):197, 2005.

van Roon D, Steenbergen B: The use of ergonomic spoons by people with cerebral palsy: effects on food spilling and movement kinematics, *Dev Med Child Neurol* 48(11):888, 2006.

CHAPTER 19

EATING DISORDERS

The latest edition of the *Diagnostic and Statistical Manual of Mental Disorders,* the *DSM-IV-TR* (APA, 2000), describes three categories of eating disorders: **anorexia nervosa (AN)**, **bulimia nervosa (BN)**, and **eating disorders not otherwise specified (EDNOS)**. AN and BN are at least 2 to 3 times as common among females as among males, although binge eating disorder (BED), an EDNOS, appears to be more equally distributed between genders (Ackard et al., 2007; Hudson et al., 2007). The lifetime prevalence of AN, BN, and BED among women in the United States and other industrialized countries has been estimated at 0.5% to 0.6%, 1.1% to 2.8%, and 3.3%, respectively (Hudson et al., 2007).

Characteristics of Eating Disorders

AN is characterized by "a refusal to maintain a minimally normal body weight" (i.e., being 15% or more below ideal body weight); body image disturbances (e.g., misperceptions of body size or shape or denial of the degree of underweight present); serious fear of gaining weight or becoming fat, even though underweight; and amenorrhea for at least three menstrual cycles in a girl or woman who has previously menstruated (APA, 2000). Inclusion of amenorrhea as a diagnostic criterion has been questioned because it excludes males and premenarchal females from a diagnosis of AN. Amenorrhea is not a sensitive indicator of the amount of weight loss, and it does not provide much information about the extent of the disease, coexisting problems, or the likely prognosis (Wilfley et al., 2007). Anorectic behaviors are divided into restrictive (practices that limit energy intake) and purging (practices meant to remove food from the body, such as self-induced vomiting and laxative and diuretic abuse). An affected individual may exhibit one or both types of behavior (APA, 2000). A significant weight loss is not required for AN to be present; girls who do not follow the normal pattern of weight gain during adolescence can be more than 15% underweight and meet the criteria for AN.

BN is characterized by recurrent (at least twice per week for 3 months) binge eating, defined as eating much more during some period of time than a normal person would and feeling a loss of control over behavior at the same time. BN may take a purging form, with self-induced vomiting or use of laxatives in an effort to control weight, or a nonpurging form, where fasting and heavy exercise predominate (APA, 2000). Individuals with BN may or may not be underweight.

Another category, "eating disorders not otherwise specified" (EDNOS), has been established for disorders that have some of the same characteristics but do not meet all the criteria for either AN or BN (APA, 2000). BED involves binge eating episodes without compensatory behaviors, such as purging or exercise. People with BED eat so much within a finite period, e.g., 2 hours, that they are uncomfortable, and they often eat alone when they binge because of embarrassment over their behavior. Binge eating in BED occurs at least twice per week, and bingeing is followed by feelings of guilt, depression, or disgust. AN and BN are usually diagnosed in teenagers or very young adults, whereas BED may be diagnosed much later in adulthood (APA, 2000; Jacobi et al., 2004; Wilson et al., 2007).

The *DSM-IV-TR,* which describes the criteria for eating disorders and other disruptions of mental health, is under revision, with the new edition due to be published in 2012. The criteria for eating disorders will surely be revised in the new edition, and EDNOS is one of the diagnoses most likely to be altered (Wilfley et al., 2007). As many as 60% of eating disorders diagnosed fall into this category, resulting in a very heterogeneous group of patients brought together in one diagnosis (Fairburn et al., 2007).

Risk Factors for Development of Eating Disorders

Risk factors for developing eating disorders include gender, ethnicity, early childhood eating and gastrointestinal problems, elevated weight and shape concerns, negative self-evaluation, sexual abuse and other adverse experiences, and general psychiatric morbidity (Jacobi et al., 2004). Cultural factors (e.g., society's emphasis on thinness as desirable and beautiful) probably play a role. Repeated dieting, overweight, internalization of the belief that thinness is ideal, and body image dissatisfaction are associated with eating disorders (Jacobi et al., 2004; Striegel-Moore and Bulik, 2007). AN and BN, but not BED, appear to be less common among African-American and Hispanic women than Caucasian women (Taylor et al., 2007). Twin studies suggest that 48% to 76% of cases of AN and 50% to 83% of BN can be explained by heritability (Striegel-Moore and Bulik, 2007). Molecular genetic studies have identified polymorphisms (different alleles) of several genes, most notably those for particular central serotonin and dopamine receptors, likely to be related to AN and BN (Bulik et al., 2007).

Numerous hormonal abnormalities are observed in eating disorders. Levels of estradiol and testosterone are reduced, and those of growth hormone and ghrelin (a hormone produced primarily in the stomach that is involved in appetite control) are elevated (Misra and Klibanski, 2006). Other psychiatric disorders, including depression, chemical dependence, and personality disorders, are more frequent among individuals with eating disorders than the general population (Wilson et al., 2007).

The "female athlete triad" is a term given to the relationships among energy availability, menstrual function, and bone mineral density (BMD) (ACSM, 2007). Athletes are at special risk for inadequate energy intake and/or excessive energy expenditure with abnormally low body fat, amenorrhea or disordered menstrual function, and low BMD. Coaches, trainers, and parents of teenaged athletes need to be aware of the problem and involved in helping athletes to achieve normal body weights and bone status. Male athletes, particularly those for whom lower weights are an advantage (e.g., cross-country runners) or whose sport requires them to "make weight" (e.g., wrestlers), are also at risk for disordered eating (Baum, 2006).

Prevention and Treatment

Obsession with slimness is widely promoted by the media, and efforts to combat the problem focus on developing a realistic view of attractiveness and a healthy attitude about weight.

Treatments used in eating disorders include individual psychotherapy, family therapy, and cognitive behavioral therapy (Wilson et al., 2007). Family therapy appears to be most successful in younger patients with AN and those who have been ill a relatively short time (Wilson et al., 2007). Cognitive behavioral therapy strives to help the affected individual identify faulty and maladaptive thinking and alter the maladaptive thoughts and behaviors. In BN it is effective in achieving remission in 30% to 50% of cases, and many of the others have some improvement (Wilson et al., 2007). It is also used in both AN and BED (Wilson et al., 2007). Selective serotonin reuptake inhibitors (SSRIs), particularly fluoxetine (Prozac), have been used in treatment of BN, but whether they are effective is a subject of controversy (Shapiro et al., 2007; Wilson et al., 2007). SSRIs have been associated with an increase in suicidal thoughts in young people up to 24 years of age. Anyone taking these drugs and their families or caregivers should be educated about the risk of the drug, and the patient should be carefully monitored. With the exception of fluoxetine, which is approved for treatment of major depression in children, SSRIs are only approved for use in pediatric patients for treatment of obsessive-compulsive disorder (http://www.fda.gov/cder/drug/antidepressants/antidepressants_label_change_2007.pdf).

Nutrition Assessment and Care

The SCOFF is a simple tool developed in Great Britain for screening individuals for eating disorders (Luck et al., 2002). It consists of five questions:

- Do you make yourself **S**ick because you feel uncomfortably full?
- Do you worry you have lost **C**ontrol over how much you eat?
- Have you recently lost more than **O**ne stone (14 lb [6.3 kg]) in a 3-month period?
- Do you believe yourself to be **F**at when others say you are too thin?
- Would you say that **F**ood dominates your life?

With two abnormal responses the SCOFF had a sensitivity of 84.6% and a specificity of 89.6% in detecting eating disorders (Luck et al., 2002). For those patients identified as having an eating disorder, Box 19-1 provides a guide to structure the nutrition assessment. Individuals with eating disorders may be deficient in any or all nutrients, depending on the severity and duration of their symptoms. Goals of care are for the individual to change weight gradually (if underweight), change eating behaviors in an incremental manner until food intake patterns are normal, separate eating behaviors from feelings and psychologic issues, learn to maintain a weight that is healthful without using abnormal food- and weight-related behaviors, and develop more effective coping skills to deal with stress and conflict.

Box 19-1   Assessment of Eating Disorders

Anthropometric Data

Height, weight, BMI

Optional: skinfold measurements, body composition

History

Weight and Activity History

What was your maximum weight and your height at the time of that weight? When was that?

What is the least you have weighed in the past year? When was that?

What would you like to weigh?

Are you trying to lose weight now?

How often do you exercise? How long at a time?

What kinds of exercise/sports do you participate in (e.g., running/jogging, dance/ballet, gymnastics, team sports, swimming)?

Do you exercise to lose weight?

Diet History

What did you eat or drink in the past 24 hours?

Is your intake in the past 24 hours similar to your usual intake? (Discuss current dietary practices: ask for specifics—amounts, food groups, fluids, restrictions.)

Do you use calorie counting or fat gram counting? Do you have taboo foods (foods you avoid)?

Do you ever binge eat (eat so much at one time that you are uncomfortable)? If so, how often? How much? What kinds of things make you start to binge?

Do you ever vomit after eating? How often? How long after meals?

Do you ever use diuretics, laxatives, diet pills, or ipecac to try to control your weight? How often? How much?

Describe you normal bowel habits. Do you have constipation or diarrhea?

Relevant Health History

When did menses begin? Are cycles regular? When was the last menstrual period?

Continued

Box 19-1   Assessment of Eating Disorders—cont'd

Do you smoke, use drugs, drink alcohol? How often and how much?

Physical and Laboratory Signs

Problems Related to Purging

Fluid and electrolyte imbalances: hypokalemia, hyponatremia, hypochloremic acidosis, dehydration; T wave inversions and depressed ST segment on ECG

Russell sign (calluses or scarring on the dorsal surfaces of fingers or hand from self-induced vomiting; scratches on the palate

Parotid gland enlargement, giving face a "chipmunk" appearance

Tissue damage related to chronic vomiting: dental enamel erosion, upper gastrointestinal bleeding related to esophagitis or esophageal tears (Mallory-Weiss tears)

Problems Related to Restriction of Food Intake

General: fatigue, weakness, pallor

Cardiovascular: sinus bradycardia, other dysrhythmias, orthostatic hypotension; heart failure related to thiamin and/or protein-energy deficits

Gastrointestinal: delayed gastric emptying, gastric dilation, constipation, abnormal liver function tests (usually related to fatty liver)

Hematologic: anemia, especially iron deficiency; leukopenia

Endocrine: amenorrhea, osteopenia

Neurologic: cortical atrophy; confusion, ataxia, abnormal ocular movements (Wernicke encephalopathy related to thiamin deficiency)

Temperature regulation: hypothermia, cold extremities, acrocyanosis

Ophthalmic: keratomalacia (corneal damage usually related to vitamin A deficiency)

Hair: hair loss (AN), change in hair texture

Box 19-1   Assessment of Eating Disorders—cont'd

Problems Related to Restriction of Food Intake

Skin: lanugo (soft, downy body hair, seen in AN), dry skin, cheilitis (cracking at corner of mouth), dermatitis related to micronutrient deficiencies, including zinc, niacin (pellagra), pyridoxine, essential fatty acids

---

Data from Birmingham CL, Gritzner S: Heart failure in anorexia nervosa: case report and review of the literature, *Eat Weight Disord* 12(1):e7, 2007; Committee on Adolescence: Identifying and treating eating disorders, *Pediatrics* 111(1):204, 2003; Cooney TM, Johnson CS, Elner VM: Keratomalacia caused by psychiatric-induced dietary restrictions, *Cornea* 26(8):995, 2007; Heath ML, Sidbury R: Cutaneous manifestations of nutritional deficiency, *Curr Opin Pediatr* 18(4):417, 2006; Kleinman RE, editor: *Pediatric nutrition handbook*, ed 5, Elk Grove Village, Ill, 2004, American Academy of Pediatrics; Misra M et al: Effects of anorexia nervosa on clinical, hematologic, biochemical, and bone density parameters in community-dwelling adolescent girls, *Pediatrics* 114(6):1574, 2004; Peters TE et al: A case report of Wernicke's encephalopathy in a pediatric patient with anorexia nervosa—restricting type, *J Adolesc Health* 40(4):376, 2007; Roberts CM et al: Malnutrition and a rash: think zinc, *Clin Exp Dermatol* 32(6):654, 2007; Strumia R: Dermatologic signs in patients with eating disorders, *Am J Clin Dermatol* 6(3):165, 2005.

AN, Anorexia nervosa; *BMI,* body mass index; *ECG,* electrocardiogram.

Intervention and education. Care of the patient includes correction of nutritional deficits and electrolyte abnormalities; individual and family counseling; nutrition education; modeling of healthful eating and activity patterns, coping strategies, and assertiveness skills; and monitoring the patient's status and responses to therapy. Intervention requires a team approach, with psychologic, medical, and nutritional expertise. A registered dietitian should be involved in the assessment, intervention, and education of all individuals with eating disorders (ADA, 2006).

Medical nutrition therapy. Medical nutrition therapy involves nutrition education that focuses on an understanding of normal nutrition needs, meal planning, developing regular eating patterns, and discouraging dieting (ADA, 2006). The long-term goal is for weight to be at least 85% to 90% of that expected for height. However, nutritional rehabilitation must go hand in hand with appropriate psychotherapy. In programs where medical nutrition therapy was initiated first, or used in preference to psychotherapy, dropout rates were as high as 100% (Wilson et al., 2007).

In moderate undernutrition (weight 75% to 85% of desirable), vital signs are frequently unstable. Physical activity can be restricted until vital signs stabilize and there is no bradycardia. Patient–health care team contracts are established, setting out the goals for weight gain and the rate of gain. If treatment is done on an outpatient basis, patients are seen frequently by the team, possibly in a day treatment program.

In severe malnutrition (<75% of desirable body weight), hospitalization is usually required, especially if vital signs are unstable (e.g., orthostatic hypotension), bradycardia is present, and electrolyte and other laboratory values are abnormal. Meals and snacks should be supervised to ensure that they are consumed and that food is not discarded or vomited, and the client should be observed for at least 90 minutes after eating. Bathroom visits should also be supervised to prevent purging or surreptitious exercising, and the client should not be allowed to visit the bathroom for at least 30 minutes after a meal. Enteral tube feeding or total parenteral nutrition (TPN; see Chapters 8 and 9) is normally reserved for severe, life-threatening malnutrition and is never used as a punishment for failing to eat. Hospitalization goals are to stop weight loss and begin to achieve weight gain, to stabilize vital signs and correct serum chemistry values, and to begin the process of helping the patient to recognize and consume a healthful diet.

For all degrees of undernutrition the following guidelines apply (Rock and Curran-Celentano, 1996):

- Patient food preferences should be accommodated as much as possible, especially early in treatment. People with eating disorders usually have foods that are considered "bad" or are feared. Including these foods in the diet early in treatment may cause excessive stress. These foods can be introduced later in treatment, when the patient has developed trust that the health care team will not let her or him lose control of eating and gain excessive weight.
- Adequate vitamins and minerals should be provided in the diet, or supplements should be used, with special attention given to zinc, calcium, iron, thiamin, and folic acid. Severely malnourished individuals, who are at risk of refeeding syndrome, generally need vitamin-mineral supplementation, with special care given to ensuring that adequate thiamin is consumed.
- Patients usually deny hunger. They need adequate supervision to prevent the overuse of chewing gum, diet soft drinks, and

foods modified to be low in energy, which may help them to avoid feelings of hunger.

Refeeding syndrome. All severely malnourished individuals are at risk of the refeeding syndrome, which is characterized by sodium and water retention with edema and risk of heart failure that is worsened by cardiac atrophy; hypokalemia and hypomagnesemia as these ions move inside the cells during nutritional repletion; hypophosphatemia as additional phosphate is required for metabolism of glucose; and depletion of thiamin, a cofactor in glycolysis (Stanga et al., 2007). Refeeding should be gradual, with the initial energy intake well below the estimated needs and increases as tolerated. Serum levels of potassium, magnesium, and phosphate should be monitored frequently (at baseline, 4 to 6 hours after treatment begins, and daily thereafter in the severely depleted individual). Supplemental potassium, magnesium, and phosphate, as well as a multimineral supplement providing 100% of the Dietary Reference Intake (DRI) and a vitamin supplement providing 200% of the DRI, are recommended. Thiamin depletion is especially likely as energy metabolism increases and can lead to acute neurologic disorders (Wernicke syndrome); thiamin has low toxicity, and a supplement of 200 to 300 mg daily for 3 days will help to restore tissue stores (Stanga et al., 2007). The patient should be monitored for signs of gait disorders, abnormal eye movements, and confusion. Increasing edema, shortness of breath, tachypnea, or tachycardia could be signs of refeeding syndrome.

Special concerns in bulimia nervosa. Bulimic individuals may be at or even above their ideal body weights at the time they begin treatment, but they are likely to have electrolyte and other nutrient imbalances that need to be corrected. Establishing a pattern of regular eating, with dieting being discouraged, is the first step in therapy. Weight maintenance is the initial goal. Only after bulimic behaviors are under control will it be safe for the individual to undertake a weight reduction diet, if weight needs to be lost. The following measures help achieve weight maintenance and avoid bingeing (Rock and Curran-Celentano, 1996; Seidenfeld et al., 2004):

■ The client needs to avoid becoming excessively hungry. Bulimic individuals fear losing control of eating, and excessive hunger can lead to a loss of control. A diet plan with meals or snacks approximately every 3 hours (i.e., three meals and two or three snacks per day) reduces the risk of hunger. Adequate fiber and fat also help to promote satiety.

■ Education and supervision to help avoid unhealthy weight control strategies and excessive focus on body weight are needed. Excessive exercise and strategies such as calorie or fat gram counting need to be identified and corrected.

■ The patient should be helped to include forbidden or "bad" foods in the diet, using behavioral strategies (discussed below). Health care providers can help the individual to plan ways to control stimuli and to plan ahead for situations that have resulted in bingeing in the past.

■ Dietary record keeping is useful, because the patient and the health care team review the records for evidence of progress and of potential problems.

Behavioral strategies for avoiding binge eating. The patient can be taught to maintain control of eating behaviors by practicing the following habits:

■ Identify activities that can serve as distractions when temptations or negative emotions prompt a desire to binge. Excessive physical activity should be discouraged, because it is an ineffective coping mechanism, but moderate activity such as a walk with a friend can be a healthful distraction.

■ Identify cues or stimuli that lead to overeating, and alter these stimuli. For instance, if overeating is most likely to occur in the kitchen, avoid eating in the kitchen and instead eat only in the dining room.

■ Learn what an appropriate serving size is (using scales, measuring cups, or food models), and eat that amount. Many individuals with eating disorders have spent most of their lives either eating almost nothing or gorging. They may have little knowledge of normal serving sizes.

■ Eat slowly, because bingeing is associated with rapid eating.

■ Eat at regular mealtimes. Skipping meals and becoming excessively hungry may trigger bingeing.

■ Avoid repeated helpings of food. At meals, serve the food and then put leftovers away before beginning to eat. At parties, stay as far from the food as possible.

- Plan ahead for events when excessive energy intake can be expected. For instance, the individual who plans to go out for pizza with friends can reduce food intake throughout the day to compensate.
- Limit alcohol intake because it can reduce control over behavior.

Setbacks are normal and should be accepted calmly. Social situations are often stressful to people with an eating disorder. They need to practice healthy ways of coping with interpersonal interaction, rather than focusing on food. It can be helpful for the recovering binge eater to keep a dietary intake record, as well as records of any episodes of vomiting and diuretic or laxative use. Health professionals and the affected individual evaluate these records for signs of progress and to plan strategies for dealing with problems.

Lifestyle changes to correct eating disorders

Most individuals with AN and BN have misconceptions about food and nutrition, as well as about physical activity level. They need help in recognizing and selecting a nutritious diet. Initially the diet may have to be planned and served to them, with the clear expectation that all the food will be eaten. Gradually the patient can assume more responsibility for selecting an adequate diet. The goal is to establish the habit of eating a healthful diet while maintaining a balance with energy expenditure so that it will not be necessary to resort to unhealthy practices, such as self-induced vomiting or excessive exercise to control weight. Changes should be made gradually to avoid increasing stress. Foods that are most feared (usually those likely to be associated with bingeing) should be introduced only after recovery is well under way. The person with an eating disorder needs to learn a new approach to food intake, focusing on the nutritional contributions and other desirable characteristics of foods, rather than on the energy content. In regard to physical activity, the goal is for the individual to view it as a means to optimize health and receive enjoyment, rather than focusing solely on exercise as a tool for weight control.

Osteopenia

Osteopenia is common among individuals with AN or BN. It does not appear to be primarily a nutritional disorder but instead is related to the altered hormonal environment, with decreased levels of estradiol, testosterone (among females), and insulin-like growth factor–1 (IGF-1), all of which normally help stabilize bone (Misra et al., 2004; Misra and Klibanski, 2006; Naessen et al., 2006). Lean body mass and body mass index (BMI) are strongly correlated with BMD (Misra et al., 2004). Peak bone mass is reached during the teen years or in very early adulthood, and therefore osteopenia may have lifelong implications, predisposing women to fractures. Weight gain and restoration of normal menstrual cycles are likely to be the most effective remedy. Calcium and vitamin D intake should be assessed and supplements provided as needed to maintain an adequate intake (Misra and Klibanski, 2006).

Conclusion

Eating disorders often require long-term therapy (at least 1 to 2 years), and relapses frequently occur (Wilson et al., 2007). In long-term follow-up, patients with AN or BN were likely to be depressed, and mortality risk, especially mortality from suicide, was higher among those with AN than among comparable individuals without eating disorders (Berkman et al., 2007). Approaches aimed at helping young people develop realistic views of ideal weight, as well as healthy self-esteem and body image, have the potential to reduce the psychologic costs, morbidity, and mortality associated with eating disorders.

REFERENCES

Ackard DM, Fulkerson JA, Neumark-Sztainer D: Prevalence and utility of DSM-IV eating disorder diagnostic criteria among youth, *Int J Eat Disord* 40(5):409, 2007.

American College of Sports Medicine (ACSM): The female athlete triad. Position stand, *Med Sci Sports Exerc* 39(10):1867, 2007.

American Dietetic Association (ADA): Position of the American Dietetic Association: nutrition intervention in the treatment of anorexia nervosa, bulimia nervosa, and other eating disorders, *J Am Diet Assoc* 106(12): 2073, 2006.

American Psychiatric Association (APA): *Diagnostic and statistical manual of mental disorders, text revision (DSM-IV-TR)*, ed 4, text revision, Washington, DC, 2000, The Association.

Baum A: Eating disorders in the male athlete, *Sports Med* 36(1):1, 2006.

Berkman ND, Lohr KN, Bulik CM: Outcomes of eating disorders: a systematic review of the literature, *Int J Eat Disord* 40(4):293, 2007.

Bulik CM et al: The genetics of anorexia nervosa, *Annu Rev Nutr* 27:263, 2007.

Fairburn CG et al: The severity and status of eating disorder NOS: implications for DSM-V, *Behav Res Ther* 45(8):1705, 2007.

Hudson JI et al: The prevalence and correlates of eating disorders in the National Comorbidity Survey Replication, *Biol Psychiatry* 61(3):348, 2007.

Jacobi C et al: Coming to terms with risk factors for eating disorders: application of risk terminology and suggestions for a general taxonomy, *Psychol Bull* 130(1):19, 2004.

Luck AJ et al: The SCOFF questionnaire and clinical interview for eating disorders in general practice: comparative study, *BMJ* 325(7367): 755, 2002.

Misra M et al: Effects of anorexia nervosa on clinical, hematologic, biochemical, and bone density parameters in community-dwelling adolescent girls, *Pediatrics* 114(6):1574, 2004.

Misra M, Klibanski A: Anorexia nervosa and osteoporosis, *Rev Endocr Metab Disord* 7(1-2):91, 2006.

Naessen S et al: Bone mineral density in bulimic women—influence of endocrine factors and previous anorexia, *Eur J Endocrinol* 155(2):245, 2006.

Rock CL, Curran-Celentano J: Nutritional management of eating disorders, *Psychiatr Clin North Am* 19(4):701, 1996.

Seidenfeld ME, Sosin E, Rickert VI: Nutrition and eating disorders in adolescents, *Mt Sinai J Med* 71(3):155, 2004.

Shapiro JR et al: Bulimia nervosa treatment: a systematic review of randomized controlled trials, *Int J Eat Disord* 40(4):321, 2007.

Stanga Z et al: Nutrition in clinical practice—the refeeding syndrome: illustrative cases and guidelines for prevention and treatment, *Eur J Clin Nutr* 62(6):687, 2008.

Striegel-Moore RH, Bulik CM: Risk factors for eating disorders, *Am Psychol* 62(3):181, 2007.

Taylor JY et al: Prevalence of eating disorders among Blacks in the National Survey of American Life, *Int J Eat Disord* 40(suppl):S10, 2007.

Wilfley DE et al: Classification of eating disorders: toward DSM-V, *Int J Eat Disord* 40(suppl):S123, 2007.

Wilson GT, Grilo CM, Vitousek KM: Psychological treatment of eating disorders, *Am Psychol* 62(3):199, 2007.

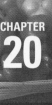

PEDIATRIC DISORDERS

Many nutrition needs of infants and children with disease-related nutritional impairments have been discussed previously in the relevant chapters. This chapter describes nutrition problems in selected disorders that either occur only in pediatrics or are likely to cause significant nutrition problems early in life. Cystic fibrosis and cerebral palsy, two other long-term problems that become apparent during childhood, are discussed in Chapters 15 and 18, respectively.

Low Birthweight Infants

Newborn infants can be classified by their gestational ages and their birthweights. ("Gestational age" is the time elapsed between the first day of the last normal menstrual period and the day of delivery. "Postmenstrual age" is the gestational age plus the time elapsed after birth [chronologic age] [Committee on Fetus and Newborn, 2004]. Thus the postmenstrual age of an infant born 5 weeks ago at 32 weeks of gestation is 37 weeks.) Term infants are born at 37 weeks of gestation or greater, and preterm or premature infants are those born before 37 weeks of gestation. Term and preterm infants are **small for gestational age (SGA**; body weight <10th percentile for gestational age), appropriate for gestational age (AGA; body weight between the 10th and 90th percentiles for gestational age), or large for gestational age (LGA; weight >90th percentile for gestational age). **Low birthweight (LBW)** infants are those with birthweights less than 2500 g. This includes many, although not all, preterm infants, as well as term infants who are SGA. LBW infants can be stratified as moderately LBW, with birthweights between 2500 and 1500 g; **very low birthweight (VLBW)** infants, with birthweights less than 1500 g, and **extremely low birthweight (ELBW) infants**, weighing less than 1000 g at birth. About 8% of all births in the United States are LBW, and 12.5% are preterm (Matthews and Dorman, 2007). The smaller and the more premature the infant, the lower the survival rate, the more likely the infants will have long-term sequelae, and the greater the nutritional risk (Martin et al., 2006). The following list provides some of the factors contributing to nutrition problems:

- *Decreased nutrient stores*: Most fat, glycogen, and minerals— such as iron, calcium, phosphorus, and zinc—are deposited during the last 8 weeks of pregnancy. Thus preterm infants have increased potential for hypoglycemia, rickets, and anemia.
- *Increased energy and nutrient needs for growth*: The LBW infant requires approximately 105 to 140 kcal/kg/day, compared with about 108 kcal/kg/day for the term neonate. Needs for protein and other nutrients are also increased when expressed per kg body weight (Kleinman, 2004).
- *Immature mechanical function of the gastrointestinal (GI) tract*: A coordinated suck-swallow-breathing function may not be present in the preterm infant, particularly those born before 32 weeks of gestation (Lau et al., 2003). Delayed gastric emptying and poor intestinal motility are common in preterm infants.
- *Reduced digestive capability*: Preterm infants have a smaller pool of bile salts, which are required for fat digestion and absorption, than do term infants. Production of pancreatic amylase and lipase, enzymes involved in carbohydrate and fat digestion, is also reduced. Lactase levels are low until about 34 weeks of gestation.
- *Immature lungs with increased work of breathing and increased energy needs*: A tachypneic infant, with a respiratory rate greater than 60 breaths/min, cannot be safely nipple-fed, nor can an infant requiring mechanical ventilation.
- *Potential for heat loss*: Preterm infants have a large body surface area in relation to body weight, as well as little subcutaneous fat to provide insulation. Loss of heat increases energy needs.
- *Susceptibility to **necrotizing enterocolitis (NEC)***: NEC is a serious disease of the GI tract that can result in intestinal perforation and even death. It affects about 6% to 10% of LBW infants. The risk of developing NEC is increased by prematurity, asphyxia, catheterization of the umbilical arteries, congenital heart disease, exchange transfusion for severe hyperbilirubinemia, or myelomeningocele (Martin et al., 2006).

Treatment

Immaturity of the lungs (particularly inadequate surfactant production, resulting in respiratory distress syndrome [RDS]) is a significant problem for many preterm infants. Surfactant replacement, oxygen therapy, and mechanical ventilation are mainstays of treatment.

Nutrition Assessment and Care

A thorough nutrition assessment should be performed as described in Chapter 2. Initial and ongoing nutrition assessment is summarized in Tables 20-1 and 20-2. Weight, length, head circumference, and weight-for-length should be plotted on growth curves derived from LBW infants without major illnesses or from intrauterine growth data. Some commonly used charts may be found in Kleinman (2004), Fenton (2003), and Ehrenkranz et al. (1999). The intrauterine growth curves do not allow for the weight loss that occurs in the early neonatal period, and therefore the 1- and 2-week measurements may fall below the birth percentile when plotted on the curve. A commonly accepted goal is that the infant would receive adequate nutrients to enable growth to occur as rapidly as it would have in the uterus, or approximately 15 g/kg/day (Martin et al., 2006; Moyer-Mileur, 2007).

Intervention and family education
Nutrition support
Total parenteral nutrition.   Virtually all ELBW infants and many other LBW and preterm infants require total parenteral nutrition (TPN; Martin et al., 2006). Severe RDS, congenital bowel anomalies (e.g., intestinal atresia, where some portion of the lumen of the bowel fails to form), and NEC are examples of some of the conditions necessitating TPN. It may be delivered through an umbilical artery catheter, a central venous catheter inserted into the subclavian vein, a peripherally inserted central catheter (PICC), or a peripheral vein (see Chapter 9).

Amino acid requirements for tissue synthesis and energy production are very high in fetal life, and administering glucose alone, without amino acids, to the LBW infant results in loss of protein and failure to synthesize new tissue. Early initiation of amino acid–containing solutions, as soon as the first day of life, helps to prevent negative nitrogen balance and improve growth. Amino acids delivered at 2.5 to 3.5 g/kg/day are recommended for LBW

Table 20-1 Anthropometric Assessment of LBW Infants

Parameter	Frequency	Technique/Comments
Anthropometric Measurements		
Weight	Daily	Weigh nude on calibrated electronic scales, record measurement to nearest 0.1 kg; use bed scales for very sick infants who cannot be moved. Measurement altered by changes in fluid balance. Regain of birthweight should be complete in 2-2.5 wk, and there should be steady gain after that in infants without major illnesses.
Length	Weekly	Use plastic recumbent measuring board, not measuring tape. Knees should be straight and feet at 90-degree angle. Record to the nearest 0.1 cm. Requires 2 examiners to measure accurately.
Head circumference	Weekly[*]	Measure with a paper measuring tape positioned firmly around the head above the supraorbital ridges, at the most prominent part of the frontal bulge anteriorly, and over the part of the occiput that gives the maximum circumference. Record to the nearest 0.1 cm.
Abdominal circumference	Every 8 hr or as indicated	Measure with a paper measuring tape before feeding and at the end of expiration and record to the nearest 0.1 cm; location of the measurement must be agreed on within the neonatal unit, usually either at the umbilicus or 1 cm above the umbilicus. Used as a measure of enteral feeding tolerance. Affected by time elapsed since defecation.

Data from Ehrenkranz RA et al: Longitudinal growth of hospitalized very low birth weight infants, *Pediatrics* 104(2 pt 1):280, 1999; Kleinman RE, editor: *Pediatric nutrition handbook*, ed 5, Elk Grove Village, Ill, 2004, American Academy of Pediatrics; Mihatsch WA, Hogel J, Pohlandt F: The abdominal circumference to weight ratio increases with decreasing body weight in preterm infants, *Acta Paediar* 93(2):273, 2004; Moyer-Mileur LJ: Anthropometric and laboratory assessment of very low birth weight infants: the most helpful measurements and why, *Semin Perinatol* 31(2):96, 2007.

LBW, Low birthweight.

[*]More frequently in infants with rapidly increasing head size, particularly if >1.25 cm/wk.

Table 20-2   Suggested Metabolic Monitoring Schedule for VLBW Infants Receiving Parenteral or Enteral Nutrition Support

Parameter	Parenteral Nutrition		Enteral Nutrition	
	Initial Phase*	Stable Phase†	Initial Phase*	Stable Phase†
Intake and output	Daily	Daily	Daily	Daily
Glucose				
Serum	As indicated	As indicated	As indicated	As indicated
Urine	1-3 times/day	As indicated	Baseline	As indicated
Electrolytes	1-3 times/day	Every 1-2 wk	Baseline	Every 2-3 wk
Calcium, magnesium, phosphorus	2-3 times/wk	Every 1-2 wk	Baseline	Every 2-3 wk
Triglycerides	Daily during dose increase	Every 1-2 wk	As indicated	As indicated
BUN/creatinine	2-3 times/week	Every 1-2 wk	Baseline	Every 2-3 wk
Serum albumin and/or prealbumin	Baseline	Every 2-3 wk	Baseline	Every 2-3 wk
Liver enzymes	Baseline	Every 2-3 wk	Baseline	Every 2-3 wk
Alkaline phosphatase	Baseline	Every 2-3 wk	Baseline	Every 2-3 wk
Blood cell count	Baseline	Every 2-3 wk	Baseline	Every 2-3 wk
Vitamin and trace mineral status or other specific tests	As indicated	As indicated	As indicated	As indicated

Adapted from Moyer-Mileur LJ: Anthropometric and laboratory assessment of very low birth weight infants: the most helpful measurements and why, *Semin Perinatol* 31(2):96, 2007. Used with permission.

*The phase as PN solutions or enteral feedings are adjusted to meet the specific energy and nutrient needs of individual infants. This period generally lasts for <1 week for parenteral nutrition support and 7-10 days for enteral nutrition support.

†The phase when the infant is in a metabolically steady state. For clinically stable infants receiving an adequate nutrient intake with desired growth, the interval between laboratory measurements may be increased beyond the above recommendations.

BUN, Blood urea nitrogen; *VLBW*, very low birthweight.

infants as soon as possible after birth, although additional research is needed to determine whether this amount is optimal (Martin et al., 2006; Denne and Poindexter, 2007).

Small amounts of enteral feedings seem to "prime" the GI tract by stimulating the GI mucosal development, GI motility, and gut hormone release. Therefore "minimal" or "trophic" enteral feedings of formula or human milk delivered at 0.5 to 24 ml/kg/day are often begun when TPN is still needed, if some GI function is present (Martin et al., 2006). An evidence-based review suggested that infants given minimal feedings progress more rapidly to full enteral feedings and have a shorter average length of stay (Tyson and Kennedy, 2005). Nevertheless, the largest clinical studies to date show a strong tendency toward an increased prevalence of NEC with minimal feedings (Tyson and Kennedy, 2005). Thus the possible benefits of minimal feeding need to be balanced against the potential risks.

LBW infants are especially vulnerable to mechanical and infectious complications of nutrient delivery. To prevent these complications, nutrition support must be carefully administered and monitored (see Chapters 8 and 9). State of hydration should be monitored continually. Fluid overload increases the workload on the heart and can interfere with normal postnatal closure of the ductus arteriosus. On the other hand, phototherapy and the use of radiant warmers increase fluid requirements because they increase insensible fluid losses. Laboratory data that are part of the continuing assessment of nutritional status and feeding tolerance include blood or serum glucose and serum electrolytes, triglycerides (if receiving lipid emulsions), calcium, phosphate, and magnesium (see Table 20-2).

Enteral tube feedings. Enteral tube feedings are used when there are GI motility (active bowel sounds or passage of stools); no excessive abdominal distention; soft, nontender abdomen (indicating no signs of peritonitis); no bilious nasogastric (NG) drainage, which would indicate abnormal bowel motility; no evidence of GI bleeding; and no signs of intestinal obstruction. Asphyxia impairs perfusion of the GI tract and is a risk factor for NEC, and therefore enteral feedings may need to be delayed in infants who have required resuscitation (Martin et al., 2006).

Enteral feedings can be delivered intermittently by means of oral-gastric (OG) or NG tubes or continuously by means of OG,

NG, or nasojejunal tubes. Gastrostomy or jejunostomy feedings are also used for some infants who require long-term enteral feeding or who have undergone abdominal surgery. Intermittent (gavage) feedings are given every 1 to 3 hours, initially over a period of approximately 20 to 25 minutes (Martin et al., 2006). There is concern that NG tubes could compromise gas exchange in small infants. For this reason, some clinicians advocate OG tubes for infants weighing less than 2 kg (Martin et al., 2006). Delayed gastric emptying in LBW infants may interfere with adequate milk or formula intake during intermittent feedings. Gastric emptying is stimulated by use of breast milk, if the mother chooses to breastfeed, and positioning the infant on his or her right side after feeding (Martin et al., 2006).

Nonnutritive feeding, or sucking a pacifier, during tube feedings appears to speed the transition to nipple feedings and shorten hospitalization in preterm infants without any adverse effects (Pinelli and Symington, 2005). In assessing the response to enteral feedings, include the anthropometric and metabolic parameters in Tables 20-1 and 20-2, as well as the infant's color, respiratory effort, oxygen saturation, and any increase in prevalence of apnea and bradycardia. The volume of gastric aspirates and occurrence of any emesis should also be noted.

Nipple feedings. Nipple feedings are used in infants with a normal respiratory rate (<60 breaths/min) and the ability to coordinate breathing, sucking, and swallowing. Usually, these infants are at least 33 to 34 weeks' postmenstrual age. However, younger infants may be able to nipple feed safely, particularly if breast fed, and some older infants may not have the necessary feeding skills (Martin et al., 2006). Evaluation by a speech therapist can aid in determination of whether an infant is ready to be fed orally and provide a guide to techniques that may be used to improve nipple-feeding efficiency and safety. Perioral and intraoral stimulation helps to desensitize the mouth and prepare the infant to begin to nipple feed (McGrath and Braescu, 2004). Nonnutritive sucking is also used to assess readiness for nipple feeding in the gavage-fed infant (Martin et al., 2006). Nonnutritive sucking may not be a close indicator of skill in nutritive sucking, but it is useful in evaluating the infant's ability to coordinate breathing and sucking and maintain oxygen saturation during sucking (McGrath and Braescu, 2004). Allowing the infant to nuzzle or suck on a pumped breast is another nonnutritive sucking opportunity for evaluating feeding readiness (Premji et al., 2004).

The VLBW infant usually remains immature in feeding skills even to the time of hospital discharge. Caregivers in the hospital can use the following measures to help the VLBW infant develop feeding skills and can teach the parents or appropriate home caregivers to use these techniques (McGrath and Braescu, 2004; Premji et al., 2004; Premji, 2005; Martin et al., 2006; Thoyre, 2007):

- Position the infant more upright than necessary for a term infant, to allow gravity to facilitate swallowing. The infant should be lightly flexed and held with the head in the midline, the back straight, and the shoulder flexed slightly forward.
- Wrap the infant securely in a blanket, and dim the lights and decrease noise, if possible, to reduce distractions during feeding.
- Observe the infant carefully for subtle signs that apnea and bradycardia are about to occur (e.g., pallor and duskiness around the mouth). Noninvasive blood gas monitoring or pulse oximetry can be helpful during feeding, but it does not take the place of an attentive observer.
- Offer nonnutritive sucking to an infant before feeding to help bring the infant to an alert state. Alternatively, put a drop of milk on the lip or stroke the cheek gently to elicit the rooting reflex.
- Keep one finger under the infant's chin, about halfway to the neck, to help stabilize the jaw and support the base of the tongue. Supporting the cheeks may also help to improve sucking, but the caregiver has to be especially carefully not to hold the cheeks too firmly, because the infant may need to be able to let the mouth open and let milk run out when trying to breathe.
- Observe carefully for choking, excessive milk running out of the mouth, or milk running from the nostrils, and discontinue the feeding if the infant is unable to recover and continue at this time.
- If the infant is breastfeeding and the nipple is very full and distended, he or she may have difficulty latching on. Expressing a little milk before the feeding can help to make the nipple more accessible for the small infant. If the nipple is not excessively full, there is no need for milk expression. Suckling to stimulate milk letdown gives the infant a brief period of nonnutritive sucking that can help him or her to organize feeding skills before

milk begins to flow. It may help if the mother holds her breast in a slightly compressed position, with the thumb on the top and her other fingers under the breast, to keep the breast away from the infant's nose and to improve access to the breast. The "football" hold, with the infant held by the arm on the same side as the breast he or she is feeding from and the head in the mother's hand, is often a very effective position for the LBW infant.

■ Observe the infant carefully to determine level of skill in self-pacing. Sucking in the mature infant takes place in short bursts, with pauses in between and interspersing of breathing with the sucking. The immature infant is apt to have dysregulated sucking, with lack of coordination of sucking, swallowing, and breathing. If the infant is having difficulty self-pacing (interrupting swallowing to breathe), provide external pacing by removing the nipple after a sucking burst to allow breathing and recovery. This can prolong the feeding and tire the infant, however, so the caregiver needs to be especially sensitive to the infant's cues.

Weigh the breastfed infant on an electronic scale before and after breastfeeding if there is concern about whether intake is adequate. The number of grams gained is approximately equal to the milliliters of milk consumed. A mechanical scale is usually not accurate enough for this type of measurement. If breastfeeding is insufficient to meet the infant's needs at first, the mother needs support and reassurance that practice improves skill for both the mother and infant. Mothers need to be cautioned to continue pumping on their regular schedules until the infant has a strong suck, feeds from both breasts at each feeding, and is consistently gaining approximately 15 to 40 g/day (Martin et al., 2006).

Milk and formulas for low-birth-weight infants. Human milk is an excellent source of antiinfective factors, long-chain fatty acids, and growth factors. Milk from mothers of preterm infants (preterm milk) has higher levels of minerals and protein than milk of mothers delivering at term (term milk). Nevertheless, levels of calcium, phosphorus, energy, zinc, and sodium in preterm milk are likely to be too low for rapidly growing premature infants (Martin et al., 2006). Commercial fortifiers containing protein, carbohydrates, lipid, minerals, and vitamins are available for addition to human milk. Infants who receive their mothers' milk have a reduced incidence of NEC compared with infants receiving a formula designed for preterm infants (Martin et al., 2006). Because of this, and because providing breast milk can strengthen the bond between the mother and her hospitalized infant, mothers of LBW infants should be encouraged to breast-feed. Most mothers of LBW infants will need to pump or hand-express milk for some time after birth until the infant is well and strong enough to suckle.

Specially prepared formulas with greater protein, mineral, vitamin, and energy content than formulas for term infants are available for preterm infants whose mothers cannot or do not wish to provide breast milk (Table 20-3). Characteristics of these formulas are as follows:

- Carbohydrate is provided by corn syrup solids or glucose oligosaccharides in addition to lactose because lactose digestion is not mature.
- Fat includes medium-chain triglycerides (MCTs; approximately 20% to 50% of total fat) in addition to long-chain triglycerides (LCTs). Use of MCTs helps to compensate for low intestinal lipase activity and bile salt release.
- Energy is concentrated into a smaller volume than in formulas for term infants (24 kcal/oz rather than 20 kcal/oz).
- Levels of minerals and protein are increased in comparison with formulas for term infants to promote growth.
- Protein is predominately in the form of whey, a more readily digestible protein than the other major milk protein, casein. Whey protein is less likely than casein to cause formation of a lactobezoar (a coalescence of indigestible material in the GI tract, usually the stomach, causing partial or complete obstruction of the tract).
- Taurine, an amino acid needed for retinal development and found in high concentrations in human milk, is included.
- Very-long–chain polyunsaturated fatty acids are included. These fatty acids (arachidonic acid, docosahexaenoic acid) are normally transferred to the fetus by way of the placenta during gestation and are found in human milk, but they are not abundant in cow's milk, which is used to make many infant formulas. These fatty acids are important in development of the central nervous system and vision.
- Carnitine, which facilitates entry of long-chain fatty acids into the mitochondria for metabolism, is included. Although adults can synthesize carnitine, the immature enzyme systems in preterm infants may result in deficiency.

Table 20-3   Comparison of Selected Nutrients in Human Milk and Formulas for LBW Infants

Content per 100 ml	Mature Preterm Human Milk*	Formulas for Hospitalized Infants		Postdischarge Formulas	
		Similac Special Care, 24 cal/oz with Iron (Abbott)	Enfamil Premature Lipil, 24 cal/oz with Iron (Mead Johnson)	Similac NeoSure (Abbott)	Enfamil Enfacare Lipil (Mead Johnson)
Energy (kcal)	67	81	81	74	73
Protein (g)	1.4	2.4	2.4	2.1	1.9
Fat (g)	3.9	4.4	4.1	4.1	3.5
Carbohydrate (g)	6.6	8.4	8.9	7.5	6.9
Vitamin A (international units)	387	1014	1008	342	300
Vitamin D (international units)	2	122	218	52	50
Vitamin E (international units)	1.1	3.2	5.1	2.7	2.7
Folic acid (mcg)	3.3	30	32	19	17
Calcium (mg)	25	146	133	78	80
Phosphorus (mg)	13	81	67	46	44
Magnesium (mg)	3.1	10	7.2	6.7	5.3
Zinc (mg)	0.3	1.2	1.2	0.9	0.8
Iron (mg)	0.1	1.5	1.4	1.3	1.2

*Compiled by Denne SC et al: Enteral nutrition. In Martin RJ, Fanaroff AA, Walsh MC, editors: *Fanaroff and Martin's neonatal-perinatal medicine*, ed 8, Philadelphia, 2006, Mosby. Formula data from www.abbottnutrition.com and www.meadjohnson.com. Accessed December 15, 2007.
LBW, Low birthweight.

Special formulas are available for LBW infants after discharge. These have higher protein, energy, and mineral contents than standard infant formulas, although they are not as high in energy as the formulas for in-hospital use (see Table 20-3). Evidence is insufficient to determine whether these formulas should be recommended for all LBW infants (Greer, 2007). However, these formulas promote faster growth in length and weight and greater bone mineral content than standard formulas (Kleinman, 2004). The discharge formulas will be provided by WIC (Women, Infants, and Children; supplemental food program) with a prescription that specifies the indication for their use, and they avoid the need for any other supplements. Infants who are at highest nutritional risk are those who are being breast-fed. Although breast milk is the ideal feeding for term infants, it is low in the mineral, vitamin, and protein content needed to promote adequate bone mineralization and growth in growing LBW infants (see Table 20-3). Using milk fortifiers is not feasible when the infant is fed at the breast. If the infant does receive some feedings of expressed breast milk (e.g., if the mother has returned to work), the feedings taken from the bottle can have a commercial fortifier added. If milk fortifiers are not used, vitamin and mineral supplements to achieve the recommended intakes for LBW infants should continue since the majority of dietary intake is from human milk (Greer, 2007).

Long-term consequences of low birthweight. Follow-up of infants born at less than 26 weeks' postmenstrual age indicates that they remain smaller in weight, height, head circumference, and body mass index (BMI) at 30 months of age than non-LBW children. The children with the most impaired growth were those whose parents reported feeding problems and those who spent the longest time on oxygen. These findings indicate a need to find ways to improve nutrition and growth in LBW survivors (Wood et al., 2003).

In marked contrast to the poor growth observed during early childhood, it appears that older children and adults who were LBW infants are at risk for disorders usually thought of as implying overnutrition. The metabolic syndrome, a constellation of findings including hypertension, altered glucose metabolism, abdominal obesity, and dyslipidemia, is more common among adults who were LBW infants, particularly infants who were SGA (Cottrell and Ozanne, 2007). It appears that early neonatal events program metabolism for life. Children who were LBW infants exhibit insulin resistance as early as 8 years of age (Toumba et al., 2005). When two groups of children who had been SGA infants (2500 to 2600 g but born at term) were studied at 6 to 8 years of age, blood pressure was significantly higher in the group that had received a nutrient-enriched formula that contained nearly 30% more protein to promote catch-up growth than in the group that had received a standard formula (Singhal et al., 2007). Achieving catch-up growth is likely to be most successful during the first year of life, and factors other than aggressive infant feeding, such as parental weight and the infant's own weight and lifestyle factors in later life, may be equal to or greater in importance than infant feeding practices during the first year of life. Therefore no evidence at the present time warrrants discouraging catch-up growth (Greer, 2007).

Cleft Lip or Palate

Cleft lip and cleft palate are two separate disorders, but they are often found together. Cleft lip varies in severity from a small notch in the lip margin to a complete separation extending into the floor of the nose. Cleft palates may be unilateral or bilateral and may involve the soft and/or hard palate. Deformed or absent teeth are common, especially with cleft palate. A submucous cleft is a defect in the hard palate that is covered by an intact soft palate. It may be missed at birth because the signs are subtle. Possible causes of clefts include maternal drug or alcohol exposure, nutritional factors (e.g., inadequate folate), or genetic factors. Pierre Robin sequence or complex is a syndrome associated with cleft palate in which the lower jaw is unusually small or is set back from the upper jaw, and the tongue is displaced backward.

Treatment

Treatment needs depend on the severity of the defect. The complete treatment program for the child with a cleft lip or palate may require years of special treatment by a team consisting of a pediatrician, plastic surgeon, otolaryngologist, pediatric dentist, prosthodontist, orthodontist, speech therapist, geneticist, medical social worker, psychologist, nurse, and dietitian. The initial surgical repair of cleft lip usually occurs at about 2 to 3 months of age, and this repair may be revised one or more times later. A cleft palate is usually closed by 9 to 12 months of age to aid in development of normal speech (Behrman et al., 2004).

Nutrition Assessment and Care

The primary problem of an infant with cleft lip or palate is inefficient feeding, caused by difficulty making an adequate seal so that efficient sucking can be accomplished and regurgitation of the milk through the nose (Reid et al., 2006; Masarei et al., 2007). Delayed growth may be seen (Box 20-1), especially in infants with larger defects and those with Pierre Robin sequence, who are especially likely to have inefficient sucking because of difficulty in maintaining an open airway while feeding (Reid et al., 2006). Anthropometric measurements should be plotted on the standard growth charts (see Appendix D on Evolve) at every health visit to identify deficits and determine whether additional intervention is needed.

Intervention and family education

Feeding problems. Breastfeeding is often successful with a cleft lip, because the soft tissue of the breast helps to block the defect in the lip. Some children with cleft palate can also be breast-fed (Garcez and Giugliani, 2005). For those infants who are not breast-fed, special feeding equipment is available. An obturator (soft plastic shield) may be used to cover a cleft palate during feeding, but a soft nipple with an enlarged feeding hole on a pliable bottle may be just as effective (Glenny et al., 2004; Kleinman, 2004). Several versions of the nipple and bottle are available commercially (e.g., Haberman feeder, Mead Johnson cleft palate feeder, and Pigeon bottle; information is available from the Cleft Palate Foundation at www.cleftline.org). The individuals involved in feeding the infant need instruction on safe feeding practices (Glenny et al., 2004; Kleinman, 2004):

- Be patient in feeding the infant. Do not rush, leave the infant alone with a propped bottle, or put an older infant to bed with a bottle.
- Hold the infant in a more upright position than for a typical newborn so that gravity assists in swallowing. In particular, do not place an infant with Pierre Robin sequence in a horizontal position during feeding. Infants with cleft palates are at risk for pulmonary aspiration during feeding. Observe the infant carefully for choking, difficulty breathing, or cyanosis during a feeding.

Box 20-1   Assessment in Vulnerable Infants and Children

Undernutrition/Inadequate Growth

History

Cleft palate: ↓ intake related to poor suck and increased work of feeding

SCD: impaired absorption related to hypoxia; ↑ needs related to frequent infections; ↑ resting energy expenditure; inadequate intake related to chronic pain (especially abdominal)

Physical examination

Poor weight gain; length or height <5th percentile for age

Vitamin Deficiencies

A

History

SCD: ↑ needs related to increased RBC turnover, frequent infections, inflammation

Physical examination

Poor growth, possibly dry skin (xerosis)

Laboratory analysis

Serum retinol <20 mcg/dl

D

History

SCD: inadequate intake related to avoidance of dairy products (perhaps because of lactose intolerance); little vitamin D formation in skin related to little sun exposure and dark skin

Laboratory analysis

↓ Bone mineral density

Folate

History

SCD: ↑ needs for RBC synthesis

Physical examination

Pallor, fatigue

Box 20-1 Assessment in Vulnerable Infants and
Children—cont'd

Laboratory analysis
↓ Hct, ↑MCV, ↓ serum and RBC folate

Mineral Deficiency
Calcium
History
SCD: inadequate intake related to avoidance of dairy products

Laboratory analysis
↓ Bone mineral density

Fluid Volume Deficit
History
SCD: hot environment, heavy exercise, acute illness with vomiting or diarrhea

Physical examination
↓ Skin turgor; dry, sticky mucous membranes

Laboratory analysis
↑Serum sodium, BUN; ↑Hct

BUN, Blood urea nitrogen; *Hct,* hematocrit; *MCV,* mean corpuscular volume; *RBC,*
red blood cell; *SCD,* sickle cell disease.

■ Squeeze the bottle gently and rhythmically (not continuously), trying to follow the infant's sucking rhythm. The Pigeon bottle has an adjustable regulator for milk flow.
■ Try angling the nipple to the side of the mouth to allow the infant to use the gum to help compress the nipple.
■ Burp the infant often because the defect causes more air swallowing than in the normal infant. Even older infants will need to stop during the feeding and burp.
■ Avoid tension on the sutures in the immediate postoperative period. Breastfeeding appears to cause less tension than spoon feeding the infant during this period.

Sickle Cell Disease

Although sickle cell disease (SCD) is not only a pediatric illness, the topic is included in this chapter because children with SCD are especially likely to have nutritional deficits and growth failure. SCD is a genetically transmitted disorder in which the person has an abnormal form of hemoglobin (Hgb S). This disorder is found predominantly among individuals with African ancestry. Hgb S causes the red blood cell (RBC), which is normally a flexible biconcave disk, to form a rigid sickle shape. The RBCs are prone to hemolysis, and their rigid shape also causes them to occlude the small vessels. Many complications associated with SCD (e.g., retinopathy, necrosis of the femoral head, splenic infarction with resulting impaired immune function, liver and kidney dysfunction, stroke) are related to ischemia caused by these occlusions. Infections and chronic pain are common problems in SCD. Acute chest syndrome (development of a new pulmonary infiltrate, fever, respiratory symptoms) can result from viral or bacterial infection, but it is frequently associated with vascular occlusion in the lung. It can progress to adult (acute) respiratory distress syndrome. Episodes of acute anemia can be life threatening. Acute anemia results either from increased hemolysis, pooling of large amounts of blood cells and platelets in the spleen (splenic sequestration), or aplastic crisis (shortened RBC life span without a compensatory increase in reticulocyte formation, usually resulting from a viral infection) (Behrman et al., 2004).

Treatment

Hydroxyurea, an antineoplastic agent, is used to decrease hemolysis and the need for transfusion in adult patients, but no long-term studies of safety and efficacy in children have been done (Behrman et al., 2004). Pharmacologic therapy is given as needed for infections and pain relief. RBC transfusions are administered in acute anemia, and splenectomy may be performed if splenic sequestration has occurred or the spleen is markedly enlarged. Individuals who have had splenectomy remain on long-term prophylactic antibiotic treatment. Organ damage (liver or kidney failure) is treated as appropriate. Cholecystectomy may be required for bilirubin gallstones (caused by excessive hemolysis) and hip replacement for femoral head necrosis. Bone marrow transplantation is currently the only curative form of treatment.

Nutrition Assessment and Care

Children with SCD are especially likely to have height and weight below average for age and decreases in subcutaneous fat and muscle mass. These nutrition problems may contribute to delayed puberty (Kleinman, 2004). A thorough nutrition assessment should be done as described in Chapter 2. Common findings in SCD are outlined in Box 20-1.

Intervention and education

Fluid needs. Maintaining adequate hydration is the most important measure to reduce the risk of vascular occlusion (Kleinman, 2004). The person with SCD frequently is unable to form concentrated urine and consequently may excrete 2 L or more of urine per day. Table 8-3 provides estimated maintenance fluid needs. The family (and the child, as he or she becomes old enough) should be taught what normal fluid intake should be, based on weight, as well as the need to avoid vigorous physical activity, increase fluid intake during (moderate) physical activity and fever, replace fluid losses promptly during episodes of vomiting or diarrhea (contact the health care provider immediately if oral fluid replacement is unsuccessful), and avoid exposure to the sun or excessive heat. In addition, they should be taught to recognize signs of dehydration (thirst, dry mucous membranes, poor skin turgor, and sunken eyes and fontanel in infants). The family should keep oral rehydration solutions available and should be taught to give them frequently in small amounts if fluid deficits occur.

Energy and protein needs. Resting energy needs and protein requirements are increased in SCD (Barden et al., 2000; Akohoue et al., 2007). Energy intake should be adequate to maintain a normal rate of growth and development (see standardized growth charts in Appendix D on Evolve). The biologic parents' heights should be obtained and used as a guide to the growth expected from the child. Frequent assessment of length or height, weight, head circumference (in children <3 years), and pubertal status (of children >10 years) is a guide to determining whether nutrition needs are met or the energy intake goal needs to be higher. Intensive nutrition counseling and follow-up may be adequate to improve intake for many children. Modular products supplying protein and/or energy can be added to foods and beverages if necessary to increase nutrient density (see Table 8-2). Some children may benefit from use of age-appropriate oral supplements.

Vitamin and mineral needs. Numerous vitamin and mineral deficits have been observed in children with SCD, including zinc, calcium, folate, and vitamins A, D, E and B_6 (Nelson et al., 2002; van der Dijs et al., 2002; Buison et al., 2004; Schall et al., 2004; Kawchak et al., 2007). Supplementation at levels higher than the Dietary Reference Intake (DRI) may be necessary to achieve adequate nutritional status (van der Dijs et al., 2002). An increase in folate needs may be related to increased needs for RBC formation, since RBC life span is decreased by ongoing hemolysis (Behrman et al., 2004). Iron supplements should be used only if iron deficiency is documented (i.e., low serum ferritin levels and increased total iron-binding capacity). Iron overload may occur in these patients with continual release of iron from RBC.

Vitamins A and E are antioxidants, and SCD is a condition in which oxidative stress appears to be increased (Akohoue et al., 2007). Counseling should include information about good dietary sources of antioxidants, such as polyunsaturated oils and deep green and yellow vegetables (see Appendix B on Evolve). Supplements may also be needed.

Intake of milk products is likely to be low among African Americans because lactose intolerance is common. Calcium and vitamin D supplements are needed if dietary intake of these nutrients cannot be optimized.

Conclusion

Nutrition problems that arise out of childhood disorders and diseases not only raise acute issues but also may pose threats to long-term health. In the case of cleft lip or palate, feeding difficulties may be severe in the young infant, but they resolve after surgery. In LBW infants and in children with SCD, on the other hand, nutrition-related problems may last a lifetime. How to best promote growth in vulnerable LBW infants while minimizing the risk of promoting the metabolic syndrome is one pressing concern that requires further research.

REFERENCES

Akohoue SA et al: Energy expenditure, inflammation, and oxidative stress in steady-state adolescents with sickle cell anemia, *Pediatr Res* 61(2):233, 2007.

Barden EM et al: Total and resting energy expenditure in children with sickle cell disease, *J Pediatr* 136(1):73, 2000.

Behrman RE, Kliegman RM, Jenson HB, editors: *Nelson textbook of pediatrics*, ed 17, Philadelphia, 2004, Saunders.

Buison AM et al: Low vitamin D status in children with sickle cell disease, *J Pediatr* 145(5):622, 2004.

Committee on Fetus and Newborn: American Academy of Pediatrics. Policy statement: age terminology during the perinatal period, *Pediatrics* 114(5):1362, 2004.

Cottrell EC, Ozanne SE: Developmental programming of energy balance and the metabolic syndrome, *Proc Nutr Soc* 66(2):198, 2007.

Denne SC, Poindexter BB: Evidence supporting early nutritional support with parenteral amino acid infusion, *Semin Perinatol* 31(2):56, 2007.

Ehrenkranz RA et al: Longitudinal growth of hospitalized very low birth weight infants, *Pediatrics* 104(2 pt 1):280, 1999.

Fenton TR: A new growth chart for preterm babies: Babson and Benda's chart updated with recent data and a new format, *BMC Pediatr* 3:13, 2003.

Garcez LW, Giugliani ER: Population-based study on the practice of breastfeeding in children born with cleft lip and palate, *Cleft Palate Craniofac J* 42(6):687, 2005.

Glenny AM et al: Feeding interventions for growth and development in infants with cleft lip, cleft palate or cleft lip and palate, *Cochrane Database Syst Rev* (3):CD003315, 2004.

Greer FR: Post-discharge nutrition: what does the evidence support? *Semin Perinatol* 31:89, 2007.

Kawchak DA et al: Adequacy of dietary intake declines with age in children with sickle cell disease, *J Am Diet Assoc* 107(5):843, 2007.

Kleinman RE, editor: *Pediatric nutrition handbook*, ed 5, Elk Grove Village, Ill, 2004, American Academy of Pediatrics.

Lau C, Smith EO, Schanler RJ: Coordination of suck-swallow and swallow respiration in preterm infants, *Acta Paediatr* 92(6):721, 2003.

Martin RJ, Fanaroff AA, Walsh MC, editors: *Fanaroff and Martin's neonatal-perinatal medicine,* ed 8, Philadelphia, 2006, Mosby.

Masarei AG et al: The nature of feeding in infants with unrepaired cleft lip and/or palate compared with healthy noncleft infants, *Cleft Palate Craniofac J* 44(3):321, 2007.

Matthews TJ, Dorman MF: *Infant mortality statistics from the 2004 period linked birth/infant death data set. National vital statistics reports*, vol 55, no 15, Hyattsville, Md, 2007, National Center for Health Statistics.

McGrath JM, Braescu AV: State of the science: feeding readiness in the preterm infant, *J Perinat Neonatal Nurs* 18(4):353, 2004.

Moyer-Mileur LJ: Anthropometric and laboratory assessment of very low birth weight infants: the most helpful measurements and why, *Semin Perinatol* 31(2):96, 2007.

Nelson MC et al: Vitamin B6 status of children with sickle cell disease, *J Pediatr Hematol Oncol* 24(6):463, 2002.

Pinelli J, Symington A: Non-nutritive sucking for promoting physiologic stability and nutrition in preterm infants, *Cochrane Database Syst Rev* (4):CD001071, 2005.

Premji SS: Enteral feeding for high-risk neonates: a digest for nurses into putative risk and benefits to ensure safe and comfortable care, *J Perinat Neonatal Nurs* 19(1):59, 2005.

Premji SS, McNeil DA, Scotland J: Regional neonatal oral feeding protocol: changing the ethos of feeding preterm infants, *J Perinat Neonatal Nurs* 18(4):371, 2004.

Reid J, Kilpatrick N, Reilly S: A prospective, longitudinal study of feeding skills in a cohort of babies with cleft conditions, *Cleft Palate Craniofac J* 43(6):702, 2006.

Schall JI et al: Vitamin A status, hospitalizations, and other outcomes in young children with sickle cell disease, *J Pediatr* 145(1):99, 2004.

Singhal A et al: Promotion of faster weight gain in infants born small for gestational age: is there an adverse effect on later blood pressure? *Circulation* 115(2):213, 2007.

Thoyre SM: Feeding outcomes of extremely premature infants after neonatal care, *J Obstet Gynecol Neonatal Nurs* 36(4):366, 2007.

Toumba M et al: Evaluation of the auxological and metabolic status in prepubertal children born small for gestational age, *J Pediatr Endocrinol Metab* 18(7):677, 2005.

Tyson JE, Kennedy KA: Trophic feedings for parenterally fed infants, *Cochrane Database Syst Rev* (3):CD000504, 2005.

van der Dijs FP et al: Optimization of folic acid, vitamin B(12), and vitamin B(6) supplements in pediatric patients with sickle cell disease, *Am J Hematol* 69(4):239, 2002.

Wood NS et al: The EPICure study: growth and associated problems in children born at 25 weeks of gestational age or less, *Arch Dis Child Fetal Neonatal Ed* 88(6):F492, 2003.

APPENDIXES LIST

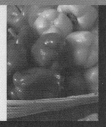

Please access your Student Resources on Evolve® at http://evolve.elsevier.com/Moore/nutritional/ for these resources

GLOSSARY

achalasia: Incomplete relaxation of the lower esophageal sphincter after swallowing.

acute-phase reactant: A protein synthesized and released by the liver in increased quantities in response to injury, trauma, inflammation, or infection, e.g., C-reactive protein, fibrinogen, serum amyloid A, and α_1-acid glycoprotein.

Adequate Intake (AI): A recommendation for the level of intake of a nutrient. The AI is assigned, rather than a Recommended Dietary Allowance (RDA), when the nutrient intake recommended is believed to cover the needs of almost all of the population, but nutrient needs cannot be quantified as precisely as those for an RDA.

alcohol abuse: Heavy drinking with an increasing tolerance for ethanol but no withdrawal symptoms when drinking stops.

alcoholism: A strong craving for ethanol, associated with increasing tolerance to alcohol's intoxicating effects and symptoms of withdrawal when drinking is discontinued.

alternative medical therapies: A group of diverse medical and health care systems, practices, and products that are not presently considered to be part of conventional medicine but are used in place of conventional therapies. An example is the use of diet and meditation to treat cancer rather than conventional surgical, radiation, and chemotherapy treatments.

anabolism: Formation of new body tissue.

anemia of chronic disease: An anemia observed in some patients affected by cancer, renal failure, and other chronic illnesses in which the bone marrow fails to produce adequate red blood cells, even though iron stores may be normal. The anemia is often normocytic (normal-sized cells), rather than microcytic, as in iron deficiency.

anorexia nervosa (AN): A psychiatric eating disorder often resulting in extreme thinness. The affected person usually has a strong aversion to food intake and a distorted body image.

anthropometric measurements: Measurements of the designated aspects of the human body, such as height and weight.

antioxidant: Any of various substances (e.g., beta-carotene, vitamin C, vitamin E) that inhibit oxidation or reactions promoted by oxygen and peroxides and apparently protect the living body from the deleterious effects of free radicals.

attention-deficit/hyperactivity disorders (ADHDs): A set of related disorders characterized by focusing on irrelevant stimuli, impulsive behavior, inconsistency, and lack of persistence. Overactivity may be a feature of the disorder in some individuals.

basal energy expenditure: Amount of energy required to maintain the critical life processes (e.g., breathing, beating of the heart) in an individual at rest, in a comfortable thermal environment, and after an overnight fast. Usually used as a synonym for basal metabolic rate and resting metabolic rate.

body mass index (BMI): An indication of the appropriateness of a person's weight for height, which correlates relatively well with measures of body fat. BMI is usually calculated as the person's weight (in kilograms) divided by the height (in meters) squared.

bulimia nervosa (BN): A psychiatric eating disorder characterized by repeated episodes of bingeing on large amounts of foods, followed by efforts to rid the body of the food by self-induced vomiting or abuse of laxatives and diuretics. Also known as the binge-purge syndrome.

cancer cachexia: A severe form of cancer-related malnutrition associated with a poor prognosis and characterized by anorexia, early satiety, weight loss, anemia, weakness, and muscle wasting.

carbohydrate counting: A technique for planning the diet in diabetes that focuses on the carbohydrate content of foods consumed.

carotenes: Another term for carotenoids.

carotenoids: A group of pigments (yellow, orange, or red) found in plant and animal products. Beta-carotene, lutein, cryptoxanthin, and zeaxanthin are examples of carotenoids. All carotenoids have some vitamin A activity, but beta-carotene is the primary vitamin A precursor.

catabolism: Breakdown of body tissues.

celiac disease (nontropical sprue or gluten-sensitive enteropathy): A disorder characterized by impaired absorption and steatorrhea.

It results from intestinal mucosal damage caused by an immune reaction to the gliadin fraction of the gluten protein or closely related proteins.

chylomicron: A lipoprotein formed in the intestine after consumption of fat. It transports the fat from the intestinal cell into the lymph and from there into the blood.

colostrum: The milk produced for about the first 3 to 5 days after birth. Colostrum is yellowish, rich in immunoglobulins and lymphocytes, and higher in protein than mature human milk.

complementary medical therapies: A group of diverse medical and health care systems, practices, and products that are not presently considered to be part of conventional medicine but are used together with conventional therapies. An example is the use of aromatherapy to relieve discomfort following surgery.

complete protein: A protein that contains all the essential amino acids in sufficient amounts and in proportion to one another so that it can support growth and maintenance of tissues.

Crohn disease: A form of inflammatory bowel disease that can affect any portion of the gastrointestinal tract and can extend through all layers of the bowel. It is often associated with severe chronic diarrhea, nutritional deficits, and weight loss.

cystic fibrosis (CF): A disease resulting from a defect in the cystic fibrosis transmembrane conductance regulator (CFTR) gene. This defect prevents the formation of CFTR, a protein involved in chloride transport across cell membranes in the body. It results in several problems, including thickened mucous secretions in the lungs, which interfere with lung function and promote respiratory infections, and pancreatic insufficiency.

cytokines: Immunoregulatory proteins, such as the interleukins, tumor necrosis factor, and interferon, that are secreted by cells, especially those of the immune system.

Daily Value (DV): A reference value used in nutrition labeling of foods. The DV, which is based on the Recommended Dietary Allowance (RDA), provides a guideline to the amount of a particular nutrient that the daily diet should contain. On the label, information for most nutrients is expressed in both units of weight (g or mg) and %Daily Value (DV).

dehydration: A deficit of body fluid.

Dietary Guidelines for Americans: Guidelines written in lay language that are intended to help Americans optimize their health and reduce nutrition-related health risks.

Dietary Reference Intakes (DRIs): Guidelines for nutrient intake for the healthy population. The DRIs contain two types of measures, the Recommended Dietary Allowances (RDAs) and Tolerable Upper Intake Levels. The DRIs do not focus merely on preventing deficiency diseases but quantify the relationship between nutrients and risk of disease, e.g., calcium and osteoporosis. The DRIs include important nonnutrients found in food, such as fiber.

dumping syndrome: A common side effect of gastric bypass or gastrectomy. It occurs because stomach contents pass into the small bowel rapidly. Nutrients that raise the osmotic concentration within the small bowel substantially, such as simple carbohydrates, draw fluid into the bowel and cause a reduction in the circulating blood volume. The symptoms include dizziness, sweating, nausea, weakness, tachycardia, and diarrhea.

dysphagia: Difficulty in swallowing.

eating disorders not otherwise specified (EDNOS): A category of disorders of eating that do not meet the criteria for any specific eating disorder.

elemental formulas: Liquid diets containing nutrients in a form easy to digest, absorb, and assimilate (e.g., hydrolyzed protein and/or free amino acids). These are commonly used for individuals with digestive or absorptive disorders. Also known as predigested or oligomeric formulas.

enteral feedings: Feedings delivered into any part of the gastrointestinal tract. Enteral feedings are given either by mouth or by tube.

erythropoietin: A hormone produced by the kidney that stimulates red blood cell formation.

essential amino acids (EAAs): Amino acids that cannot be synthesized in the body in the amounts needed for the building of tissues and therefore must be provided by the diet.

Estimated Average Requirement (EAR): The average daily nutrient intake that is believed to meet the requirements of half the healthy individuals in a life-stage or gender group.

extremely low birthweight (ELBW): Weighing less than 1000 g at birth.

failure to thrive: Failure of an infant to regain birth weight by 3 weeks of age, or continuous weight loss or failure to gain weight at the appropriate rate during infancy or childhood.

fetal alcohol syndrome (FAS): A constellation of congenital abnormalities that results from alcohol intake during pregnancy. Features of FAS may include microcephaly (abnormally small head circumference), prenatal and postnatal growth failure, mental retardation, facial abnormalities, cleft palate, skeletal-joint abnormalities, abnormal palmar creases, cardiac defects, and behavioral abnormalities. The only known preventive measure is to avoid drinking alcohol during pregnancy.

food hypersensitivity: An immunologic (allergic) reaction to ingestion of a food or food additive. Symptoms can include anaphylaxis, failure to thrive (in infants and children), vomiting, abdominal pain, diarrhea, rhinitis, sinusitis, otitis media, cough, wheezing, rash, urticaria, and atopic dermatitis.

food jags: Periods during which young children consume only one or two foods for several days. This behavior is normal unless it lasts more than a few days.

free redicals: A highly reactive chemical that often contains oxygen and is produced when molecules are split to give products that have unpaired electrons (a process called oxidation). Free radicals can damage important cellular molecules such as DNA or lipids or other parts of the cell.

functional food: A foodstuff (e.g., a fortified food or a dietary supplement) that is held to provide health or medical benefits in addition to its basic nutritional value; also known as a nutraceutical.

gastroesophageal reflux disease (GERD): Reflux of stomach contents into the esophagus.

gastroparesis: Partial paralysis of the stomach; the condition is common among individuals with long-standing diabetes and is associated with postprandial nausea, vomiting, and abdominal distention.

gestational diabetes mellitus (GDM): Diabetes that first becomes evident during pregnancy.

gliadin: A part of the gluten protein, found in wheat. Closely related proteins (prolamins) are found in rye and barley. An immune reaction to the prolamins causes damage to the intestinal mucosa in susceptible individuals.

gluten: A protein found especially in wheat that gives dough a sticky texture.

glycemic index: Ratio between the change in the blood glucose concentration produced by consuming some food, compared with the change produced by some reference carbohydrate (usually white bread or glucose).

hemochromatosis: A genetic disorder in which excessive iron is stored in various organs—especially the liver, pancreas, heart, gonad, skin, and joints—disrupting organ function.

hemoglobin A_{1c} (Hb A_{1c}): Hemoglobin with glucose molecules attached; it is increased by elevated blood glucose over the life span of the red blood cells and serves as an indicator of blood glucose concentrations over a period of several weeks to a few months.

hepatic encephalopathy: A disorder resulting from accumulation of toxic substances in the blood as a result of liver failure. It is characterized by memory loss, personality change, tremors, and a decrease in the level of consciousness. The affected person may progress to stupor and coma.

hepatitis: An inflammation of the liver caused by a virus, toxin, obstruction, parasite, or drug.

high-biologic-value (HBV) proteins: Proteins of high quality that promote positive nitrogen balance; believed to be effective in maintenance and synthesis of tissues.

high-density lipoprotein (HDL): A lipoprotein formed in the liver to transport cholesterol from the tissues to the liver for metabolism. This function makes HDL protective against heart disease, and thus the HDL cholesterol is considered "good" cholesterol.

hydrogenated fat: Fat to which hydrogen atoms have been added to remove some of the double bonds. Hydrogenation converts the fats from liquids to solids (e.g., shortening or margarine) and increases the number of *trans* molecules in the fat.

hyperemesis gravidarum: Severe nausea and vomiting that may continue throughout pregnancy.

hypermetabolism: Abnormally increased energy expenditure, as occurs in sepsis or following injuries such as burns.

hyperoxaluria: Excessive loss of oxalates in the urine.

impaired glucose tolerance (IGT): Having a glucose concentration ≥ 140 mg/dl (≥ 7.8 mmol/L) and <200 mg/dl (<11.1 mmol/L) 2 hours after ingestion of a 75-g glucose load; a risk factor for later development of diabetes mellitus.

incomplete protein: A protein lacking in one or more essential amino acids and therefore lacking in the ability to maintain normal growth and maintenance of tissues.

inflammatory bowel disease (IBD): Two types of inflammatory processes, Crohn disease and ulcerative colitis, that affect the gastrointestinal tract. Crohn disease can affect any part of the gastrointestinal tract and can extend through all layers of the bowel. Ulcerative colitis is primarily a disease of the large bowel, and it affects only the intestinal mucosa and the submucosal layer. The most common symptom is chronic bloody diarrhea. Nutritional deficits are common, especially in Crohn disease, where malabsorption and weight loss may be severe.

insulin resistance: Reduced sensitivity to insulin by the body's insulin-dependent processes (such as muscle glucose uptake, lipolysis, and inhibition of glucose production by the liver). Occurs in type 2 diabetes but also in individuals that are not diabetic.

isoflavones: Compounds found in soy that have mild estrogen-like effects.

ketogenic diet: A high-fat diet that stimulates ketone production.

leptin: The product of the *ob* gene. Leptin is released by adipose (fat) tissue, and it appears to provide a mechanism for the adipose tissue to communicate with the central nervous system and contribute to the control of food intake and energy metabolism.

lipodystrophy syndrome: A group of side effects of antiretroviral therapy for HIV infection that include high triglyceride levels in the blood, diabetes, and redistribution of fat in the body resulting in changes in body conformation and that are believed to result especially from treatment with protease inhibitors.

lipoproteins: Lipid-protein complexes.

low birthweight (LBW): Weighing less than 2500 g (5.5 lb) at birth.

low-density lipoproteins (LDLs): Lipoproteins that have a very high content of cholesterol, which the LDLs deposit in the tissues. The cholesterol in LDL is associated with increased likelihood of developing atherosclerosis, making LDL cholesterol the so-called "bad" cholesterol in causation of heart disease.

malnutrition: Poor nutritional status (either undernutrition or overnutrition). It can result from inadequate intake, disorders of digestion or absorption, or excessive intake of nutrients.

medical nutrition therapy: Nutrition assessment, planning, intervention, and guidance provided by a nutrition professional.

medium-chain triglyceride (MCT): A triglyceride (consisting of glycerol bound to three fatty acids) in which the fatty acids are 8 to 12 carbons in length. MCTs are most often used in the nutrition care of people with limited digestive and absorptive ability.

metabolic equivalent (MET): One MET is the energy required while sitting quietly—for example, while reading a book.

metabolic syndrome: A condition characterized by insulin resistance and defined as having three or more of the following characteristics: (1) waist circumference >102 cm (men) or >88 cm (women), (2) blood pressure of at least 130/85 mm Hg, (3) fasting serum glucose level of at least 110 mg/dl (6.1 mmol/L); (4) serum triglyceride level of at least 150 mg/dl, and (5) high-density lipoprotein (HDL) cholesterol level of less than 40 mg/dl in men or 50 mg/dl in women. The metabolic syndrome is a risk factor for cardiovascular disease. Also known as the insulin resistance syndrome or syndrome X.

micelle: A combination of bile salts and fat in which the bile emulsifies fat into very small particles to increase its exposure to digestive enzymes and to enhance its solubility so that it can be absorbed by the intestinal mucosa.

monounsaturated fatty acid: A fatty acid with one carbon-carbon double bond.

MyPyramid: A graphic and interactive plan, consistent with the Dietary Guidelines for Americans, that provides an individualized guide regarding food consumption and activity goals.

necrotizing enterocolitis (NEC): An intestinal disorder most often occurring in preterm infants. On x-ray, gas can be seen between the layers of the intestine; in severe cases, intestinal perforation and peritonitis are present.

nephrolithiasis: Formation of calculi (stones) in the kidney.

nephrotic syndrome: A condition in which there is damage to the basement membrane of the nephrons. The syndrome is characterized by loss of protein in the urine, edema, and decreased serum albumin concentrations.

nitrogen balance: The relationship between the amount of nitrogen (from proteins or amino acids) consumed and the amount excreted. Balance is positive if more nitrogen is consumed than excreted and negative if more nitrogen is excreted than consumed.

nonessential amino acid: An amino acid that can be synthesized in the body in amounts sufficient to maintain tissue and sustain growth.

nonnutritive feeding: Sucking a pacifier.

nutraceutical (also nutriceutical): A foodstuff (e.g., a fortified food or a dietary supplement) that is held to provide health or medical benefits in addition to its basic nutritional value; also known as a functional food.

nutrition assessment: The process used to evaluate nutritional status, identify malnutrition, and determine which individuals need aggressive nutrition support.

nutrition care process: A process consisting of four steps (nutrition assessment, nutrition diagnosis, nutrition intervention, and nutrition monitoring and evaluation) and designed to provide a framework for delivery of nutrition care to individuals, groups, or communities in order to facilitate the delivery of quality care by the nutrition professional, generate useful outcomes data, and demonstrate the value of professional nutrition care.

nutrition support: The provision of specially formulated and/or delivered parenteral or enteral nutrients to maintain or restore optimal nutritional status.

nutrition quackery: Promotion of misconceptions about food and nutrition. An example is the idea that certain foods or dietary supplements have "fat-burning" properties.

omega-3 fatty acid (n-3 fatty acid): A fatty acid with a carbon-carbon double bond three carbons from the omega (methyl group) end of its chain. These fatty acids have been reported to reduce serum triglyceride concentrations and to reduce the aggregation of platelets, resulting in a reduced risk of myocardial infarction (heart attack). Fish from cold waters are generally rich in omega-3 fatty acids; canola oil is another source.

osmolality: The property of a solution that depends on the concentration of solute (the number of osmotically active particles) per kilogram of solvent (usually water).

pancreatitis: Inflammation, edema, and necrosis of the pancreas as a result of digestion of the organ by pancreatic enzymes.

parenteral feedings: Delivery of nutrients by the intravenous route.

phytochemical: A chemical component of a plant, especially one having health-protective effects.

pica: The consumption of substances usually considered nonfoods (e.g., clay) or of excessive amounts of food products low in nutrients (e.g., ice, cornstarch).

polymeric formulas: Liquid diets used for oral supplementation or enteral tube feeding. Polymeric formulas contain intact (not predigested) carbohydrates, proteins, and fats.

polyunsaturated fatty acid: A fatty acid containing more than one carbon-carbon double bond.

prebiotic: A food ingredient that benefits the host by selectively stimulating the growth or the activity of one or a limited number of nonpathogenic bacteria in the colon.

preeclampsia: A syndrome characterized by hypertension, albuminuria, and excessive edema. Also called pregnancy-induced hypertension or toxemia.

pregnancy-induced hypertension (PIH): A syndrome characterized by hypertension, albuminuria, and excessive edema. Also called preeclampsia or toxemia.

probiotic: Live microorganisms that confer a health benefit on the host, improving immune and nonimmune mechanisms of resistance to infection in the intestine.

protein-energy malnutrition (PEM): Undernutrition resulting from inadequate intake, digestion, or absorption of protein or calories. There are two forms, kwashiorkor and marasmus, and a combined form, referred to as marasmic kwashiorkor. PEM is also known as protein-calorie malnutrition (PCM).

Recommended Dietary Allowance (RDA): An amount of a nutrient estimated to meet the biologic needs of almost all (97% to 98%) of the healthy population. The RDA is one of the measures included in the Dietary Reference Intakes (DRIs).

refeeding syndrome: A potential complication of refeeding of the severely malnourished individual. During refeeding, especially with high-carbohydrate feedings, insulin levels rise and cellular uptake of glucose, water, phosphorus, potassium, and other nutrients is stimulated. Serum levels of phosphorus, potassium, magnesium, and other minerals or electrolytes subsequently fall if close attention is not paid to their replacement. Refeeding syndrome is characterized by cardiac dysrhythmias, congestive heart failure, hemolysis, muscular weakness, seizures, acute respiratory failure, and a variety of other complications, including sudden death.

respiratory quotient (RQ): The ratio of the carbon dioxide produced to the oxygen consumed in a given unit of time.

resting energy expenditure (REE): Amount of energy required to maintain the vital life processes (e.g., breathing, circulation) at rest in an overnight-fasted condition and in a comfortable environmental temperature.

sensitivity: The probability that a test indicates a nutrient deficiency, given that the person actually does have a deficiency.

short bowel syndrome: Varying degrees of impaired digestion and absorption resulting from surgical removal of parts of the intestines.

small for gestational age (SGA): Exhibiting intrauterine growth restriction; low birth weight and length for the infant's gestational age.

specificity: The probability that a test indicates no nutrient deficiency, given that the person does not have a deficiency.

steatorrhea: Loss of excess fat in the stools.

systemic inflammatory response syndrome (SIRS): A severe systemic response to a condition (e.g., trauma, infection, burn) that provokes an acute inflammatory reaction.

therapeutic lifestyle changes (TLC): A systematic approach to correction of dyslipidemia and reduction of risk of heart disease including dietary changes to reduce saturated and *trans* fat intake to <10% of total energy intake and cholesterol intake to <200 mg/day; adjustment of energy intake to maintain or reduce weight; regular physical activity; and recommendations to consider consuming increased viscous fiber, plant sterols/stanols, and soy protein.

thermic effect of food (TEF): Production of body heat as a result of food intake; the energy required to digest and absorb food and transport nutrients to the cells. TEF accounts for approximately 10% of daily energy needs. Also referred to as diet-induced thermogenesis.

Tolerable Upper Intake Level (UL): The upper limit of intake associated with a low risk of adverse effects in almost all members of a given population. The UL is one of the measures included in the Dietary Reference Intakes (DRIs).

trans fatty acid: A fatty acid formed especially when unsaturated oils are partially hydrogenated to make them harder. Increased intake is associated with elevated serum cholesterol.

type 1 diabetes mellitus: Previously known as insulin-dependent diabetes; characterized by insulin deficiency, which results from destruction of the beta cells of the pancreas, usually by an autoimmune process. Classic symptoms include excessive hunger and thirst and weight loss.

type 2 diabetes mellitus: Previously known as non–insulin-dependent diabetes; characterized by insulin resistance, or decreased tissue uptake of glucose in response to insulin, along with inability to secrete enough insulin to compensate for the insulin resistance.

ulcerative colitis: A form of inflammatory bowel disease that usually involves only the large bowel and primarily affects the mucosal and submucosal layers of the intestine.

unsaturated fatty acid: A fatty acid that does not contain the maximum possible number of hydrogen atoms, allowing it to have carbon-carbon double bonds. Monounsaturated fatty acids have one double bond and polyunsaturated fatty acids have more than one double bond.

very low birthweight (VLBW): Weighing less than 1500 g at birth.

very–low-density lipoprotein (VLDL): Lipoprotein formed in the liver to transport lipids made in the liver to other body cells. Most of their lipid content is in the form of triglycerides, but they also transport cholesterol.

visceral fat: Fat located in proximity to the abdominal visceral organs. Visceral fat lies deeper in the body than the subcutaneous abdominal adipose tissue.

weight cycling: Also known as "yo-yo" dieting, occurs when individuals repeatedly lose and regain weight.

Index